Essential Urology

CURRENT CLINICAL UROLOGY

Eric A. Klein, MD, SERIES EDITOR

***Essential Urology:** A Guide to Clinical Practice,* edited by **Jeannette M. Potts,** 2004

***Management of Prostate Cancer,** Second Edition,* edited by **Eric A. Klein,** 2004

***Management of Benign Prostatic Hypertrophy**,* edited by **Kevin T. McVary,** 2004

Laparoscopic Urologic Oncology, edited by **Jeffrey A. Cadeddu,** 2004

***Essential Urologic Laparoscopy:** The Complete Clinical Guide,* edited by **Stephen Y. Nakada,** 2003

***Pediatric Urology**,* edited by **John P. Gearhart,** 2003

***Urologic Prostheses:** The Complete Practical Guide to Devices, Their Implantation, and Patient Follow-Up,* edited by **Culley C. Carson, III,** 2002

***Male Sexual Function:** A Guide to Clinical Management,* edited by **John J. Mulcahy**, 2001

Prostate Cancer Screening, edited by **Ian M. Thompson, Martin I. Resnick, and Eric A. Klein,** 2001

***Bladder Cancer:** Current Diagnosis and Treatment,* edited by **Michael J. Droller,** 2001

***Office Urology:** The Clinician's Guide,* edited by **Elroy D. Kursh and James C. Ulchaker,** 2001

***Voiding Dysfunction:** Diagnosis and Treatment,* edited by **Rodney A. Appell,** 2000

Management of Prostate Cancer, edited by **Eric A. Klein,** 2000

ESSENTIAL UROLOGY

A GUIDE TO CLINICAL PRACTICE

Edited by

JEANNETTE M. POTTS, MD

Glickman Urological Institute, Cleveland Clinic Foundation, Cleveland, OH

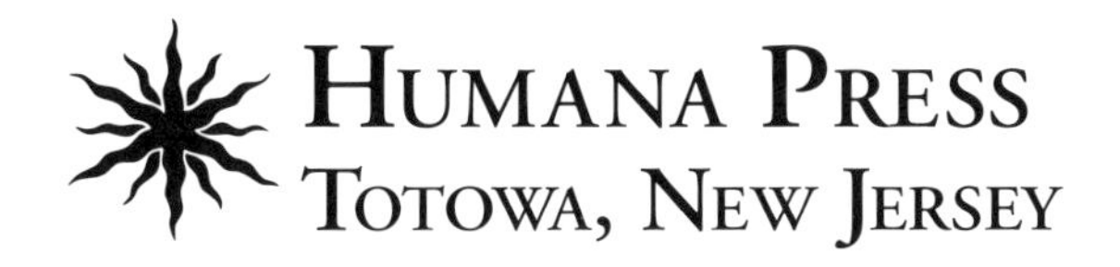

999 Riverview Drive, Suite 208
Totowa, New Jersey 07512

www.humanapress.com

For additional copies, pricing for bulk purchases, and/or information about other Humana titles, contact Humana at the above address or at any of the following numbers: Tel.: 973-256-1699; Fax: 973-256-8341, E-mail: humana@humanapr.com; or visit our Website: http://humanapress.com

Production Editor: Robin B. Weisberg
Cover illustration layout by Jeannette M. Potts. Cover illustration by Michelle Wolf. Cover design by Patricia F. Cleary.

This publication is printed on acid-free paper. ∞
ANSI Z39.48-1984 (American National Standards Institute) Permanence of Paper for Printed Library Materials.

Printed in the United States of America. 10 9 8 7 6 5 4 3

E-ISBN 1-59259-737-8

Library of Congress Cataloging-in-Publication Data

Essential urology : a guide to clinical practice / edited by Jeanette M. Potts.
p. ; cm. -- (Current clinical urology)
Includes bibliographical references and index.
ISBN 1-58829-109-X (alk. paper)
1. Genitourinary organs--Diseases.
[DNLM: 1. Urologic Diseases. 2. Urogenital Diseases. WJ 140 E78 2004] I. Potts, Jeanette M. II. Series.
RC871.E883 2004
616.6--dc22

2003016746

Dedication

To my children, Bradley and Ellen,
and to my mentors, Jonathan Ross, MD and Elroy Kursh, MD

Preface

As a medical urologist with a background in family medicine, I have enjoyed the overlapping aspects of urology and primary care. Urological diseases are often brought to the attention of primary care providers who must then diagnose and manage these disorders. *Essential Urology: A Guide to Clinical Practice* is intended to provide support to primary care physicians through its review of common genitourinary problems. It is meant to enhance the recognition of urological disease as well as outline current management strategies.

Disorders of the urinary tract may be encountered during pregnancy, either as a maternal diagnosis or as a fetal anomaly detected *in utero*. Children as well as adults require screening and monitoring of genitourinary disorders, some of which are gender-specific. Urinary tract infections may be manifestations of risk factors, anatomical or functional abnormalities, specific to age and/or gender. These issues are presented in this text. Hematuria, frequently encountered in the primary care setting as an incidental finding, is discussed in a comprehensive chapter, followed by related chapters detailing urological imaging studies and the evaluation and management of nephrolithiasis, respectively. Urinary function is addressed in the chapters reviewing female incontinence, interstitial cystitis, and bladder outlet obstruction secondary to benign prostatic hyperplasia. Screening for urological cancers, particularly prostate and bladder cancers, is reviewed. We have included a chapter summarizing complementary therapies in urology and a chapter that introduces alternative approaches to frequently diagnosed abacterial prostatitis/pelvic pain syndrome. Finally, we address the quality-of-life impact and medical significance of erectile dysfunction and its treatment.

Essential Urology: A Guide to Clinical Practice addresses various life stages and respective urological conditions and should be a valuable resource to family practitioners, internists, pediatricians, obstetricians, physician's assistants, and nurse clinicians.

Jeannette M. Potts, MD

Contents

Contributors

JOSEPH B. ABDELMALAK, MD • *Glickman Urological Institute, Cleveland Clinic Foundation, Cleveland, OH*
JOSEPH BASLER, MD • *Division of Urology, University of Texas Health Science Center at San Antonio, San Antonio, TX*
ELLIOT FAGELMAN, MD • *Department of Urology, St. Luke's-Roosevelt Hospital Center, College of Physicians and Surgeons, Columbia University, New York, NY*
RICHARD W. GRADY, MD • *Department of Urology, Children's Hospital and Regional Medical Center, University of Washington School of Medicine, Seattle, WA*
ELROY D. KURSH, MD • *Glickman Urological Institute, Cleveland Clinic Foundation, Cleveland, OH*
MILTON M. LAKIN, MD • *Section of Medical Urology, Glickman Urological Institute, Cleveland Clinic Foundation, Cleveland, OH*
JOHN C. LIESKE, MD • *Division of Nephrology, Department of Medicine, Mayo Clinic and Medical School, Rochester, MN*
KEVIN R. LOUGHLIN, MD • *Division of Urology, Department of Surgery, Brigham and Women's Hospital, Harvard Medical School, Boston, MA*
FRANKLIN C. LOWE, MD, MPH • *Department of Urology, St. Luke's-Roosevelt Hospital Center, College of Physicians and Surgeons, Columbia University, New York, NY*
BRIDGIT MENNITE, BS • *University of Albany, Albany, NY*
DROGO K. MONTAGUE, MD • *Center for Sexual Function, Glickman Urological Institute, Cleveland Clinic Foundation, Cleveland, OH*
MARK J. NOBLE, MD • *Glickman Urological Institute, Cleveland Clinic Foundation, Cleveland, OH*
KENNETH M. PETERS, MD • *Department of Urology, William Beaumont Hospital, Royal Oak, MI*
JEANNETTE M. POTTS, MD • *Section of Medical Urology, Glickman Urological Institute, Cleveland Clinic Foundation, Cleveland, OH*
RAYMOND R. RACKLEY, MD • *Glickman Urological Institute, Cleveland Clinic Foundation, Cleveland, OH*
MARTIN I. RESNICK, MD • *Department of Urology, University Hospitals of Cleveland, Case Western Reserve University, Cleveland, OH*
MARTIN B. RICHMAN, MD • *Department of Urology, University Hospitals of Cleveland, Case Western Reserve University, Cleveland, OH*
JONATHAN H. ROSS, MD • *Section of Pediatric Urology, Glickman Urological Institute, The Children's Hospital at the Cleveland Clinic, Cleveland Clinic Foundation, Cleveland, OH*
JOSEPH W. SEGURA, MD • *Departments of Urology and Surgery, Mayo Clinic and Medical School, Rochester, MN*
IAN M. THOMPSON, MD • *Division of Urology, University of Texas Health Science Center at San Antonio, San Antonio, TX*
SANDIP P. VASAVADA, MD • *Glickman Urological Institute, Cleveland Clinic Foundation, Cleveland, OH*

Value-Added eBook/PDA

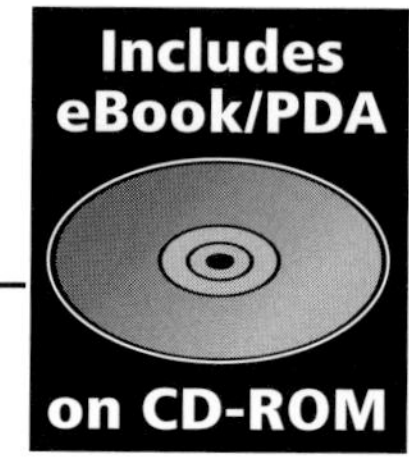

This book is accompanied by a value-added CD-ROM that contains an Adobe eBook version of the volume you have just purchased. This eBook can be viewed on your computer, and you can synchronize it to your PDA for viewing on your handheld device. The eBook enables you to view this volume on only one computer and PDA. Once the eBook is installed on your computer, you cannot download, install, or e-mail it to another computer; it resides solely with the computer to which it is installed. The license provided is for only one computer. The eBook can only be read using Adobe® Reader® 6.0 software, which is available free from Adobe Systems Incorporated at www.Adobe.com. You may also view the eBook on your PDA using the Adobe® PDA Reader® software that is also available free from Adobe.com.

You must follow a simple procedure when you install the eBook/PDA that will require you to connect to the Humana Press website in order to receive your license. Please read and follow the instructions below:

1. Download and install Adobe® Reader® 6.0 software
   You can obtain a free copy of Adobe® Reader® 6.0 software at www.adobe.com
   *Note: If you already have Adobe® Reader® 6.0 software, you do not need to reinstall it.
2. Launch Adobe® Reader® 6.0 software
3. Install eBook: Insert your eBook CD into your CD-ROM drive
   PC: Click on the "Start" button, then click on "Run"
   At the prompt, type "d:\ebookinstall.pdf" and click "OK"
   *Note: If your CD-ROM drive letter is something other than d: change the above command accordingly.
   MAC: Double click on the "eBook CD" that you will see mounted on your desktop.
   Double click "ebookinstall.pdf"
4. Adobe® Reader® 6.0 software will open and you will receive the message
   "This document is protected by Adobe DRM" Click "OK"
   *Note: If you have not already activated Adobe® Reader® 6.0 software, you will be prompted to do so. Simply follow the directions to activate and continue installation.
   Your web browser will open and you will be taken to the Humana Press eBook registration page. Follow the instructions on that page to complete installation. You will need the serial number located on the sticker sealing the envelope containing the CD-ROM.

If you require assistance during the installation, or you would like more information regarding your eBook and PDA installation, please refer to the eBookManual.pdf located on your CD. If you need further assistance, contact Humana Press eBook Support by e-mail at ebooksupport@humanapr.com or by phone at 973-256-1699.

1 Management of Urological Problems During Pregnancy

A Rationale and Strategy

Kevin R. Loughlin, MD

CONTENTS

INTRODUCTION

The pregnant patient presents unique management problems to the urologist. Attention must be given to the unique physiological changes that occur throughout pregnancy and the impact that diagnostic, and therapeutic maneuvers may have on the fetus must also be considered. In this review, I will discuss the common urological problems that occur during pregnancy and outline an approach to their management.

From: *Essential Urology: A Guide to Clinical Practice*
Edited by: J. M. Potts © Humana Press Inc., Totowa, NJ

PHYSIOLOGICAL ALTERATIONS DURING PREGNANCY

Changes occur in the cardiovascular, respiratory, hematological, gastrointestinal, and renal systems during pregnancy. Total blood volume increases by 25 to 40% by the end of pregnancy *(1)*. This is predominantly a consequence of a 50% rise in plasma volume that begins in the first trimester and reaches a peak between 24 and 28 wk gestation *(2)*. A smaller increase of approx 15% occurs in red blood cell volume, and the consequence of this hemodilution is a fall in hematocrit. This hemodilution results in an increase of the free fraction of protein-bound drugs that can alter their effects and toxicity *(3–5)*.

The cardiovascular system during pregnancy becomes hyperdynamic to meet increased metabolic demands. Cardiac output is increased by 30 to 50% by the third trimester *(1)* with a redistribution of cardiac output that effects increased blood flow to the placenta, uterus, skin, kidneys, and mammary glands. Simultaneously, systemic vascular resistance is reduced as a result of vascular relaxation caused by increased progesterone and prostacyclin *(6,7)*.

The gravid uterus may cause compression of the great vessels during the second half of pregnancy. This can result in reduced aortic blood flow below the level of obstruction as well as decreased cardiac output when venous return is impaired *(5)*.

The respiratory system is also dramatically affected during pregnancy. One of the most crucial changes is a 20% reduction in functional residual capacity by the fifth month of pregnancy *(8)*. This phenomenon, coupled with a 15% increase in oxygen consumption, causes the pregnant mother to be at increased risk of becoming hypoxemic during periods of hypoventilation. Pregnant women have a more rapid rate of decline in PaO_2 than nonpregnant women *(9)*. Aside from the proportionally greater increase in plasma volume as compared with red cell volume, which results in the so-called physiological anemia of pregnancy, other critical hematologic changes occur. Most importantly, the blood of the pregnant patient becomes hypercoagulable. This is to the result of several activities, the first being an increase in factors VII, VIII, X, and fibrinogen during pregnancy *(10)*. In addition, the fibrinolytic activity of the plasma is depressed *(11,12)*, as well as both a reduction of the velocity of venous blood flow in the lower extremities and a rise in venous pressure *(12,13)*. All of these factors contribute to a significantly increased risk of venous thromboembolism in the pregnant woman. This risk appears to be greatest in the third trimester or immediately postpartum and has been estimated to be five to six times greater than for nongravid, nonpuerperal women *(11)*.

There are no prospective series of the use of prophylactic anticoagulation in patients undergoing surgery during pregnancy. However, some investigators *(11,14)* have advocated the use of low-dose heparin (which does not cross the placenta) in pregnant women who have a history of thromboembolism.

The gastrointestinal tract also undergoes alterations during pregnancy. Progesterone inhibits gastric and intestinal motility and relaxes the gastroesophageal sphincter *(10)*. In addition, the gravid uterus displaces the abdominal contents upward toward the diaphragm, which may compromise the competence of the gastroesophageal sphincter further. It has also been shown that a delay in gastric emptying begins as early as 8 to 11 wk gestation *(15)* and that placental secretion of gastrin, which starts in the first trimester, lowers the pH of gastric secretions *(10)*. All of these factors contribute to an increased risk of perioperative aspiration in the pregnant patient.

Important physiological changes are also known to occur throughout the urinary tract during pregnancy. The renal calyces, pelves, and ureters dilate significantly beginning

Table 1
Physiological Changes of Pregnancy

System	*Change*	*Clinical implications*
Cardiovascular	Uterine compression of vena cava	Decreased cardiac output Increase in venous stasis in lower extremities.
Respiratory	Decrease in FRC; Increase in oxygen consumption	Increased risk of perioperative hypoxemia
Hematologic	Increase in clotting factors and hypercoagulability	Increased rate of thromboembolism
Gastrointestinal	Decreased gastric motility and reduced competency of gastroesophageal sphincter.	Increased risk of aspiration.
Renal	Dilation of collecting system; Increase in glomerular filtration rate	Increased risk of pyelonephritis Changes in renal clearance of some drugs

Modified from Barron *(10)* and Loughlin *(24)*.
FRC, functional residual capacity.

in the first trimester *(16)*. The cause of the dilation is probably both humoral and mechanical. Hsia and Shortliffe *(17)* have also demonstrated in an animal model that hydronephrosis in pregnancy may be the result of increased urinary tract compliance. Schulman and Herlinger *(18)* reviewed 220 excretory urograms performed during pregnancy and found the right side to be the more dilated side in 86% of the cases. The relative urinary stasis that occurs may explain why pregnant women have a higher incidence of pyelonephritis associated with bacteriuria than nonpregnant females.

Other renal changes that occur include a 30 to 50% increase in glomerular filtration rate and renal plasma flow during pregnancy *(10)*. Therefore, normal ranges for serum creatinine and blood urea nitrogen are about 25% lower during gestation. Because of the increase in renal hemodynamics, medications administered in the perioperative setting may undergo rapid urinary excretion and dosage adjustment may, therefore, become necessary. In addition to upper tract changes, pregnancy causes changes in the bladder and urethra. Pregnancy induces a significant (greater than 50%) decrease in the contractile response of the rabbit bladder to phenylephrine *(19)*. The increased compliance and decreased responsiveness to α-adrenoceptor stimulation of both bladder neck and urethra that occurs during pregnancy may explain the stress urinary incontinence associated with pregnancy *(20–22)*. The physiological alterations observed in pregnancy and their impact in the surgical patient are outlined in Table 1 *(23,24)*.

ACUTE ABDOMEN AND SURGICAL CONSIDERATIONS DURING PREGNANCY

Making the correct diagnosis of the acute abdomen in the pregnant patient can be a daunting challenge. The incidence of nonobstetrical surgery during pregnancy is approx 1 in 500 deliveries *(25)*. Appendicitis is the most common cause of nonobstetrical surgery (1 in 1500 to 6600 deliveries; refs. *26,27*) followed by intestinal obstruction (1 in 2500 to 3500 deliveries; ref. *28*) and cholecystitis (1 in 1000 to 10,000 deliveries; refs. *25,29*). Drago et al. *(30)* reviewed their own experience and others in the literature and found the incidence of urolithiasis in pregnancy to be 1 in 1500 deliveries, which is the same as in the nonpregnant female.

However, pregnancy-specific causes of abdominal pain during pregnancy are much more common than the aforementioned problems. For example, ectopic pregnancy occurs in every 1 in 300 pregnancies; placental disruption occurs in every 1 in 100 pregnancies *(31)*.

Smoleniec and James *(32)* have emphasized that two important clinical effects of increased uterine growth during pregnancy are the displacement of the appendix upward above the iliac crest and the separation of the viscera from the anterior abdominal wall, which may result in a decrease of somatic pain. These factors can make the evaluation of the acute abdomen during pregnancy extremely treacherous. Silen *(33)* pointed out that as a consequence of the cephalad displacement of the appendix, cholecystitis, right pyelonephritis, and appendicitis may be extremely difficult to differentiate during pregnancy. The optimal time to perform nonobstetrical surgery during pregnancy appears to be the second trimester. There is an increased risk of miscarriage during the first trimester *(25,34)* and an increased risk of premature labor during the last trimester *(34)*.

ANESTHETIC CONSIDERATIONS DURING PREGNANCY

The goal of anesthetic management of the pregnant patient is maternal safety and fetal well-being. Gestation is associated with a decrease in drug requirements for both general and regional anesthesia. Palahniuk and associates *(35)* have reported a 25 to 40% reduction in minimal alveolar concentrations by using halothane and isoflurane during ovine pregnancy. This is most likely because of the sedative effects of progesterone and the increased levels of endogenous opiates *(36,37)*.

The requirement for local anesthetics is also reduced early in the first trimester of pregnancy *(38)*. Progesterone induced enhancement of membrane sensitivity to local anesthetics has been proposed as the most likely mechanism for this observation *(39)*. Further decreases in drug requirements for spinal or epidural anesthesia occur with advancing gestation because epidural venous engorgement reduces the volume of cerebrospinal fluid and the epidural space. This vascular engorgement also increases the risk of unintended intravascular injection of local anesthetic.

Diazepam should not be given during pregnancy because two retrospective studies have demonstrated an association between maternal diazepam use and occurrence of cleft lip and/or palate in their progeny *(40,41)*.

URINARY TRACT INFECTIONS AND ANTIBIOTIC USE DURING PREGNANCY

The prevalence of bacteriuria among pregnant women has been published as ranging from 2.5 to 11% *(42)* with most investigators reporting a prevalence between 4 to 7% *(43)*. This is similar to the prevalence of bacteriuria among other sexually active women of childbearing age. Recurrent episodes of bacteriuria are more common among pregnant women who have bacteriuria documented at their initial prenatal evaluation *(44)*. Unfortunately, the presence of symptoms traditionally associated with urinary tract infections has a low predictive value for identifying pregnant women with bacteriuria

Table 2
Potential Toxicity of Antimicrobial Drugs During Pregnancy

	Potential toxicity	
Drug	*Fetal*	*Maternal*
Penicillin	No known toxicity	Allergy
Cephalosporins	No known toxicity	Allergy
Erythromycin base	No known toxicity	Allergy
Sulfonamides	Kernicterus hemolysis (G6PD)	Allergy
Nitrofurantoin	Hemolysis (G6PD)	Interstitial pneumonia neuropathy
Aminoglycosides	Central nervous system toxicity ototoxicity	Ototoxicity; nephrotoxicity
Metronidazole	—	Blood dyscrasia
Clindamycin	—	Pseudomembranous colitis; allergy
Isoniazid	Neuropathy; seizures	Hepatotoxicity
Tetracycline	Tooth dysplasia; inhibition of bone growth	Hepatotoxicity; renal failure
Chloramphenicol	Gray syndrome	Marrow toxicity
Trimethoprim-Sulfamethoxazole	Folate antagonism	Vasculitis
Quinolones	Abnormality of bone growth	Allergy

Modified after Loughlin *(24)*.

(45). Therefore, it is generally accepted that all pregnant women should be screened with quantitative urine cultures. The purpose of screening programs is to prevent the complications associated with bacteriuria in pregnancy. There is an association between the presence of bacteriuria in the first trimester and the subsequent development of acute pyelonephritis. Kass and associates reported that 20 to 40% of women with untreated bacteriuria will subsequently develop pyelonephritis *(45–47)*. Zinner and Kass *(43)* have stated that 1 in 3000 pregnant women with pyelonephritis will eventually develop end-stage renal disease.

Maternal bacteriuria also is associated with adverse consequences for the fetus. There is an increased risk of prematurity in pregnant women with pyelonephritis *(48)*. However, it is not clear whether treatment of asymptomatic urinary tract infections during pregnancy reduces the incidence of prematurity. It appears that increased risk of prematurity occurs mainly in women who have underlying renal involvement *(49)*. The real rationale for aggressive antibiotic treatment of bacterial cystitis during pregnancy is to prevent upper-tract infection and its potential sequelae.

Antibiotic use during pregnancy must be based on the knowledge of potential increased drug clearance caused by increased maternal glomerular filtration rate as well as the potential drug-specific toxicities to the fetus. Table 2 is modified after Loughlin *(24)* and Krieger *(43)* and lists the potential toxicity of antibiotics to the mother and fetus.

Kunin *(50)* has recommended that all pregnant women should be screened by quantitative urine cultures at their first prenatal visit, preferably in the first trimester. Most investigators recommend an antibiotic course of 7 to 10 d for urinary tract infections in pregnancy. If there is demonstration of persistent bacteriuria during pregnancy, there is an increased risk of structural urinary tract abnormalities, and a thorough urological evaluation should be performed postpartum. Quinolones have been shown to cause cartilage erosion in animal studies and are contraindicated during pregnancy *(51)*.

HYDRONEPHROSIS AND RENAL RUPTURE IN PREGNANCY

Dilation of the upper urinary tract occurs commonly in pregnancy. Dilation starts at 6 to 10 wk of gestation and is present in approx 90% of women by the third trimester. Both mechanical as well as hormonal factors likely contribute to the "physiological" hydronephrosis of pregnancy, although the mechanical factors appear to be far more important. Although dilation of the upper urinary tract is common, spontaneous rupture of the kidney or collecting system is rare. These have been 17 cases of spontaneous rupture of the collecting system or renal parenchyma *(52,53)*. Of these, five occurred in the second trimester and 12 occurred during the third trimester or immediately postpartum.

In six of the seven reported cases of spontaneous rupture of the renal parenchyma, a nephrectomy was performed. The seventh patient died before surgery could be performed. It would seem prudent to individualize the care of these patients based upon the degree of extravasation and presence of stable vital signs. In most patients, an attempt at conservative treatment with ureteral stent drainage appears reasonable. Rupture of the renal parenchyma with significant perinephric hemorrhage presents a cogent case for immediate flank exploration. If catheter drainage is unsuccessful, then open exploration, including drainage and repair, should be performed. Nephrectomy should only be performed if more conservative measures are unsuccessful.

RENAL CALCULI DURING PREGNANCY

As has been mentioned previously, it has been estimated that renal calculi occur in 1 in 1500 pregnancies *(30)*. Most stones are diagnosed during the second and third trimesters of pregnancy *(54–56)*.The initial management should be conservative because 50 to 80% of stones diagnosed during pregnancy will pass spontaneously *(57,58)*. Urinary stones, however, can jeopardize the pregnancy by causing significant fever or pain, and stones have also been reported as causing initiation of premature labor *(59,60)*.

The incidence of renal calculi is the same in pregnant women as it is in nonpregnant females *(61)*. Because of the increase in glomerular filtration rate, the filtered trace of sodium, calcium, and uric acid increases during pregnancy. Sodium excretion is unchanged because of increased tubular reabsorption, but there is an increase in uric acid excretion *(61)*. Calcium excretion can double during pregnancy *(62)*. This is because there is increased gastrointestinal absorption of calcium as the result of an increase in plasma 1,25 dihydroxy-D3. More calcium is absorbed than is required for the fetal skeleton *(61)*.

If initial conservative therapy of urolithiasis fails, then intervention of some type is indicated. However, because of the presence of hydronephrosis of pregnancy, the documentation of urolithiasis during pregnancy may not always be straightforward. Hendricks et al. *(57)* have reported that ultrasound alone confirmed the diagnosis of urinary stones in 47% of their patients. In symptomatic patients, where ultrasound was not diagnostic, they advocated a limited excretory urogram, which would normally expose the fetus to only 0.4 to 1.0 rad. Stothers and Lee *(63)* reported that ultrasound had a 34% sensitivity rate and an 86% specificity rate for stone detection in a symptomatic patient.

The use of radiation for diagnostic studies during pregnancy has been and remains controversial. Swartz and Reichling *(64)* noted the first trimester as the most significant risk period for limited ionizing radiation exposure during pregnancy. After that time, birth defects and spontaneous abortion were felt to be unlikely. However, sobering data are available that would suggest that, as urologists, we should make every effort to avoid fetal exposure to even low doses of radiation. Harvey and associates *(65)* have reported a case-control study investigating the relationship between prenatal x-ray exposure and subsequent childhood cancer. This was a retrospective study of twins born in Connecticut during a 40-yr period. Twins were chosen because a limited abdominal plain film was used to diagnose the presence of a twin gestation. It was estimated that the radiation dose to the fetus ranged from 0.16 to 4 rads, with an average dose of 1 rad, which is similar to the exposure of a limited intravenous pyelogram. Statistical analysis revealed a 1.6 relative risk of leukemia, a 3.2 relative risk of solid childhood cancers, and an overall risk of 2.4 for all childhood malignancies. Other studies *(66,67)* also have suggested a relationship between fetal irradiation and subsequent childhood malignancy. It would therefore seem prudent for the urologist to avoid any radiation to the fetus during gestation, unless the radiographic study will leave a major impact on the care of the mother.

Although radiographic studies may continue to be required in some cases of renal colic during pregnancy, technological advances are making reliance on radiography less compelling. The limitations of transabdominal ultrasound in the diagnosis of ureteral stones in pregnancy have been well described *(58,62)* However, the use of Doppler ultrasound has been reported as increasing the accuracy of diagnosing ureteral stones *(68,69)*. Doppler ultrasound has been applied to assess the mean intrarenal resistive index as a means of differentiating upper tract dilation from functional obstruction *(70)*. Hertzberg et al. *(71)* have demonstrated that the mean intrarenal resistive indices in pregnant women without urinary obstruction (physiologic hydronephrosis) was the same as in nonpregnant women without obstruction.

Another technological advance that may enhance the management of ureteral stones in pregnancy without the use of x-ray is the use of the vaginal ultrasound probe. Preliminary experience at our institution suggests that the vaginal ultrasound probe enhances the diagnosis of distal ureteral calculi that may be missed by transabdominal ultrasound alone in both pregnant and nonpregnant patients *(72)*.

If initial conservative therapy of urolithiasis fails, then intervention of some type is indicated. Our own experience with placement of internal urinary stents has been quite favorable *(73)*. Denstedt and Razvi *(74)* have stated that a potential drawback of stent placement in pregnancy is the need for x-ray confirmation of stent placement. However, we now use ultrasound alone to guide and confirm ureteral stent placement during pregnancy *(75)*. Jarrard et al. *(76)* have reported a similar experience.

If a ureteral stent cannot be passed successfully from below using ultrasound guidance, then either ureteroscopic stone removal or placement of a percutaneous nephrostomy tube should be considered. Several investigators have reported on the use of a percutaneous nephrostomy for treatment of renal colic during pregnancy *(74,75,77–79)*. Placement of the nephrostomy tube can be achieved with local anesthesia under ultrasound guidance. The experience with nephrostomy tubes in pregnancy has generally been satisfactory, although Kroovand *(55)* cautions that nephrostomy tubes may result in a higher risk of infection and more patient discomfort than internal stents. Denstedt and Razvi *(74)* advocate the placement of a percutaneous nephrostomy tube rather than an internal stent in the pregnant patient with urosepsis to ensure adequate drainage. Although there have been reports of successful percutaneous nephrolithotomy in pregnancy *(79,80)*, we agree with Kroovand *(55)* that because of prolonged anesthesia requirements and the potential harmful effects of ionizing radiation that such procedures are rarely indicated during pregnancy.

A common complication of both ureteral stents and nephrostomy tubes has been stone encrustation *(73,*78). This may be exacerbated by hyperuricosuria and hypercalciuria that may occur during pregnancy *(81,82)*. The optimal interval for stent or nephrostomy tube changes in pregnancy has not been determined. However, it would appear reasonable to encourage good hydration in all pregnant patients with stents or nephrostomy tubes and to consider tube changes at least every 8 wk during pregnancy.

However, both ureteral stents and nephrostomy tubes may cause the patient discomfort. Some investigators have advocated ureteroscopic stone removal during pregnancy *(83,84)*. If uteroscopy is used, it should be used without fluoroscopy *(85)*. Extracorporeal shock wave lithotripsy has not been approved for use during pregnancy, and a recent report demonstrates intrauterine growth retardation after exposure to extracorporeal shock wave lithotripsy (ESWL) in an animal model *(86)*. However, a recent report showed no birth defects in the children of six women who had inadvertently undergone ESWL during the first month of pregnancy *(87)*. Nonetheless, the current recommendation is that no pregnant women should undergo ESWL. In a small percentage of patients, open surgical removal of stones may be necessary.

PLACENTA PERCRETA INVADING THE URINARY BLADDER

The placenta, normally confined to the decidual lining of the uterine cavity, can in some instances invade the muscular wall of the uterus, a condition known as placenta accreta. Less common is placenta increta, in which placental cotyledons become intertwined with the muscular stroma of the uterus. Placenta percreta, in which the trophoblastic tissues penetrate the serosa of the uterus and may extend directly to adjacent structures, including the bladder, is even more rare and potentially life threatening. We have reported our own experience with three cases of placenta percreta invading the urinary bladder and 10 other cases previously reported in the literature *(88)*. All of these cases had a previous history of cesarean section and all presented with hematuria. Any case of placenta percreta with invasion into the bladder presents the potential for massive blood loss, which the surgical team needs to anticipate. In any woman with a previous history of cesarean section, who presents with hematuria during pregnancy, the diagnosis of placenta percreta should be considered. Ultrasound evaluation is extremely valuable. If cystoscopy is performed, the bladder lesion should not be biopsied, as severe bleeding may occur.

UROLOGICAL CANCER DURING PREGNANCY

It has been estimated that the incidence of malignancy in pregnancy is approx 1 in 1000 *(89)*. Although Gleicher et al. *(90)* have stated that pregnancy and cancer are the only two biological conditions in which antigenic tissue is tolerated by a seemingly intact immune system, there does not seem to be any increased incidence of cancer in pregnancy as compared with nonpregnant women of reproductive age *(91)*.

Walker and Knight *(92)* have reviewed the subject of renal cell carcinoma in pregnancy. They emphasize in their literature review that renal adenocarcinoma is the most common renal neoplasm in pregnancy, accounting for almost 50% of renal malignancies, with angiomyolipoma being second. The most common symptom of renal cell carcinoma in pregnancy is a palpable mass, which occurred in 88% of patients; hematuria was noted in 47% of the patients. The diagnostic workup is tailored to limit radiation exposure to mother and child. Abdominal ultrasound and magnetic resonance imaging can adequately identify and stage a solid renal mass in most cases without exposing the mother or fetus to radiation *(93)*. Management of the solid renal mass during pregnancy should be based on the premise that the urologist's primary responsibility is to the mother. Surgery in the first trimester will result in fetal loss, whereas surgery in the third trimester usually will result in survival of both mother and fetus. When planning management in an individual case, two important facts should be given consideration. First, the doubling time of renal carcinoma has been estimated to be 300 d *(94)*. Second, with improved perinatal care, fetal survival continues to improve. At 28 wk gestation, neonatal survival rates of over 90% can be expected *(95,96)*. With these caveats, it would seem advisable to operate on all women with a solid renal mass diagnosed in the first trimester. If the mass is diagnosed in the second trimester, it would seem reasonable to continue the pregnancy to 28 wk gestation, test for fetal lung maturity, and then perform a radical nephrectomy with delivery of the infant if labor ensues. Successful cases of simultaneous cesarean section and radical nephrectomy have been reported at 28 wk gestation *(97)*. If a solid renal mass is diagnosed in the third trimester, it is reasonable, after documenting fetal lung maturity, to proceed with radical nephrectomy. Obviously, the cases will be individualized to some extent, based on the wishes and concerns of the mother and other family members.

Ten cases of transitional cell carcinomas of the bladder have been reported during pregnancy *(98–104)* All pregnant patients with hematuria should have their upper tracts evaluated with renal ultrasound. It should be noted that four patients with bladder cancer during pregnancy reported in the literature were initially thought to have vaginal bleeding rather than gross hematuria. Our own experience and others suggest that a well-performed bladder ultrasound may obviate the need for cystoscopy *(105)*. Successful transurethral resection of bladder tumors can be accomplished during pregnancy and should be performed if a bladder tumor is found. Pheochromocytoma during pregnancy presents an interesting challenge to the obstetrical and surgical team. Pheochromocytoma in pregnancy is most dangerous if it remains undiagnosed *(106–111)*. In these circumstances, maternal mortality exceeds 50% *(112–114)*. Deaths have been caused primarily by malignant hypertensive crisis and/or shock, which is most often precipitated by delivery. The signs and symptoms of pheochromocytoma during pregnancy are essentially no different than in the nonpregnant patient. The patients most often present with severe preeclampsia or typical attacks of paroxysmal hypertension, sweating, and tachycardia. McCullough *(115)* has emphasized that supine hypertension is an important clue to pheochromocytoma in the pregnant patient. Plasma catecholamines and/or urinary metanephrines and vanillylmandelic acid are measured to document the presence of pheochromocytoma. Radiographic localizing studies can be modified during pregnancy. Greenberg et al. *(116)* have reported the use of magnetic resonance imaging as an alternative to computed tomography scanning for localization of pheochromocytoma during pregnancy. We have successfully used abdominal ultrasound to document the presence of pheochromocytoma during pregnancy. At the present time, there are no reports on the use of meta-(I-131) iodobenzylguanidine during pregnancy.

After the diagnosis of pheochromocytoma has been established, the α-adrenergic blockade should be instituted. Because of the potential mutagenic effects of phenoxybenzamine, prazosin is considered the α-blocker of choice during pregnancy. Beta blockade may also be necessary, but may slow fetal heart rate and increase myometrial contractility *(113,114)*. Usually, it is safest to proceed with surgical resection regardless of the gestational age of the fetus. With accurate preoperative diagnosis and proper pharmacologic management, mother and child have a good prognosis for survival is surgery if performed in the third trimester.

Janetschek et al. *(111)* have recently reported two successful cases of the laparoscopic removal of pheochromocytomas during pregnancy. The patients underwent surgery at 16 and 20 wk of gestation. Another case by Aishima et al. *(115)* has reported the laparoscopic removal of an adrenal during pregnancy because of Cushing's syndrome. However, further reports and wider experience will be necessary before the laparoscopic approach to the adrenal during pregnancy becomes the standard of care.

PREGNANCY AFTER URINARY DIVERSION

Successful pregnancies and deliveries have been reported after both continent and standard urinary diversions *(115–120)*. It has been recommended that the mode of delivery should be guided by obstetric indications *(116)*, although vaginal delivery has been accomplished in the majority of these patients. If a cesarean section is necessary, a urologist should be available to the obstetrical team for consultation. Patients with urinary diversions do not appear to be at greater risk for urinary tract infections during pregnancy than the average patient *(117)*. The physiological changes that occur during pregnancy usually do not compromise the continence mechanisms in patients with either urinary or fecal continent diversions *(119–121)*.

Hill and Kramer *(122)* reported the management of pregnancy after augmentation cystoplasty in 15 patients. They found urinary tract infection or pyelonephritis in 9 of the 15 patients and premature labor occurred in 4 patients. Their recommendation was that a vaginal delivery could be performed in patients without a history of bladder neck reconstruction. However, if the patient has a history of placement of an artificial sphincter or bladder neck reconstruction, cesarean section should be performed.

PREGNANCY AFTER RENAL TRANSPLANTATION

Murray and associates *(123)* reported the first successful pregnancy following renal transplantation. It has been estimated that pregnancy occurs in 1 of 200 women of reproductive age on dialysis and 1 in 50 women of childbearing age after successful renal transplantation. Complications during pregnancy are more common in renal transplant patients. Complications that are more likely to occur include urinary tract infections, preeclampsia, premature delivery, premature rupture of membranes, premature onset of labor, and babies that are small for their gestational age *(124)*. Approximately 9% of patients will experience an episode of acute rejection during pregnancy, which is comparable with that of the nonpregnant population *(124)*. There does appear to be an increased risk of premature delivery in renal transplant patients, which may be the result of pregnancy-induced hypertension, worsening renal function, or fetal distress *(122)*. The commonly used immunosuppressive drugs, such as prednisone, azathioprine, and cyclosporine A, present potential teratogenic risks *(125,126)*. However, fetal malformation caused by immunosuppressive drugs appears to be rare and does not contraindicate maintenance of maternal immunosuppression.

PREGNANCY AND URINARY INCONTINENCE

There are three areas of interest regarding pregnancy and urinary incontinence. First, if the patient has had anti-incontinence surgery before surgery does it alter the obstetrical management? Second, what influence, if any, does pregnancy have on urinary incontinence during gestation? Third, how does pregnancy impact postpartum continence rates? The answer to the first question is that cesarean section appears to be the preferred method of delivery in women who have undergone previous anti-incontinence surgery. A report by Dainer et al. *(127)* of a cohort of pregnant women who had undergone previous anti-incontinence surgery demonstrated a 73% postpartum continence status in women who had vaginal deliveries compared with a 95% continence rate in those managed by cesarean section ($p = 0.0344$)

The second issue is what effect does the state of pregnancy itself have on continence mechanisms? The answer is that urinary incontinence during pregnancy appears to be quite common. Mason et al. *(128)* reviewed the literature and found the prevalence of stress incontinence reported to be between 20 and 67%. They followed this with a questionnaire to over 1000 of their own patients and corroborated that 59% of the women responding confirmed stress incontinence during pregnancy, and in 31%, it persisted after delivery.

The third issue of postpartum incontinence is complex and is probably affected by multiple factors. As mentioned above, vaginal deliveries are associated with a higher rate of stress incontinence than cesarean sections. However, at least one study suggests *(129)* that birth weight per se is not predictive of postpartum incontinence.

THE UROLOGIST IN THE DELIVERY ROOM

Bladder injury has been reported to occur in 4 to 14% of women undergoing cesarean section *(130–133)*. Injuries to the bladder dome are easily recognized and repaired. However, injuries to the bladder base, which are more often associated with repeat cesarean sections, can transect the entire trigone and present a more difficult operative challenge. In managing such injuries, the ureteral orifices should be identified and catheterized before repair of the bladder.

Ureteral injuries occur during 1 in 1000 cesarean deliveries *(131–133)*. Most often, ureteral injuries occur during efforts to control bleeding from the lateral extension of the uterine incision. When repairing ureteral injuries in these circumstances, the urologist should control the bleeding, obtain adequate exposure, and check for other unrecognized injuries to the urinary tract *(134)*. The use of a ureteral catheter and suprapubic tube is preferable in most cases. The preferred operation in most circumstances is a ureteroneocystostomy with a psoas hitch *(135)*.

CONCLUSION

In summary, the entire range of urological problems from urinary tract infections to malignancy can be encountered during pregnancy. Following the principles outlined above, it should be possible to manage all of these problems in a rational manner while minimizing morbidity and mortality to mother and fetus.

REFERENCES

1. Lee MM, Taylor SH, Scott DB, et al. A study of cardiac output at rest during pregnancy. J Obstet Gynaecol Br Commonwealth 1967; 74:319–328.
2. Lund CJ, Donovan JC. Blood volume during pregnancy. Am J Obstet Gynecol 1967; 98: 393–408.
3. Steinberg ES, Santos AC. Surgical anesthesia during pregnancy. Int Anesthesiol Clin 1990; 28: 58–66.
4. Dean M, Stock B, Patterson RJ. Serum protein binding of drugs during and after pregnancy in humans. Clin Pharmacol Ther 1980; 28: 257–261.
5. Santos AC, Pederson H, Harmon TW, et al. Does pregnancy alter the systemic toxicity of local anesthetics? Anesthesiology 1989; 70: 991–995.
6. Veland K, Parer JT. Effects of estrogens on the cardiovascular system of the ewe. Am J Obstet Gynecol 1966; 96: 400–406.
7. Goodman RP, Killam AP, Brash AR, Branch RA. Prostacyclin production during pregnancy: Comparison of production during normal pregnancy and pregnancy complicated by hypertension. Am J Obstet Gynecol 1982; 142: 817–822.
8. Prowse CM, Gaensler EA. Respiratory and acid-base changes during pregnancy. Anesthesiology 1965; 26: 381–392.
9. Archer GW, Marx GF. Arterial oxygenation during apnea in parturient women. Br J Anaesth 1974; 46: 358–360.
10. Barron WM. Medical evaluation of the pregnant patient requiring nonobstetric surgery. Clin Perinatol 1985; 12(3):481–496.
11. Hathaway WE, Bonnar J. Perinatal Coagulation. Grune and Stratton, New York, NY, 1978, pp. 27–51.
12. Letsky E. The hematological system. In: Hytten F, Chamberlain G, eds. Clinical Physiology in Obstetrics. Blackwell Scientific Publications, Oxford, England, 1980, pp. 43–78.
13. de Swiet M. The cardiovascular system. In: Hytten F, Chamberlain G, eds. Clinical Physiology in Obstetrics. Blackwell Scientific Publications, Oxford, England, 1980, pp. 3–42.
14. Kakkar VV. The current status of low-dose heparin in the prophylaxis of thrombophlebitis and pulmonary embolism. World J Surg 1978; 2: 3–13.
15. Simpson KH, Stakes AF, Miler M. Pregnancy delays Paracetamol absorption and gastric emptying in patients undergoing surgery. Br J Anaesth 1988; 60: 24–27.
16. Lindheimer MD, Katz AI. The renal response to pregnancy. In: Brenner BM, Rector RC, eds. The Kidney, 2nd Ed. W.B. Saunders Co., Philadelphia, PA, 1981, pp. 1762–1819.
17. Hsia TY, Shortliffe LM.: The effect of pregnancy on rat urinary tract dynamics. J Urol 1995; 154 (2pt2) 684–689.
18. Schulman A, Herlinger H. Urinary tract dilatation in pregnancy. Br J Radiol 1975; 48: 638–645.
19. Tong YC, Wein AC, Levin RM. Effects of pregnancy on adrenergic function in the rabbit urinary bladder. Urodyn 1992; 11: 525–533.
20. Foldspang A, Mommsen A, Law GW, Elving L. Parity as a correlate of adult female urinary incontinence prevalence. J. Epidemiol Common Health 1992; 46: 595–600.
21. Viktrup L, Lose G, Rolff M, Barfoed K. The symptom of stress incontinence caused by pregnancy or delivery in primiparas. Obstet Gynecol 1992; 79: 945–949.
22. Lee JG, Wein AJ, Levin RM. Effects of pregnancy on urethral and bladder neck function. Urology 1993; 42: 747–752.
23. Barron WM. The pregnant surgical patient: Medical evaluations and management. Ann Intern Med 1984; 101: 683–691.
24. Loughlin KR. Caring for your pregnant patient. Contemp Urol 1992; 4: 22–38.
25. Kammerer WS. Non-obstetric surgery during pregnancy. Med Clin North Am 1979; 6: 1157–1164.
26. Babaknia A, Hossein P, Woodruff JD. Appendicitis during pregnancy. Obstet Gynaecol 1977; 50: 40–44.

27. Horowitz MD, Gomez GA, Santiesteban R, Burkett G. Acute appendicitis during pregnancy. Arch Surg 1985; 120: 1362–1367.
28. Welch JP. Miscellaneous causes of small bowel obstruction. In: Wekh J, ed. Bowel Obstruction: Differential Diagnosis and Clinical Management. W.B. Saunders Co., London, England, 1990, pp. 454–456.
29. Woodhouse DR, Haylen B. Gallbladder disease complicating pregnancy. Aust NZ J Obstet Gynaecol 1985; 25: 223–237.
30. Drago JR, Rohner TJ Jr, Chez RA. Management of urinary calculi in pregnancy. Urology 1982; 20: 578–581.
31. Setchell M. Abdominal pain in pregnancy. In Studd J, ed. Progress in Obstetrics and Gynaecology, Vol. 6. Churchill Livingstone, London, England, 1987, pp. 87–99.
32. Smoleniec J, James D: General surgical problems in pregnancy. Br J Surg 1990; 77: 1203–1204.
33. Silen W. Cope's Early Diagnosis of the Acute Abdomen, 17th Ed. Oxford University Press, New York, NY, 1987, pp. 210–213.
34. Hull LM, Johnson CE, Lee RA. Cholecystectomy in pregnancy. Obstet Gynecol 1975; 9: 291–293.
35. Palahniuk RJ, Schneider SM, Eger EI. Pregnancy decreases the requirements for inhaled anesthetic agents. Anesthesiology 1974; 41: 82–83.
36. Merryman W: "Progesterone" anesthesia in human subjects. J Clin Endocrinol Metab 1954; 14: 1567–1568,.
37. Lyreras S, Nyberg F, Lindberg B, Terenius L. Cerebrospinal fluid activity of dynorphin-converting enzyme at term pregnancy. Obstet Gynecol 1988; 72: 54–58.
38. Fagraeus L, Urban BJ, Bromage PR. Spread of epidural analgesia in early pregnancy. Anesthesiology 1983; 58: 184–187.
39. Datta S, Lambert DH, Gregus J. Differential sensitivities of mammalian nerve fibers during pregnancy. Anesth-Analg 1983; 62: 1070–1072.
40. Safra M, Oakley GP. Association between cleft lip with or without cleft palate and prenatal exposure to diazepam. Lancet 1975; 2: 478–480.
41. Saxen I, Saxen L. Association between maternal intake of diazepam and oral clefts. Lancet 1975; 2: 498.
42. Krieger JN. Complications and treatment of urinary tract infections during pregnancy. Urol Clin North Am 1986; 13(4):685–693.
43. Sweet RL. Bacteriuria and pyelonephritis during pregnancy. Semin Perinatol 1977; 1: 25–40.
44. Kass EH. A symptomatic infection of the urinary tract. Trans Assoc Am Phys 1956; 69: 56–63.
45. Kass EH. The role of unsuspected infection in the etiology of prematurity. Clin Obstet Gynecol 1973; 16: 134–152.
46. Norden CW, Kass EH. Bacteriuria of pregnancy: a critical appraisal. Ann Rev Med 1968; 19: 431–470.
47. Zinner SH, Kass EH. Long term (10–14 years) follow-up of bacteriuria of pregnancy. N Engl J Med 1971; 285: 820–824.
48. McFadyen IR, Eykyn SJ, Gardner NH. Bacteriuria in pregnancy. J Obstet Gynaecol Br Commonwealth 1973; 80: 385–405.
49. Zinner SH. Bacteriuria and babies revisited. N Engl J Med 1979; 300: 853–855.
50. Kunin, CM. The Concepts of "significant bacteria" and asymptomatic bacteria, clinical syndromes and the epidemiology of urinary tract infections. In: Detection, Prevention and Management of Urinary Tract Infections, 4th Ed. Lea and Febiger, Philadelphia, PA, 1987, pp. 57–124.
51. The Medical Letter. 1991; 33 (849): 71–73.
52. Oesterling JE, Besinger, RE, Brendler CB. Spontaneous rupture of the renal collecting system during pregnancy: successful management with a temporary ureteral catheter. J Urol 1988; 140: 588–590.
53. El Halabi DAR, Humayun MS, Sharhaan JM. Spontaneous rupture of hydronephrotic kidney during pregnancy. Br J Urol 1991; 67(2):219–220.
54. Mostwin J. Surgery of the kidney and ureter in pregnancy. In: Marshall F, ed. Operative Urology. W.B. Saunders Co., Philadelphia, PA, 1991, pp. 108–113 .
55. Kroovand RL. Stones in pregnancy and in children. J Urol 1992; 148: 1076–1078.
56. Lattanzi DR, Cook WA. Urinary calculi in pregnancy. Obstet Gynecol 1980; 56: 462–466.

57. Hendricks SK, Russ SO, Krieger JN. An algorithm for diagnosis and therapy of management and complications of urolithiasis during pregnancy. Surg Gynecol Obstet 1991; 172: 49–54.
58. Rodriguez PN, Klein AS. Management of urolithiasis during pregnancy. Surg Gynecol Obstet 1988; 166: 103–106.
59. Colombo PA, Pitino R, Pascalino MC, Quoronta S. Control of uterine contraction with tocolytic agents. Ann Obstet Gynecol Med Perinatal 1981; 102: 431–440.
60. Broaddus SB, Catalano PM, Leadbetter GW, Mann LI. Cessation of premature labor following removal of distal ureteral calculus. Am J Obstet Gynecol 1982; 143: 846–848.
61. Gorton E, Whitfield HN. Renal calculi in pregnancy. Br J Urol 1997; 56(1):4–9.
62. Maikranz P, Lindheimer M, Coe F. Nephrolithiasis in pregnancy. Balliere's Clin Obstet Gynecol 1994; 8: 375–380.
63. Stothers L, Lee LM. Renal colic in pregnancy. J Urol 1992; 148: 1383–1387.
64. Swartz HM, Reichling BA. Hazards of radiation exposure for pregnant women JAMA 1978; 239: 1907–1908.
65. Harvey EB, Boice JD, Honeyman M, Flannery JT. Prenatal x-ray exposure and childhood cancer in twins. N Engl J Med 1985; 312: 541–545.
66. MacMahon B. Prenatal x-ray exposure and childhood cancer. J Natl Cancer Inst 1962; 28: 1173–1191.
67. Mole RH. Antenatal irradiation and childhood cancer: Causation or coincidence? Br J Cancer 1974; 30: 199–208.
68. Burge HJ, Middleton WD, McClennan BL, Dildebolt CF. Ureteral jets in healthy subjects and in patients with unilateral ureteral calculi, comparison with color Doppler US. Radiology 1991; 180: 437–442.
69. Platt JF, Rubin JM, Ellis JH. Acute renal obstruction: Evaluation with intrarenal duplex Doppler and conventional US. Radiology 1993; 186: 685–688.
70. Platt JF, Rubin JM, Ellis JH, DiPietro MA. Duplex Doppler US of the kidney: differentiation of obstructive from non-obstructive dilation. Radiology 1989; 171: 515–517.
71. Hertzberg BS, Carroll BA, Bowie JD, et al. Doppler US assessment of maternal kidneys: Analysis of intrarenal resistivity indexes in normal pregnancy and physiologic pelvicaliectasis. Radiology 1993; 186: 689–692.
72. Laing FC, Benson CB, DiSalvo DN, Brown DL, Frates MC, Loughlin KR. Detection of distal ureteral calculi by vaginal ultrasound. Radiology 1994; 192(2): 545–548.
73. Loughlin KR, Bailey RB Jr. Internal ureteral stents for conservative management of ureteral calculi during pregnancy. N Engl J Med 1986; 315: 1647–1649.
74. Denstedt JD, Razvi H. Management of urinary calculi during pregnancy. J Urol 1992; 148: 1072–1075.
75. Gluck CD, Benson, Bundy AL, Doyle CJ, Loughlin KR. Renal sonography for placement and monitoring of ureteral stents during pregnancy. J Endourol 1991; 5: 241–243.
76. Jarrard DJ, Gerber GS, Lyon ES. Management of acute ureteral obstruction in pregnancy utilizing ultrasound-guided placement of ureteral stents. Urology 1993; 42: 263–268.
77. Horowitz E, Schmidt JD. Renal calculi in pregnancy. Clin Obstet Gynecol 1985; 28: 324–338.
78. Rodriguez PN, Klein AS. Management of urolithiasis during pregnancy. Surg Gynecol Obstet 1988; 166: 103–106.
79. Kavoussi LR, Albala DM, Basler JW, Apte S, Clayman RV. Percutaneous management of urolithiasis during pregnancy. J Urol 1992; 148: 1069–1071.
80. Holman E, Toth C, Khan MA. Percutaneous nephrolithotomy in late pregnancy. J Endourol 1992; 6: 421–424.
81. Boyle JA, Campbell S, Duncan AM, Greig WR, Buchanan WW. Serum uric acid levels in normal pregnancy with observations on the renal excretion of urate in pregnancy. J Clin Pathol 1966; 19: 501–503.
82. Gertner JM, Coustan DR, Kliger AS, Mallette LE, Ravin N, Broaddus AE. Pregnancy as state of physiologic absorptive hypercalciuria. Am J Med 1986; 81: 451–456.
83. Vest JM. Ureteroscopic stone manipulation during pregnancy. Urology 1990; 35: 250–252.
84. Rittenberg MH, Bagley DH. Ureteroscopic diagnosis and treatment of urinary calculi during pregnancy. Urology 1988; 32: 427–428.
85. Shokei AA, Mutabagani H. Rigid ureterscopy in pregnant women. Br J Urol 1998; 81: 678–681.

86. Smith DP, Graham JB, Prystowsky JB, Dalkin BL, Nemcek AA. The effects of ultrasound-guided shock waves during early pregnancy in Sprague-Dawley rats. J Urol 145: Abstract 180, presented at American Urological Association Meeting, Toronto, Canada, June, 1991.
87. Agari MA Sutarinejad MR, Hosseini Sy, Dadkhah F. Extracorporated Shock wave lithotripsy of renal cauli during early pregnancy. BJU Int 1999; 84: 615–617.
88. Litwin MS, Loughlin KR, Benson CB, Droege GF, Richie JP. Placenta percreta invading the urinary bladder. Br J Urol 1988; 64: 283–286.
89. Williams SF, Bitran JD. Cancer and pregnancy. Clin Perinatol 1985;12:609–623.
90. Gleicher N, Deppe B, Cohen CJ. Common aspects of immunologic tolerance in pregnancy and malignancy. Obstet Gynecol 1979; 54: 335–342.
91. Nieminen N, Remes N. Malignancy during pregnancy. Acta Obstet Gynecol Scand 1970; 49: 315–319.
92. Walker JL, Knight EL: Renal cell carcinoma in pregnancy. Cancer 1986; 58: 2343–2347.
93. Weinreb JC, Brown CE, Lowe TW, Cohen JM, Erdman WA. Pelvic masses in pregnant patients: MR and US imaging. Genit Radiol 1986; 159: 717–724.
94. Rabes HM. Growth kinetics of human renal adenocarcinoma In: Sufrin G, Beckley SA, eds. Renal Adenocarcinoma, Vol. 49, VICC Technical Report Series, Geneva International Union Against Cancer, Geneva, Switzerland, 1980, 78–95.
95. Herschel M, Kennedy JL, Kayne HL, Henry M, Cetrulo CL. Survival of infants born at 24 to 28 weeks gestation. Obstet Gynecol 1982; 60: 154–158.
96. Amon E. Limits of fetal viability. Obstet Gynecol Clin N Am 1988; 15:321–338.
97. Kobayashi T, Fukuzawa S, Muira K, et al. A case of renal cell carcinoma during pregnancy: simultaneous cesarean section and radical nephrectomy. J Urol 2000; 163: 1515–1516.
98. Bendsen J, Muller EK, Povey G. Bladder tumor as apparent cause of vaginal bleeding in pregnancy. Acta Obstet Gynecol Scand 1985; 64: 329–330.
99. Cruickshank SH, McNellis TM. Carcinoma of the bladder in pregnancy. Am J Obstet Gynecol 1983; 145: 768–770.
100. Fehrenbaker LG, Rhoads JC, Derby DR. Transitional cell carcinoma of the bladder during pregnancy: case report. J Urol 1972; 108: 419–420.
101. Keegan GT, Farkowitz MJL. Transitional cell carcinoma of the bladder during pregnancy: a case report. Tex Med 1982; 78: 44–45.
102. Sheffrey JB: Prolapsed malignant tumor of the bladder as a complication of pregnancy. Am J Obstet Gynecol 1946; 51: 910–911.
103. Choate JW, Thiede HA, Miller, HC. Carcinoma of the bladder in pregnancy: report of three cases. Am J Obstet Gynecol 1964; 90: 526–530.
104. Gonzalez-Blanco S, Mador DR, Vickar DB, McPhee M. Primary bladder cancer presenting during pregnancy in three cases. J Urol 1989; 141: 613–614.
105. Benacerraf BR, Kearney GP, Gittes RF. Ultrasound diagnosis of small asymptomatic bladder carcinoma in patients referred for gynecological care. J Urol 1984; 132: 892–893.
106. Burgess GE III. Alpha blockade and surgical intervention of pheochromocytoma in pregnancy. Obstet Gynecol 1978; 53: 266–270.
107. Schenker JG, Grant M. Pheochromocytoma and pregnancy: an updated appraisal. Aust NZ J Obstet Gynaecol 1982; 22: 1–10.
108. Manger WM, Gifford RW, Hoffman BB. Pheochromocytoma: a clinical and experimental overview. Curr Prob Cancer 1985; 9: 1–89.
109. Wagener GW, Van Rendborg LC, Schaetzing A. Pheochromocytoma in pregnancy. A case report and review. S Afr J Surg 1981; 19: 251–255.
110. Griffin J, Brooks N, Patricia F. Pheochromocytoma in pregnancy: diagnosis and collaborative management. South Med J 1984; 77: 1325–1327.
111. Janetschek G, Finkenstedt G, Gasser R, et al. Laparoscopic surgery for pheochromocytoma: adrenalectomy, partial resection, excision of paragangliomas. J Urol 1998; 160: 330–334.
112. Mitchell SZ, Frelich JD, Brant D, Flynn M. Anesthetic management of pheochromocytoma resection during pregnancy. Anesth Anal 1987; 66: 478–480.
113. Aishma M, Tanaka M, Haraoka M, Naito S. Retroperitoneal laparascopic adrenalectomy in a pregnant woman with cushing's syndrome. J Urol 2000;164: 770–771.

114. Greenberg RE, Vaughan ED Jr, Pitts WR Jr. Normal pregnancy and delivery after ileal conduit urinary diversion. J Urol 1981; 125: 172–173.
115. McCullough DL. Pheochromocytoma. In: Resnick MI, Karsh E, eds. Current Therapy in Genitourinary Surgery. C.V. Mosby Co. Toronto, Philadelphia, 1987, pp. 4–7.
116. Greenberg M, Moawad A, Weities B. Extraadrenal pheochromocytoma: detection during pregnancy using MR imaging. Radiology 1986, 161: 475–476.
117. Bravo RH, Katz M. Ureteral obstruction in a pregnant patient with an ileal loop conduit. A case report. J Reprod Med 1983; 28: 427–429.
118. Barrett RJ, Peters WA. Pregnancy following urinary diversion. Obstet Gynecol 1983; 62: 582–586.
119. Akerlund S, Bokstrom H, Jonson O, Kock NG, Wennergren M. Pregnancy and delivery in patients with urinary diversion through the continent ileal reservoir. Surg Gynecol Obstet 1991; 173: 350–352.
120. Ojerskog B, Kock NG, Philipson BM, Philipson M. Pregnancy and delivery in patients with a continent ileostomy. Surg Gynecol Obstet 1988; 167: 61–64.
121. Kennedy WA, Hensle TW, Reiley EA, Fox HE, Haus T. Pregnancy after orthotopic continent urinary diversion. Surg Gynecol Obstet 1993; 177: 405–409.
122. Hill DE, Kramer SA. Management of pregnancy after augmentation cystoplasty. J Urol 1990; 144: 457–459.
123. Murray JE, Reid DE, Harrison JH, Merrill JP. Successful pregnancies after human renal transplantation. N Engl J Med 1963; 269: 341–343.
124. Lau RJ, Scott JR. Pregnancy following renal transplantation. Clin Obstet Gynecol 1985; 28: 339–350.
125. Fine RN. Pregnancy in renal allograft recipients. Am J Nephrol 1982; 2: 117–121.
126. Pickrell MD, Sawers R, Michael J. Pregnancy after renal transplantation: severe intrauterine growth retardation during treatment with cyclosporine A. Br Med J 1988; 296: 825.
127. Dainer M, Hall CD, Choen J. Bhutian: pegnancy following incontinence surgery. Int Urogynecol J Pelvic Floor Dystruration 1998; 916: 385–390.
128. Mason L, Glenn S, Walton I, Appleton C. The prevalence of stress incontinence during pregnancy and following delivery. Midwifery 1999; 15: 120–128.
129. Kirue S, Jenson H, Agger AO, Rasmussen KL. The influence of infant birth weight on post partum stress incontinence in obese women. Arch Gynecol Obstet 1997; 259: 143–145.
130. Raghaviah NV, Devi AI. Bladder injury associated with rupture of the uterus. Obstet Gynecol 1975; 46: 573–575.
131. Eisenkop SM, Richman R, Platt LD. Urinary tract injury during cesarean section. Obstet Gynecol 1983; 60: 591–593.
132. Michal A, Begneaud WP, Hawes TP Jr. Pitfalls and complications of cesarean section hysterectomy. Clin Obstet Gynecol 1969; 12: 660–663.
133. Barclay DL. Cesarean hysterectomy: a thirty year experience. Obstet Gynecol 1970; 35: 120–123.
134. Loughlin KR. The urologist in the delivery room. Urol Clin North Am 2002; 29:705–708.
135. Meirow D, Moriel EZ, Zilberman M, Farkas A. Evaluation and treatment of iatrogenic ureteral injuries during obstetric and gynecologic operations for nonmalignant conditions. Surg Gynecol Obstet 1994; 178: 144–148.

2 Pediatric Potpourri

Jonathan H. Ross, MD

Contents

PAINLESS SCROTAL MASSES

The differential diagnosis of a painless scrotal mass includes a hernia, hydrocele, varicocele, epididymal cyst, and paratesticular and testicular tumors. The most important element in making the diagnosis is the physical exam. A hernia is usually a soft scrotal mass that extends up the inguinal canal. Often gas-filled loops of bowel can be appreciated on palpation. With the child calm, the mass can usually be reduced into the abdomen through the internal ring. A hydrocele is appreciated as a fluid-filled mass, which may be soft or firm. It generally surrounds the testis, although it may occur in the cord above the testicle. Hydroceles in children are usually communicating, and sometimes the fluid can be forced back into the abdomen with gentle compression. But even when this is not possible, a communication is usually present. In large hydroceles, the testicle can be difficult to palpate. Generally, it is in a posterior-dependent position in the scrotum and can be felt through the hydrocele fluid in this location. Because testis tumors can occasionally present with an acute hydrocele, an ultrasound should be obtained if the testis cannot be felt. Discrete masses within or adjacent to the testicle are worrisome because they raise the possibility of a tumor that may be malignant. Fortunately, scrotal malignancies are extremely rare. Most discrete scrotal masses in boys are epididymal cysts. These are felt as small firm spherical masses associated with the epididymis, usually at the upper pole of the testis. One should confirm on physical exam that the mass

From: *Essential Urology: A Guide to Clinical Practice*
Edited by: J. M. Potts © Humana Press Inc., Totowa, NJ

is separate from the testicle itself, and by transillumination that it is cystic. If either of these characteristics is uncertain, an ultrasound will resolve the issue. A varicocele is a distended group of scrotal veins that usually occurs on the left side. In the upright position it has the appearance and feel of a "bag of worms." It should reduce significantly in size in the recumbent position. In the unusual circumstance that the venous distension persists with the patient supine, the abdomen should be imaged to rule out a tumor impinging venous drainage from the retroperitoneum.

Hydroceles and hernias occur when the processus vaginalis fails to obliterate after testicular descent. The processus vaginalis is a tongue of peritoneum that descends into the scrotum adjacent to the testicle during fetal development. If it persists after birth, then peritoneal fluid can travel back and forth through this connection resulting in a communicating hydrocele. The fluid is of no consequence in itself, but if the connection increases in size over time, intestines and/or omentum may travel through it. When this occurs, the entity is considered a hernia. Most hydroceles present at birth will resolve by 1 yr of age. The parents should be told the signs of a hernia (an intermittent inguinal bulge), and unless this occurs, the patient may be safely observed. If the hydrocele fails to resolve by 1 yr of age, it is repaired surgically to prevent the ultimate development of a clinical hernia. A connection large enough to allow more than fluid to traverse it (i.e., a hernia) will not resolve over time. Intestines may become entrapped in the hernia, creating an emergency situation. For that reason, infants and children with hernias undergo surgical repair without an interval of observation. Hydrocele and hernia repairs are essentially the same operation. They are performed on an outpatient basis through an inguinal incision. The crucial element in the repair is closure of the processus vaginalis at the internal ring. There is approximately a 1% risk of injury to the testicular vessels or vas.

Testicular tumors are rare but should be suspected whenever a mass is felt in the testicle. Many testis tumors in children are yolk sac tumors—a malignancy. However, a significant number are benign. Whenever a testis tumor is suspected, an ultrasound should be obtained. If the ultrasound confirms the presence of a testicular mass, then an alphafetoprotein (AFP) level is obtained. The AFP level will be elevated in 90% of patients with a yolk sac tumor. Virtually all children with a testicular mass require surgical exploration. If, based on the ultrasound and AFP, a yolk sac tumor is considered likely, then an inguinal orchiectomy is performed. If a benign tumor is considered possible, then an inguinal exploration is undertaken and an excisional biopsy performed. Whether the testicle is then removed or replaced in the scrotum is based on the frozen section diagnosis.

HYDRONEPHROSIS

The widespread use of prenatal ultrasound has raised new questions regarding the evaluation and management of hydronephrosis. Before the use of prenatal ultrasonography, the vast majority of patients with hydronephrosis presented with symptoms such as pain, an abdominal mass, urinary tract infection, or hematuria. However, 80 –90% of infants with hydronephrosis are now being detected prenatally. The postnatal detection rate is not significantly different from the preultrasound era, implying that the overall detection rate for these lesions is 5 to 10 times greater than previously. This raises the possibility that many of these hydronephrotic kidneys might have remained asymptomatic and unrecognized if not for prenatal ultrasound. When a patient presents with hydronephrosis and symptoms, there is little question but that the obstruction should be repaired. However, when hydronephrosis is an incidental finding on prenatal ultrasonography, the best management is less obvious.

The initial evaluation of hydronephrosis depends in part on how the patient presents. When detected prenatally, the patient generally undergoes a repeat ultrasound in the first days of life. This is important to rule out an emergent situation, such as posterior urethral valves or bilateral obstruction that would compromise overall renal function in the short term. If that is the case, immediate urological consultation is indicted. In patients with purely unilateral prenatal hydronephrosis one may defer this initial ultrasound. The most common cause of prenatally detected hydronephrosis is a ureteropelvic junction (UPJ) obstruction. Other frequent causes include megaureter, ectopic ureter, and ureterocele (Fig. 1). Vesicoureteral reflux is the primary cause of prenatally detected hydronephrosis in approx 10% of cases but also occurs frequently in these patients in association with the other anomalies. Therefore, all patients with prenatally detected hydronephrosis undergo a repeat ultrasound and voiding cystourethrogram (VCUG) in the first few weeks of life. This follow-up ultrasound is important even if an ultrasound on the first day of life was normal; the low urine output in a newborn may fail to distend an obstructed system leading to a falsely normal newborn study. The combination of ultrasound and VCUG performed by experienced radiologists can generally define the specific urologic abnormality. Patients may be placed on antibiotic prophylaxis with 10 mg/kg once daily of amoxicillin until the evaluation is completed. Once the diagnosis is made, further management depends on the specific entity that is diagnosed.

Ureteropelvic Junction Obstruction

After an ultrasound and VCUG, the majority of patients will be felt to have a UPJ obstruction. The next step in management is a diethylenetriaminepentaacetic acid or mercaptoacetyl-triglycline diuretic renal flow scan to determine the degree of obstruction as well as the relative function of the obstructed kidney. The renal flow scan can also distinguish a multicystic kidney which will not function, resulting in a photopenic region on the scan. Unobstructed or equivocal kidneys should be followed with frequent ultrasound during the first year of life (roughly every 3 mo). In many cases, the hydronephrosis will resolve. If it persists, another diuretic renal scan is obtained at 1 year. If the hydronephrosis increases during observation, then a repeat renal scan is obtained sooner.

The appropriate management of the unequivocally obstructed kidney (as defined by markedly prolonged clearance on the diuretic renal scan) is controversial. Most (but not all) authors would agree that pyeloplasty is indicated in infants with unequivocal UPJ obstruction and significantly decreased renal function on a diuretic renal scan obtained beyond the first few weeks of life. The appropriate approach in infants with unequivocal obstruction, but good renal function is less clear. When followed for several years, 25% will ultimately require surgical correction owing to the appearance of symptoms or a loss of renal function. This risk could be used to argue for early intervention or observation depending on the philosophy of the surgeon and the inclination of the parents.

Megaureter

Megaureter, as its name suggests, refers to a dilated ureter. A megaureter may be caused by high-grade reflux or by obstruction at the ureterovesical junction. In many cases, however, neither reflux nor obstruction is present and the etiology of the

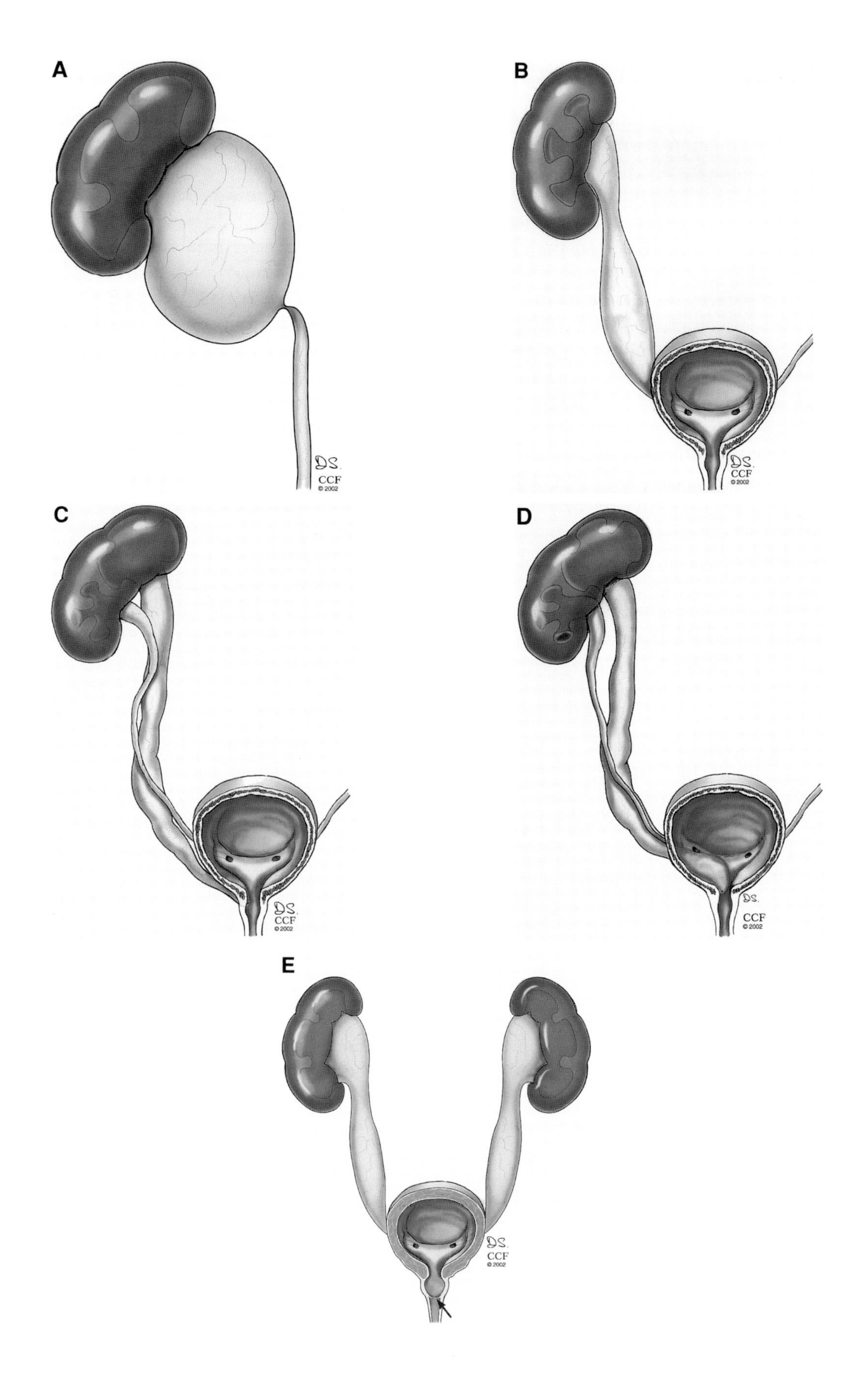
A
B
C
D
E
DS.
CCF
© 2002

dysmorphic ureter is unclear. In typical cases, the ureter is quite dilated with very little dilatation of the renal pelvis and calyces. This may be appreciated on ultrasonography or intravenous pyelography. The use of diuretic renography is not established in evaluating washout from dilated ureters, although the analog images may be evaluated to give some sense of the degree of obstruction. Even when apparently obstructed, many cases of megaureter will resolve spontaneously. Most cases are followed with periodic ultrasound. Surgical intervention is undertaken if hydronephrosis progresses, if there is deterioration in renal function, or if symptoms such as pain or urinary tract infection (UTI) develop. Early surgical intervention may be considered when there is a marked degree of intrarenal dilatation.

Upper-Pole Hydronephrosis in a Duplicated System

Upper-pole dilatation in a duplicated system is generally the result of an ectopic ureter or ureterocele. Lower-pole distension may be the result of secondary obstruction by the upper-pole ureterocele or of vesicoureteral reflux into the lower-pole moiety. These lesions can usually be well characterized by a combination of ultrasound, renal scan, and VCUG. In difficult cases, an intravenous urogram and/or cystoscopy may clarify the anatomy. Surgical intervention is usually undertaken sometime in the first months of life. Surgical options include endoscopic incision of a ureterocele, ureteral reimplantation (with excision of a ureterocele if one is present), upper-pole heminephrectomy, or upper- to lower-pole ureteropyelostomy. The choice of operation depends on the specifics of the individual anatomy.

Posterior Urethral Valves

Posterior urethral valves are an uncommon cause of neonatal hydronephrosis and represent one of the few entities for which prenatal intervention is occasionally indicated. The diagnosis must be considered in any male neonate with bilateral hydronephrosis. All such patients should undergo postnatal ultrasound and VCUG in the first few days of life. If valves are present in a term infant they may be treated with primary valve ablation. In a small or ill infant, vesicostomy may be performed, deferring valve ablation until later in life. If renal function remains poor with persistent hydronephrosis after successful valve ablation or vesicostomy, then higher diversion by cutaneous ureterostomy or pyelostomy is considered.

Multicystic Dysplastic Kidney

The options for managing a multicystic dysplastic kidney are to remove it, follow it, or ignore it. Surgical excision is supported by reports of hypertension and malignancy (both Wilms tumor and renal cell carcinoma) occurring in patients with multicystic kidneys. However, the number of reported cases is small, and the total number of multicystic kidneys, although unknown, is undoubtedly large. The risk for any given patient is probably extremely small and may not justify the surgical risk of excision. Therefore, most pediatric urologists recommend following multicystic kidneys with periodic ultrasound and blood pressure monitoring. Obviously, any patient developing

---

Fig. 1. *(Opposite page)* The differential diagnosis of hydronephrosis includes: Ureteropelvic junction obstruction **(A)**, megaureter **(B)**, ectopic ureter **(C)**, ureterocele **(D)**, and posterior urethral valves **(E)**.

hypertension or a renal mass would undergo nephrectomy. Some surgeons also remove multicystic kidneys that fail to regress. Conversely, once a multicystic kidney has regressed on ultrasound, monitoring is discontinued. However, his approach is not entirely logical. It bases management on the progression (or regression) of the cystic component of these lesions (the part that is discernible on ultrasound). Yet, the hypertension and tumors reported undoubtedly arise from the stromal component. Must patients therefore undergo periodic flank ultrasounds for life? Would it be simpler to just remove the multicystic kidney in infancy—an operation that can be performed as an outpatient through a relatively small incision? Or, given the anecdotal nature of reports of hypertension and tumors, and the difficulties of ultrasonographic follow-up, perhaps multicystic kidneys should simply be ignored. After all, that is how nearly all of them were successfully managed before the era of prenatal ultrasound (because we did not know they were there). For now, it seems that both observation and excision are reasonable options.

UNDESCENDED TESTICLES

Undescended testis is one of the most common congenital genitourinary anomalies. The incidence of undescended testis is 3% in term infants. Most undescended testes will descend spontaneously in the first months of life, and the incidence at 1 yr of age is 0.8%. An undescended testis is defined as a testis that has become arrested in its descent along the normal pathway and may be found in the abdomen, inguinal canal, at the pubic tubercle or in the high scrotum. Undescended testicles have an increased risk of developing tumors postpubertally and will not produce sperm if left in an undescended location. An undescended testicle is distinguished from the rarer ectopic testis, which is a testis that has deviated from the normal pathway of descent. Possible locations for ectopic testes include the femoral canal, perineum, prepubic space, and the contralateral scrotum.

Because most undescended testes are located in the inguinal canal, they can be evaluated on clinical exam. Impalpable testes present a more challenging problem and require a more extensive evaluation. In a child with an undescended testicle, as with any congenital anomaly, a thorough history of the pregnancy and infancy is important. The parents should also be questioned as to whether anyone has ever felt the testis. Was the undescended testis noted at birth? This is particularly important in older children who may have retractile testes. A history of the testis having been in a normal location at one time, either on examination by the primary care physician or as noted by the parents, suggests that the testis is retractile. Obviously, any history of previous inguinal surgery is important as a possible cause of secondary testicular ascent or atrophy. Although clinical hernias are uncommon in children with an undescended testis, most have a patent processus vaginalis, and a history of a hernia is important to elicit.

The physical examination of the child with an undescended testis is the most important part of the evaluation (Fig. 2). All attempts should be made to keep the child be

Fig. 2. *(Opposite page)* **(A)** To examine a child for undescended testicle, he should be placed in the frog-leg position. **(B)** The upper hand is then placed at the internal ring and brought toward the scrotum, milking the testicle down and preventing it from popping through the internal ring into the abdomen. **(C)** The lower hand can be used to push up from the scrotum to stabilize the testis, making it easier to palpate.

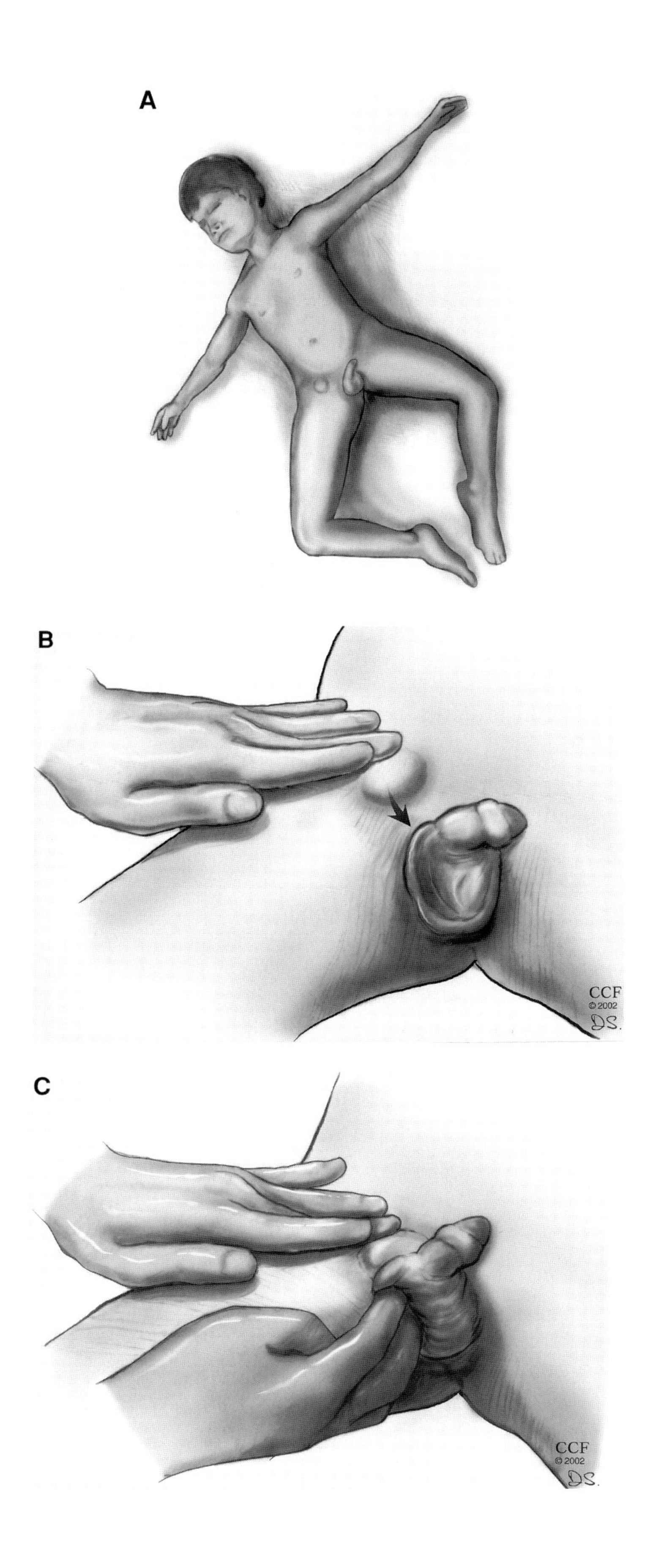
A
B
CCF
© 2002
DS.
C
CCF
© 2002
DS.

relaxed and warm during the examination. A cold room or a nervous child will exaggerate retractile testes. Before touching the child, the genitalia and inguinal region should be visually examined. Because the first touch may stimulate a cremasteric reflex, the best opportunity to see the testis in the scrotum is on initial inspection. A true undescended testis is often associated with a poorly developed hemiscrotum on the ipsilateral side. Placing the child in the frog-leg position and gently milking from the inguinal canal to the scrotum will often bring a high retractile testis down. If the testis in question can be brought down in this way and remains in the hemiscrotum without tension, then the diagnosis of a retractile testis is made. Applying a small dab of liquid soap to the examining hand can reduce friction and improve sensitivity in detecting an inguinal testis. Ectopic sites should also be palpated if no testis is felt in the inguinal region or scrotum.

The physical examination will allow for a distinction between an impalpable testis, a palpable undescended testis, and a retractile testis. In equivocal cases, re-examination at a later date will often clarify the diagnosis. When serial examinations leave the question of a retractile testis vs an undescended testis uncertain, an human chorionic gonadotropin (HCG) stimulation test may be administered. A variety of regimens may be used. We administer 500 to 2000 IU (depending on body size) every other day for a total of five doses. It is generally agreed that a retractile testis will "descend" in response to HCG stimulation. Some truly undescended testes may also descend in response to HCG, although the actual success rate is controversial. Reported success rates range from 6% to 70%. Patients with retractile testes may be reassured that no further evaluation is necessary.

In the case of a palpable undescended testis, no further evaluation is necessary unless there are other associated genital anomalies. The most important is hypospadias, which occurs in 5–10% of boys with an undescended testicle. Hypospadias in association with even one undescended testicle raises the possibility of intersex. Patients with a unilateral undescended testis and hypospadias may have mixed gonadal dysgenesis. This can be evaluated with a karyotype because these patients generally have a mosaic karyotype of 45XO/46XY. If both testes are undescended, particularly if they are impalpable, then congenital adrenal hyperplasia, or other less common forms of intersex should also be considered. In a newborn with bilateral impalpable testes, the most important abnormality to rule out is a female with congenital adrenal hyperplasia. This should definitely be considered in the newborn with bilateral impalpable testes and hypospadias, as it is the most common cause of ambiguous genitalia. However, it should also be considered in the absence of a hypospadias because androgenization can be severe in this disorder. The first steps in evaluation are a karyotype and a serum 17-hydroxyprogesterone level. This can rule out the two most common causes of ambiguous genitalia: congenital adrenal hyperplasia and mixed gonadal dysgenesis. Rarer causes of ambiguous genitalia, such as true hermaphroditism and male pseudohermaphroditism, must be considered if the child has a normal male karyotype. However, if the only genital abnormality is bilateral cryptorchidism, then a normal male karyotype is sufficient to rule out intersex.

In a boy with bilateral impalpable testes the question arises whether the testes are intra-abdominal or are absent. Bilateral anorchia can be diagnosed biochemically with an HCG stimulation test. This is accomplished by administering three doses of 1500 units of HCG on alternate days. If there is no rise in serum testosterone and baseline gonadotropin levels are elevated, then the child has anorchia and no further evaluation is necessary. If there is a rise in testosterone after the administration of HCG, then the child has at least one functioning testis—presumably intra-abdominal.

In the boy with a unilateral impalpable testis, an HCG stimulation test is obviously of no value. In these boys, and in boys with bilateral impalpable testes and a positive HCG stimulation test, further evaluation is indicated. Several radiological tests are available to identify an intra-abdominal testis. Ultrasound, computerized tomography, and magnetic resonance imaging have all been used. The accuracy of these imaging studies for localizing an intra-abdominal testis is less than 25%. Because the readily available tests are insensitive for detecting an intra-abdominal testis, they are of little benefit. In the minority of cases when a radiological study identifies an intra-abdominal testis, an operation to bring the testicle down will be required. However, the failure of any of these tests to identify a testis does not mean the testis is absent—each test has a significant false-negative rate. Therefore, a negative study also mandates an operation to locate an intra-abdominal testis or prove definitively that it is absent. Because the results of radiological tests will not alter the management, there is little value in performing them. A possible exception is the obese child whose body habitus makes physical examination of the inguinal region difficult. If ultrasound can identify an inguinal testis in such a child, then the child will be spared laparoscopy (discussed below).

The standard treatment for a palpable undescended testis is an orchidopexy. Treatment should be undertaken by 1 yr of age to maximize sperm-producing potential. Orchidopexy also places the testis in a palpable location for tumor detection, although orchidopexy does not reduce the risk of tumor formation. An impalpable testis offers more of a challenge. Approximately 50% of boys with a unilateral impalpable testis will in fact have an absent testis on that side. Because of the inability of radiological studies to reliably identify an intra-abdominal testis, an operation is required to determine the presence or absence of an impalpable testis. Historically, this has been approached through an inguinal incision. If blind-ending testicular vessels are found, then a diagnosis of a vanishing testis is made. A blind-ending vas alone is insufficient to prove testicular absence. In most cases, the vanished testis is probably the result of the intrauterine torsion of an inguinal or scrotal testis. Indeed, a tiny testicular remnant laden with brown hemosiderin pigment is often found. In that event the remnant is removed and the incision closed. If the inguinal canal is empty, then an abdominal exploration is indicated to locate an intra-abdominal testis, or confirm an absent testis. The addition of laparoscopy to the operative armamentarium has reduced the morbidity of these explorations. Before a formal operative incision, laparoscopy is performed through a supra- or infraumbilical incision. If an intra-abdominal testis is identified, then an orchidopexy is performed, which can be done laparoscopically. If blind-ending vessels are identified in the abdomen, then the procedure is terminated. If vessels are seen entering the inguinal canal, then inguinal exploration is undertaken. If a testicular remnant is identified, it is removed. If a viable testis is found, an orchidopexy is performed. Because many boys with impalpable testes will have a scrotal remnant, some authors recommend an initial scrotal exploration. If no remnant or testis is found, then laparoscopy is performed.

THE ACUTE SCROTUM

The differential diagnosis of an acute scrotum in children includes testicular torsion (torsion of the spermatic cord), torsion of the appendix testis, epididymoorchitis, hernia/hydrocele, and testis tumor. The last two do not usually present acutely but may on occasion. Findings suggestive of testicular torsion are an extremely tender high-riding testis, an absent cremasteric reflex, a cord that is thick or difficult to distinguish, and no relief of pain with elevation of the testis (as there may be in epididymitis). Although these findings are typical or suggestive of testicular torsion, their absence does not exclude the possibility. A urinalysis should always be obtained because the presence of pyuria is very suggestive of epididymoorchitis. Radionuclide testicular scan and color flow Doppler ultrasound can assist in the diagnosis of testicular torsion. On a radionuclide scan, a torsed testis will appear photopenic. In contrast, epididymoorchitis results in increased blood flow and, therefore, increased radionuclide uptake. False-positive studies may result from abscess formation or an associated hydrocele. False-negative studies may occur because of scrotal wall hyperemia or, in old torsion, from the inflammatory response. Doppler ultrasonography will demonstrate an absence of blood flow to the testis although the intratesticular vessels are small and may be difficult to assess in small children. Both studies are very operator dependent, and the availability of each is different at different institutions. Most centers currently use ultrasound because of its prompt availability.

Surgical exploration is the definitive way to diagnose testicular torsion. Because time is essential, immediate exploration is indicated in any patient suspected of having testicular torsion. Most testicles explored within 6 h of the onset of symptoms are salvaged. Most testicles explored after 24 h are not. Waiting for a nuclear scan or ultrasound to confirm the diagnosis is inappropriate. Radiographic studies should be reserved for patients who are felt to have a low likelihood of testicular torsion. As with appendicitis, occasional negative explorations are to be expected and are far better than a delayed exploration in a boy who has a torsion. At surgery, the testis is detorsed and orchidopexy or orchiectomy is performed depending on its viability (Fig. 3). Scrotal orchidopexy is also performed on the contralateral testis because of a significant incidence of metachronous contralateral torsion. Testicular torsions can also occur in the neonatal period and should be considered in a neonate with a hard scrotal mass. Although the mechanism is different in neonates than in older children, urgent urological evaluation should be obtained.

Torsion of the appendix testis also presents as an acute scrotum. The appendix testis is a small, nonfunctional piece of tissue attached to the upper pole of the testis. It is often attached by a narrow stalk and is prone to torsion (Fig. 4). Children with torsion of the appendix testis tend to be prepubertal and present with increasing pain and swelling over 1–3 d. The pain is usually not as dramatic as in testicular torsion. Many times the diagnosis of appendiceal torsion can be made on physical exam. A torsed appendix testis has a bluish hue when viewed through the scrotal skin, and a "blue dot" seen at the upper pole of the testis confirms the diagnosis. In the absence of a blue dot, the diagnosis may still be made if scrotal tenderness is isolated to a hard nodule at the upper pole of the testis in the absence of other findings suggesting torsion of the spermatic cord. However, by the time these patients present, the inflammatory response has sometimes spread throughout the hemiscrotum, making the diagnosis difficult. Doppler ultrasound can be helpful in eliminating testicular torsion by demonstrating normal blood flow to the testis, but occasionally the diagnosis can only be made by surgical exploration. When diagnosed clinically, appendiceal torsion is treated with nonsteroidal anti-inflammatory drugs, and the pain usually resolves over 7–10 d.

Epididymoorchitis is usually a bacterial infection in adolescents resulting from enteric flora or sexually transmitted organisms. Prepubertally, the inflammation may be bacte-

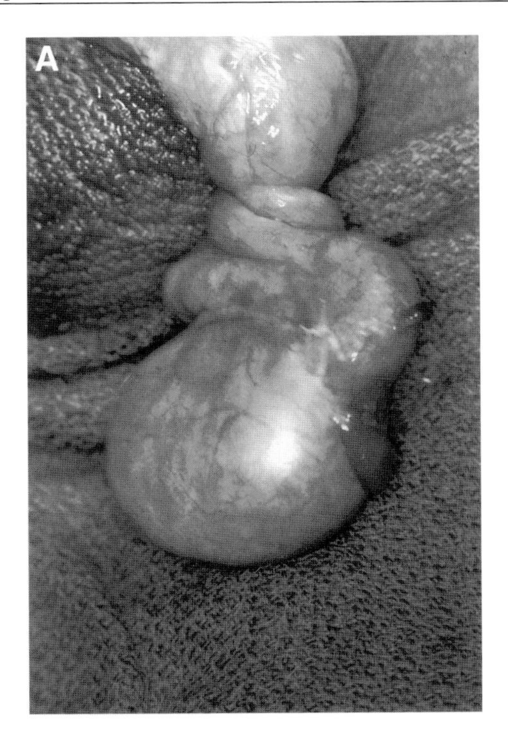

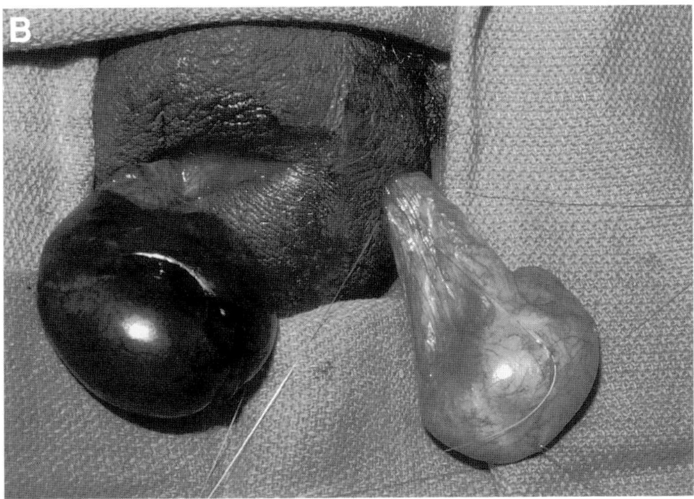

Fig. 3. (A) Intraoperative appearance of a viable torsed testicle. **(B)** A necrotic torsed right testicle and a normal left testis with pexing sutures in place.

rial or chemical. If voiding symptoms and/or pyuria are present, then epididymoorchitis is the presumptive diagnosis. Doppler ultrasound confirms good blood flow, excluding testicular torsion in equivocal cases. Treatment is usually with antibiotics against enteric organisms, although a sexually transmitted pathogen should be sought and treated in sexually active boys.

Hydroceles and hernias may present as an acute scrotal mass. Hydroceles are nontender and transilluminate. A normal testis should be palpable. In equivocal cases an ultrasound

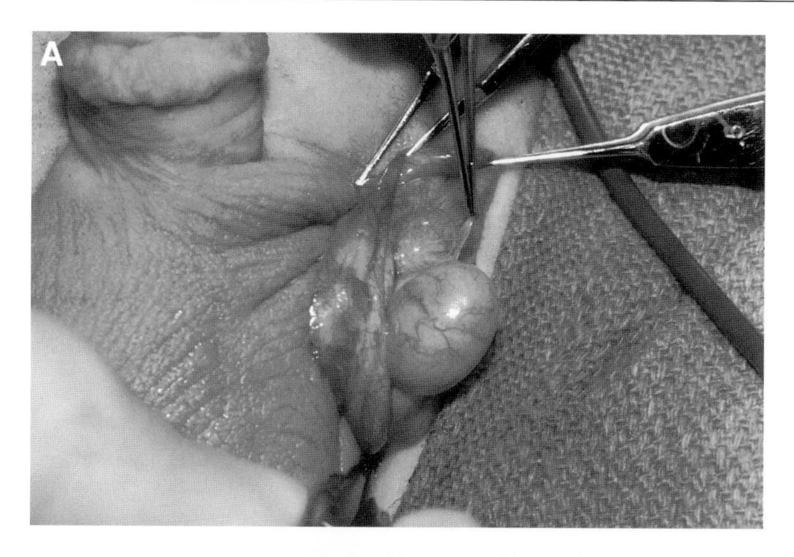

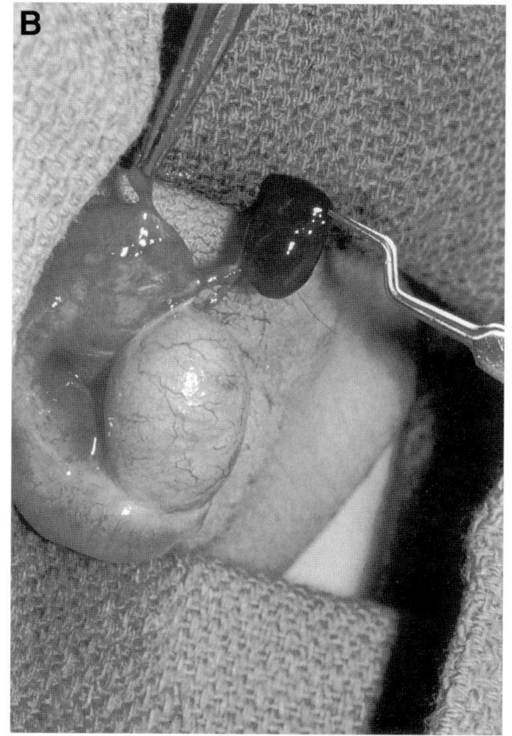

Fig. 4. (A) Normal appearance of the appendix testis (on stretch by the lower forceps). **(B)** Typical appearance of a torsed appendix testis (in bent forceps).

is diagnostic. Hernias do not transilluminate and can usually be palpated up to the inguinal ring. Bowel sounds may be auscultated. Again, ultrasound is helpful in equivocal cases. Testis tumors usually present as a scrotal mass. They are usually painless and subacute. However, pain may occur if there is hemorrhage into a tumor. This should be suspected when acute scrotal swelling occurs after apparently minor trauma.

PENIS PROBLEMS

Uncircumcised boys may develop phimosis, balanoposthitis, or paraphimosis. Phimosis is a progressive scarring of the prepuce usually caused by recurrent inflammation. The normal attachment of the foreskin to the glans penis and the normal inability to retract the foreskin in young children should not be confused with pathological phimosis. Evolution of the potential space between the glans and prepuce is a developmental phenomenon that occurs slowly after birth. Although the foreskin is rarely retractable in the newborn, by 1 yr of age 50% are retractable, and by 5 yr of age at least 90% are retractable. Virtually all foreskins become retractable in puberty. Thus, phimosis is not a pathological condition in young children unless it is associated with balanitis or, rarely, urinary retention. Failure of physicians and parents to appreciate this normal process has led to an overdiagnosis of phimosis. When truly present, phimosis may be treated with steroid cream or surgically by circumcision or prepuciotomy (incision of the scar).

Balanoposthitis refers to inflammation of the prepuce and glans penis. It generally resolves with warm baths and topical or enteral antibiotics. Paraphimosis occurs when the foreskin is retracted and not replaced over the glans penis. This leads to edema of the glans and subsequent tightening of the prepuce. A vicious cycle ensues that may require surgical intervention to correct. The problem is often iatrogenic and may be confused with balanitis.

Many penile problems may be avoided in uncircumcised boys if parents are properly educated in the care of the uncircumcised penis. The penis should be washed like any other part of the body, and the foreskin should not be retracted such that pain or preputial bleeding occurs. Forceful retraction is painful and may result in secondary phimosis. White keratin pearls that collect under the prepuce are harmless and do not need to be removed from under the unretractable foreskin. In older boys, the foreskin is easily retracted and the entire glans and preputial skin may be washed daily.

The most common complication of circumcision is meatitis, which may result in meatal stenosis. Many boys have small urethral meati. A small meatus is not necessarily a stenotic meatus. The diagnosis of meatal stenosis should only be made if the meatus is obviously scarred, or if the observed urinary stream is thin or deflected (usually upward). Meatal stenosis is easily treated with an office meatotomy using EMLA cream.

After circumcision most boys will develop penile adhesions of the shaft skin to the glans. These adhesions will resolve spontaneously as the child grows (Fig. 5). There is no need to forcibly "take-down" the adhesions. In fact, the adhesions usually recur after intentional lysis. Occasionally, boys will develop an actual skin bridge from the circumcision line to the edge of the glans. These may be divided in the office using EMLA cream.

Hypospadias refers to a condition in which the urethral meatus occurs on the underside (ventrum) of the penis. In most cases, the foreskin is incomplete ventrally, although this is not the case in about 5% of patients. Most patients with hypospadias also have chordee, that is, ventral curvature of the penis. Chordee may also occur without hypospadias. Hypospadias and chordee are contraindications to neonatal circumcision, and should be repaired at 6 to 12 mo of age.

BLADDER INSTABILITY OF CHILDHOOD

The most frequent cause of incontinence in children is bladder instability. These children present with urge incontinence and squatting behavior or "potty dancing."

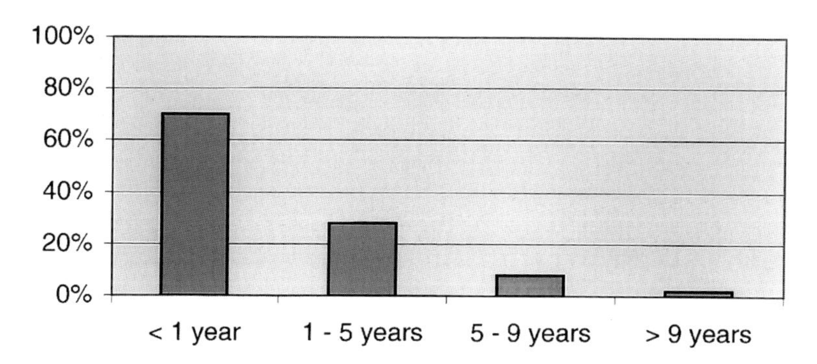

Fig. 5. The incidence of penile adhesions following neonatal circumcision as a function of age reflects the natural history of spontaneous resolution (adapted from Ponsky L, Ross JH, Knipper N, Kay R. Penile adhesions following neonatal circumcision. J Urol 2000; 164: 495–496).

Most have been wet since toilet training, although a dry period of several months after toilet training is not uncommon. Bladder instability represents a normal stage in the development of bladder control. As infants, a normal coordinated bladder contraction occurs with bladder filling. When toilet-trained, most children initially prevent wetting by activation of the external sphincter when a bladder contraction is reflexively initiated with bladder filling. Most children quickly progress to direct central inhibition of bladder contractions with filling, until an appropriate opportunity to void presents itself. A delay in this ability to centrally inhibit bladder contractions leads to the typical symptoms of bladder instability. These symptoms will resolve spontaneously but may persist for many years in some children.

Young children with typical bladder instability do not require radiographical evaluation. Boys with severe symptoms or any child with symptoms that are not improving should undergo a screening ultrasound of the kidneys and bladder. A VCUG is obtained in any child with evidence of bladder wall thickening or hydronephrosis (to rule out reflux, a neurogenic bladder, and posterior urethral valves). Urodynamics are unnecessary in children with typical bladder instability, as they will predictably reveal normal bladder compliance with uninhibited bladder contractions.

Indications to treat bladder instability include associated UTIs or vesicoureteral reflux. In the absence of these indications, treatment is initiated if the problem is causing enough psychosocial stress that the parents and/or child desire therapy. Conservative measures include timed voiding and treating any constipation that may be present as constipation is a common cause of bladder instability (Fig. 6). If conservative measures fail, then medical management is initiated. Oxybutinin chloride is prescribed at 0.5 mg/kg/d divided three times a day. Parents should be warned about the possible side effects of a dry mouth, facial flushing, heat intolerance, and constipation. Patients with associated recurrent UTIs are also placed on antibiotic prophylaxis with trimethoprim/sulfamethoxazole 0.25–0.5 cc/kg /d or nitrofurantoin 1–2 mg/kg/d. Medical therapy is discontinued every 6–12 mo to determine whether it is still required. More recently excellent results have been obtained with more intensive behavioral therapy including biofeedback aimed at improving volitional activation and relaxation of the urethral sphincter. Urethral dilation is an unproven and inappropriate therapy for pediatric voiding dysfunction.

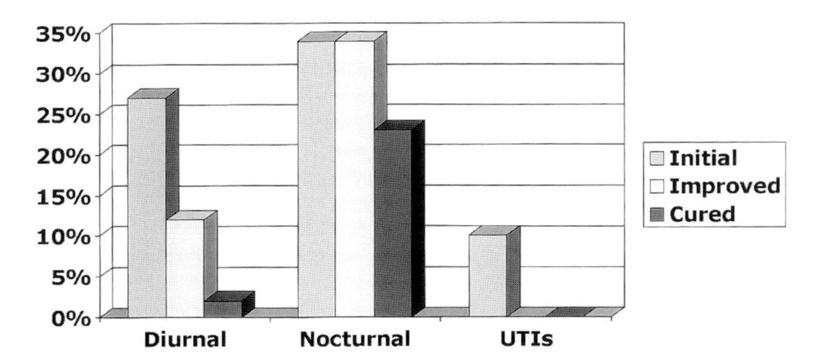

Fig. 6. The incidence of bladder problems in 234 consecutive patients presenting to a constipation clinic and the high rate of resolution of incontinence (diurnal and nocturnal) and UTIs after successful aggressive treatment of constipation in those patients. Bars refer to the incidence at presentation, at follow-up for those whose constipation is improved, and at follow-up for those whose constipation is cured. (Based on data from Loening-Baucke V. Urinary incontinence and urinary tract infection and their resolution with treatment of chronic constipation of childhood. Pediatrics 1997; 100: 228–232.)

NOCTURNAL ENURESIS

The vast majority of children with bed wetting have primary nocturnal enuresis. These are children who have wet the bed all their lives (although a dry interval of several months following toilet-training is not unusual). The diagnosis is made in the absence of any daytime symptoms or history of UTIs. The physical exam and urinalysis should be normal. A positive family history supports the diagnosis. In older children, a screening renal and bladder ultrasound may be obtained, but this is generally unnecessary.

Virtually all bed wetting will resolve spontaneously sometime before adulthood. No treatment is necessary unless the problem is distressing to the child. Treatment is discouraged in children under 6 yr of age. Treatment options include an enuresis (bed wetting) alarm, desmopressin, and imipramine. The safest, most effective, least-expensive treatment is a bed-wetting alarm. However, it requires a commitment from the child and family to use the alarm for several weeks before results are obtained. It's effectiveness can be augmented by additional behavioral approaches such as a star chart. Medications are reserved for those who fail an alarm. Two medical treatments are widely used. Nasal or oral desmopressin acetate is an expensive but relatively safe form of therapy. Treatment should be initiated with one to four puffs or one to three tablets (0.2 mg each) at bedtime. If this fails, then treatment is abandoned. The dose is raised or lowered by one puff or tablet every week or so, until the lowest effective dose is determined. Treatment should be discontinued every 6 mo to see if it is still required. Imipramine is an older medical treatment that is effective in many patients. Treatment is initiated at 25 mg at bedtime. The dose may be increased to 50 mg, and, in older children, to 75 mg, as needed. It takes several weeks to reach an optimal effect. Side effects include anticholinergic effects, alteration in sleep patterns, and behavioral changes. Parents should be warned about the risk of accidental death by overdose in younger siblings or distraught patients.

VARICOCELE

A varicocele is a varicose dilatation of the spermatic veins in the scrotum. It is recognized clinically as a "bag of worms," usually in the left hemiscrotum. Varicoceles are associated with infertility in adult men. Approximately 7% of men are infertile, half of them (approx 3% of all men) in association with a varicocele. 15% of adolescent boys and men have a varicocele. Thus, only 20% (3% of 15%) of adolescent boys and men with a varicocele will be infertile. Because adolescents will not have had a chance to test their fertility and can rarely give a reliable semen sample, selecting which varicoceles to correct is problematic. The most common indication for considering preemptive intervention is ipsilateral testicular hypotrophy, which occurs in about 50% of adolescents with a varicocele. Correction is by outpatient surgery or transvenous embolization by interventional radiology.

SUGGESTED READINGS

Brown T, Mandell J, Lebowitz RL. Neonatal hydronephrosis in the era of sonography. AJR Am J Roentgenol 1987; 148: 959.

Cendron M, Huff D, Keating MA, Snyder HM 3rd, Duckett JW. Anatomical, morphological and volumetric analysis: a review of 759 cases of testicular maldescent. J Urol 1993; 149: 570–573.

Kass EJ, Belman AB. Reversal of testicular growth failure by varicocele ligation. J Urol 1987; 137: 475–476.

Kass EJ, Stone KT, Cacciarelli AA, Mitchell B. Do all children with an acute scrotum require exploration? J Urol 1993; 150:667–669.

Laven JS, Haans LC, Mali WP, te Velde ER, Wensing CJ, Eimers JM. Effects of varicocele treatment in adolescents: a randomized study. Fertil Steril 1992; 58: 756–762.

Lee PA, Coughlin MT. Fertility after bilateral cryptorchidism. Evaluation by paternity, hormone, and semen data. Hormone Res 2001; 55: 28–32.

Loening-Baucke V. Urinary incontinence and urinary tract infection and their resolution with treatment of chronic constipation of childhood. Pediatrics 1997; 100: 228–232.

Monda JM, Husmann DA. Primary nocturnal enuresis: a comparison among observation, imipramine, desmopressin acetate and bed-wetting alarm systems. J Urol 1995; 154: 745–748.

Ponsky L, Ross JH, Knipper N, Kay R. Penile adhesions following neonatal circumcision. J Urol 2000; 164: 495–496.

Ransley PG, Dhillon HK, Gordon I, Duffy PG, Dillon MJ, Barratt TM. The postnatal management of hydronephrosis diagnosed by prenatal ultrasound. J Urol 1990; 144: 584.

Swerdlow AJ, Higgins CD, Pike MC. Risk of testicular cancer in cohort of boys with cryptorchidism. BMJ 1997; 314: 1507–1511.

3 Urinary Tract Infections in Children

Richard W. Grady, MD

CONTENTS

INTRODUCTION

Urinary tract infections (UTIs) afflict 6 million people each year and are one of the most common infectious diseases among children and adults. UTIs are the most common reason for children to see a pediatric urologist and the second most common bacterial infection in children. Urinary tract infection as a term encompasses a wide range of clinical entities, from minimally symptomatic cystitis to acute pyelonephritis.

The evaluation, management, and consequences of UTIs differ significantly between adults and children. Furthermore, variation exists in the evaluation, treatment, and management of children with UTIs despite proposals to achieve a consensus approach *(1)*. The American Academy of Pediatrics (AAP) created a subcommittee to address this. The committee's findings were published in 1999 and represent the consensus opinion of the AAP *(2)*. Current management of UTIs in children focuses on the following:

- Elimination of the acute symptoms of infection
- Prevention of recurrent UTI
- Prevention of renal scarring
- Correction of associated urologic abnormalities *(3)*

From: *Essential Urology: A Guide to Clinical Practice*
Edited by: J. M. Potts © Humana Press Inc., Totowa, NJ

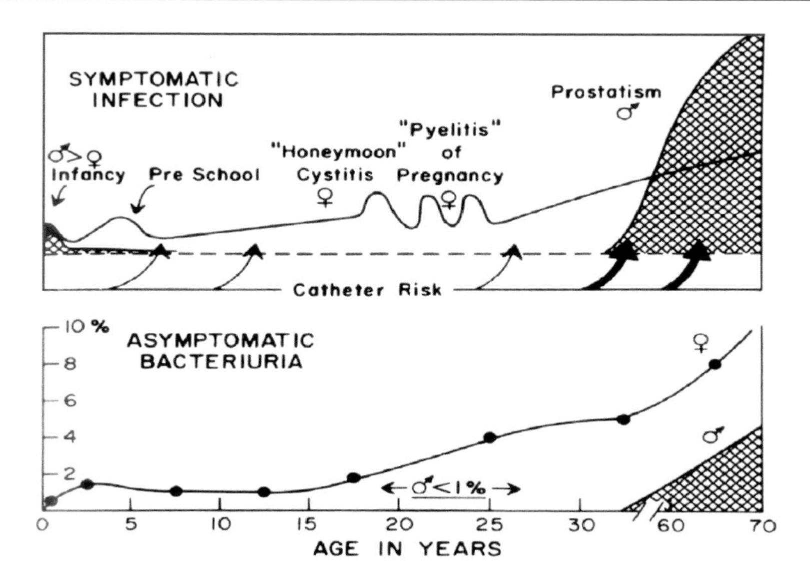

Fig. 1. The incidence of urinary tract infections.

INCIDENCE

About 2% of boys and 8% of girls experience a UTI before adolescence *(4)*. The incidence of UTI changes with age (Fig. 1; ref. *5*). During the newborn period, both males and females are at increased risk for UTI; males, in particular, are at risk in the first 3 mo of life and are three times more likely than girls to experience a UTI during this time of life *(6)*. After this time, girls are more prone to UTIs than boys, especially during the period of potty training (2–4 yr of age). The incidence of UTIs for boys remains significantly lower than for girls after the newborn period.

In the newborn period, uncircumcised males are at increased risk for UTI with a 10-fold higher incidence compared with their circumcised counterparts. Enteric bacteria commonly colonize the periurethral area of neonates and preputial skin of boys. This colonization drastically declines in the first year of life, however, making it unusual to detect after 5 yr of age except in those children prone to UTIs *(7)*. Recurrent infections occur more often in girls than in boys; 40% of girls experience a recurrence within a year of their first infection. Girls are also more prone to multiple recurrent infections *(8,9)*. By contrast, only 25% of boys will experience a recurrent UTI within the first year of life if they had a UTI early in life *(10)*. Recurrent infections are rare in boys after this period unless an underlying neurogenic or anatomic abnormality exists.

PATHOGENESIS

Enteric bacteria cause the majority of UTIs. *Escherichia coli*, in particular, causes 90% of UTIs in children. Gram-positive organisms cause 5–7% of UTIs in children. Some species, such as *Proteus mirablis*, are found more commonly in boys (approx 30% of cases; ref. *6*). In the newborn period, Group A or B streptococcus are common UTI pathogens. Hospital-acquired organisms often tend to be more aggressive (i.e., *Klebsiella* or *Serratia*) or represent opportunistic organisms (i.e., *Pseudomonas aeruginosa*; ref. *3*).

Table 1
Urinary Tract Infections Signs and Symptoms

Infants and toddlers	*Older children*
Irritability	New-onset incontinence
Fever	Foul odor to urine
Failure to thrive	Frequency/urgency
Nausea/vomiting	Pain with voiding
Diarrhea	Listlessness
Hematuria	Irritability
Foul odor to urine	Unexplained fever
	Abdominal/flank pain

It is currently believed that the majority of UTIs in infants and children occur by an ascending route of infection vs hematogenous spread. Enteric bacteria colonize the large intestine, spread to the periurethral and vaginal areas, and subsequently ascend to the urinary tract. Given the appropriate bacterial virulence factors and host environment, the bacteria reproduce and elicit a host response to cause a UTI. These bacteria colonize the periurethral area before infection in girls and the preputial area in boys. Pyelonephritis results when the bacteria possess virulence factors that allow them to ascend the urinary tract (i.e., *P. fimbriae*) or when anatomic or neurogenic abnormalities exist that predispose to upper tract infections (i.e., vesicoureteral reflux [VUR]). In the latter case, these infections are considered complicated because of the presence of anatomic or neurogenic abnormalities.

DIAGNOSIS

Because infants and young children cannot localize infections and appear to be at increased risk of renal scarring secondary to infection, the AAP issued guidelines regarding the management of UTIs in infants and young children. These guidelines specifically stated that practitioners evaluating unexplained fever in infants and young children 2 mo to 2 yr should strongly consider the possibility of a UTI *(2)*. Most emergency department protocols routinely include a urinalysis as part of the evaluation protocol for children in this age group.

Older children are able to more effectively localize the symptoms and signs of UTI. Some of the most common symptoms include dysuria, new-onset urinary incontinence, and urinary urgency (Table 1). Fever in the presence of a UTI implies kidney involvement.

Urinalysis and urine culture play a critical role in the diagnosis of UTI. Urinalysis in a young child may reveal red blood cells and leukocytes (indicated by hemoglobin and leukocyte esterase on dipstick evaluation). Infants and young children test positive less commonly for nitrites because they void so frequently.

A bacterial UTI is defined by the presence of bacteria in a urine culture. In older children, a growth of more than 10^5 colony-forming units is considered a positive culture from a clean midstream voided specimen. Urine collection from children before toilet training is problematic. To obtain the most accurate specimen, one must obtain it either from urethral catheterization or supra-pubic aspiration (SPA). Colony counts of 10^3 from urethral specimens are significant. Any growth from a specimen obtained by SPA is considered clinically important. In practice, urinary-bagged specimens are often obtained for newborns or toddlers instead because of increased ease compared with SPA or urethral catheterization. Unfortunately, these specimens are more frequently contaminated by skin flora and periurethral flora. As a result, the AAP issued the following guideline in 1999:

> *If the child (2 months to 2 years of age) is ill enough to warrant immediate antibiotic usage, the urine specimen should be obtained by SPA or urethral catheterization—not a "bagged" specimen. If an infant or young child 2 months to 2 years of age with unexplained fever is assessed as not being so ill as to require immediate antibiotic therapy, there are two options; 1) Obtain and culture a urine specimen collected by SPA or transurethral bladder catheterization, 2) Obtain a urine specimen by the most convenient means and perform a urinalysis. If the urinalysis suggests a UTI, obtain and culture a urine specimen collected by SPA or transurethral bladder catheterization; if urinalysis does not suggest a UTI, it is reasonable to follow the clinical course without initiating antimicrobial therapy, recognizing that a negative urinalysis does not rule out a UTI* (2).

To optimize the results from a bagged specimen, wash the genital skin meticulously before bag application and repeat if no voided specimen results within 3 h of bag application. Urine bags must also be removed within 15–20 min after the child voids to reduce the chance of false-positive results *(11)*.

After toilet-training, most children can provide a clean midstream catch with the assistance and supervision of their parents or caregivers. Interpretation of urine specimens from uncircumcised boys who cannot retract the foreskin can be confounded by specimen contamination from the large numbers of bacteria in the preputial folds. Urine specimens should be cooled immediately after voiding to improve the accuracy of urine culture results by reducing bacterial growth prior to inoculation on culture media *(11)*.

ACUTE MANAGEMENT

At the turn of the century, Goppert-Kattewitz noted the acute mortality of pyelonephritis in young children at 20%. Another 20% failed to recover completely and subsequently died presumably secondary to renal failure *(12)*. After sulfonamide antibiotics became available in the 1940s, mortality dropped to 2% in children hospitalized for nonobstructive UTI *(13)*. Currently, mortality secondary to UTI approaches 0% for children in the United States.

In our modern era, practice patterns for the acute treatment of UTI are subject to variation influenced by the protocol of the treating facility, which is in turn influenced by the geographic region and traditional medical opinions of the area. Because of the lack of controlled studies and well-controlled data on the acute management of UTI in children, no consensus exists on the optimal course of treatment for these children despite the AAP's published treatment guidelines in 1999. Most of these recommendations result from consensus opinion from a panel of medical experts in the field.

Initial management should include accurate diagnosis of UTI from an appropriately obtained urine specimen for urine culture and analysis. Adjunctive hematologic studies, such as a white blood cell count, C-reactive protein, and erythrocyte sedimentation rate, may be useful in some cases.

In addition, it is important to evaluate these children for urinary tract obstruction. Physical examination may reveal a palpable flank mass as the result of ureteropelvic junction obstruction, a palpable suprapubic mass secondary to posterior urethral valves, or other causes of bladder outlet obstruction. Laboratory studies may reveal an elevated serum creatinine, acidosis, or electrolyte imbalance. Symptoms of a poor urinary stream, intermittent voiding, or straining to urinate can indicate urethral obstruction.

Children who present with a febrile UTI should be treated without delay. Several retrospective studies provided evidence that a delay in treatment of greater than 4 d resulted in higher rates of renal scarring *(5)*. In contrast, initiation of treatment after only 24 h of fever has not been shown to cause an increased rate of long-term renal scarring. So, a slight delay in therapy does not adversely affect long-term outcomes *(14)*. Therapy can be initiated empirically. Antibiotic therapy can be tailored later according to the urine culture results when they become available. The initial choice of antibiotic will vary according to region. Treating physicians should be cognizant of the antibiotic resistance patterns in their geographic area and choose accordingly because bacterial resistance patterns vary by region because of differences in the use of various antibiotics. Only a few comparative, randomized studies have evaluated the safety and efficacy of antibiotics to treat children for UTI. As a consequence, the choice of antibiotic may vary by region and by treating facility. However, in many regions of the world, including the United States, ampicillin and other aminopenicillins are no longer clinically effective against many of the common bacterial pathogens that cause UTI in children *(11)*.

By convention, most children with febrile UTI have been admitted for initial inpatient therapy with intravenous antibiotics. Ampicillin and gentamicin function synergistically and have a therapeutic spectrum that covers almost all of the common bacterial pathogens that cause UTI. As a consequence, this antibiotic combination is frequently used for initial empiric antibiotic therapy. More recently, however, Hoberman and colleagues (*14*) demonstrated that outpatient oral antibiotic therapy can be effective for children with no difference in short-term treatment efficacy or long-term renal scarring compared with intravenous therapy. As a result, many health care providers now treat children with febrile UTI as outpatients. In contrast, children who appear toxic, septic, dehydrated, or unable to maintain adequate oral intake of fluids should be admitted for inpatient antimicrobial therapy and intravenous hydration. The 1999 AAP guidelines on UTI reflect this bias. They specifically recommend hospital admission for treatment until the children appear clinically improved. At that time, antibiotic therapy may be converted to an appropriate oral agent.

Current systematic reviews of the literature support a treatment course of 7–10 d duration. Treatment courses shorter than this (1–4 d) demonstrated lower cure rates. *(15)*. Longer courses of therapy result in improved outcomes in 5–21% of cases *(16)*. A test of cure (urine culture) may be performed after completion of therapy to demonstrate efficacy of therapy.

Antibiotic therapy for afebrile lower UTIs (i.e., cystitis) may be delayed until urine culture results are available with no long-term adverse consequences. In practice, most health care providers initiate empirical antibiotic therapy when these children present for treatment to reduce the associated morbidity. Common antibiotic choices for initial therapy include trimethoprim/sulfamethoxazole, nitrofurantoin, and a variety of cephalosporins. Conventional treatment duration lasts 7 to 10 d with a test of cure 1 wk after completing a course of antibiotics. For children older than 2 yr of age, short-course therapy (single dose to 2 d) also has been shown to be effective *(17)*. For single-dose therapy, slowly excreted drugs like trimethoprim/sulfamethoxazole are ideal *(11)*.

EVALUATION

After initial treatment, children should be evaluated for anatomic and functional causes that may predispose them to further UTIs. This is important for several reasons. Children with genitourinary abnormalities will have an increased incidence of recurrent UTI and an increased risk for renal damage. Up to 50% of children who have had a febrile UTI will demonstrate an anatomic abnormality. Children should also be evaluated for functional conditions that may predispose to UTI as well. Up to 70–80% of older children have a functional condition, such as detrusor instability, that contributes to increased risk for recurrent UTI.

Current recommendations from the AAP include the evaluation of all children after febrile UTI with a renal and bladder ultrasound examination and a voiding cystourethrography (VCUG). Ultrasound examination yields approx 2–8% abnormalities, including hydronephrosis, ureterocele, and posterior urethral valves. These abnormalities may be further characterized by other imaging studies, such as Lasix renography, or VCUG. Up to 50% of girls who have had a febrile UTI will demonstrate VUR on a VCUG study.

Imaging Studies

Some variation exists for the indications for imaging studies. The AAP guidelines recommend ultrasonography and VCUG for all children after the first febrile UTI *(2)*. Many experts also suggest these studies for any boy who has UTI whether associated with fever or not. Imaging studies for girls with afebrile UTI are typically not indicated. In contrast, the UTI Working Group of the Health Care Office of the European Association of Urology suggests that imaging studies be deferred until the second UTI in girls and performed after the first UTI in boys *(3)*.

Ultrasound imaging studies may be performed when convenient after initial treatment. Children should be maintained on prophylactic antimicrobial therapy until radiographic evaluation is performed to reduce the risk of UTI recurrence for those children at risk due to underlying anatomic abnormalities. In practice, children admitted for inpatient therapy often undergo ultrasonographic imaging before discharge. AAP guidelines recommend early renal and bladder ultrasound imaging if children fail to respond to antibiotic therapy within 24–48 h. Retrospective data from Bachur *(18)* suggests that the incidence of anatomic abnormalities in this patient group is not significantly different from patients who respond more rapidly to antibiotic therapy *(18)*. Before ultrasound imaging, intravenous pyelography served as the imaging study of choice to evaluate these children. Ultrasonography offers a less invasive, safer, and frequently less expensive method to evaluate these children *(2)*. This is particularly advantageous for those children who require serial imaging studies in follow-up.

Imaging voiding studies currently include VCUG or radionuclear cystography (RNC). These studies are primarily used to detect VUR. The VCUG provides information about bladder hypertrophy, urethral abnormalities (during the voiding phase), postvoid urine residual, functional bladder size, and voiding abnormalities as well. It also better characterizes the degree of VUR. As a consequence, it is the initial study of choice when evaluating children after febrile UTI. RNC has a lower radiation dose and is a more sensitive study to detect VUR. Therefore, it may be preferred for follow-up studies or in situations where the presence of VUR is being re-evaluated in children with recurrent febrile UTIs who have not previously demonstrated VUR on a VCUG. Children should remain on prophylactic antibiotic therapy until this study is performed. False-negative rates with VCUG range from 5 to 10% because of the dynamic nature of VUR. Cycling VCUG is particularly important to perform in newborns to decrease the incidence of false-negative studies. A VCUG may be performed when convenient after treatment of a febrile UTI. However, McDonald et al. (*19*) demonstrated that follow-up within 2 wk of presentation with a UTI increased patient compliance. Because of the invasive nature of this study, some children may require oral sedation with anxiolytic therapy before VCUG or RNC is performed.

[99mTc]-Dimercaptosuccinic acid (DMSA) renal scanning may be useful in the diagnosis of pyelonephritis and in the evaluation of renal scarring *(20)*. Its role in the management of patients with febrile UTI varies from institution to institution and regionally. DMSA scanning provides the most sensitive method to assess renal scarring and damage. Acute uptake defects are detectable by DMSA scanning in 50–80% of children with febrile UTI; 40–50% of these defects remain on follow-up imaging studies, indicating scar formation *(21,22)*.

Evaluation of Bladder and Bowel Function

A comprehensive history of voiding habits plays a significant role in the evaluation of children who have had a UTI. The history should include age at toilet-training, frequency of urination, presence and frequency of diurnal or nocturnal enuresis, quality of urinary stream, presence of urinary urgency, and/or curtsy (Vincent's curtsy) behavior. We use a voiding log to aid in this assessment. This log performed over a 2- to 3-d period helps further characterize voiding habits. Voiding dysfunction may manifest itself as bladder instability, producing urge incontinence, decreased sensory awareness, partial urinary retention, or a combination of these.

A bowel function history should also be obtained to assess frequency of defecation, constipation, and pain with defecation. When the history is not clear or suspicion exists, a plain radiograph of the abdomen provides an excellent method to assess the stool load in the colon. The Barr scale may be used to characterize the degree and quality of the stool load on plain radiography.

RISK FACTORS

VUR

VUR occurs when urine flows from the bladder to the upper urinary tract (Fig. 2). This anatomic abnormality allows infected urine from the bladder to reach the kidney, where it may result in pyelonephritis. VUR is the likely mechanism for the ascent of bacteria from the bladder to the kidney in approx 50% of children who develop pyelonephritis. Furthermore, some of these children also possess intrarenal reflux; this allows bacteria direct entry to the renal parenchyma to elicit a strong inflammatory response and renal scarring. Previous studies by Hodson et al. (*23*) demonstrated renal scarring secondary to sterile VUR in a pig model. This led to aggressive surgical correction of VUR in children. However, more recent clinical data in infants and children strongly suggests that reflux poses no risk for renal scarring in the absence of bacterial infection *(24,25)*. As a consequence, VUR is currently treated nonsurgically where appropriate because many children with VUR will spontaneously outgrow this condition given

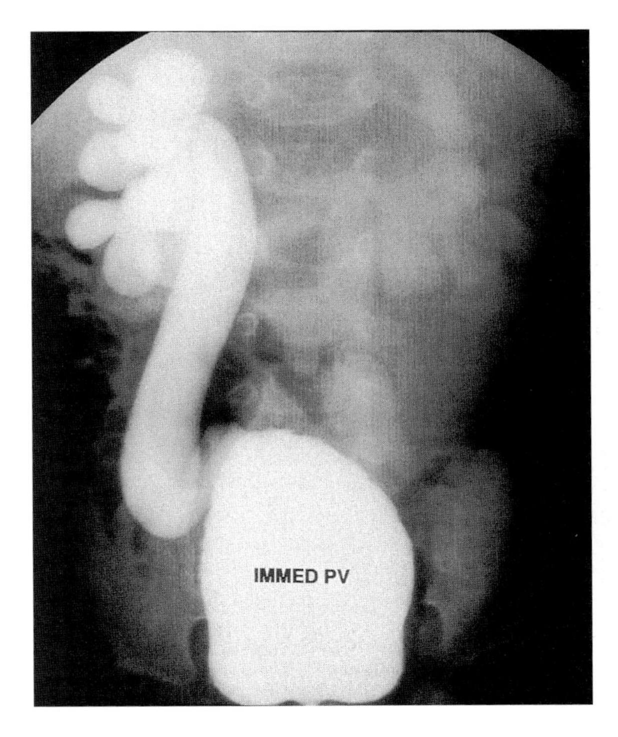

Fig. 2. A voiding cystouretrogram of a 2-yr-old boy with high-grade vesicoureteral reflux. IMMED PV, immediate post-void.

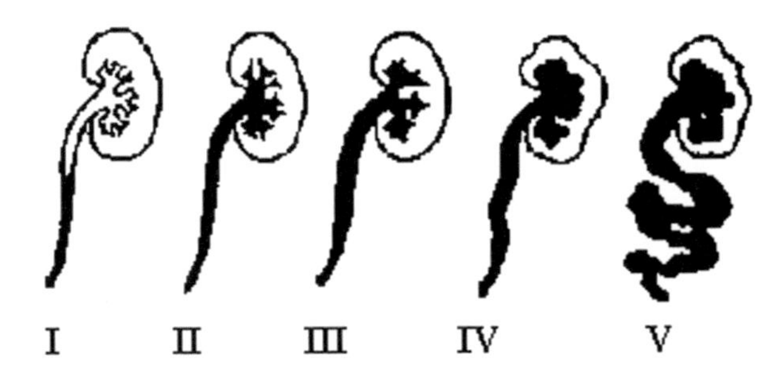

Fig. 3. International reflux study grading system for vesicoureteral reflux.

enough time *(26)*. Children may be safely treated with low-dose suppressive antibiotic therapy while they are followed conservatively for the resolution of VUR. The ideal suppressive antibiotic is low cost, has minimal effect on the gastrointestinal flora, achieves high urinary levels, and is palatable. Commonly used agents include nitrofurantoin and trimethoprim/sulfamethoxazole. The occurrence of a UTI while on suppressive antimicrobial therapy ("breakthrough UTI") is an indication for surgical or endoscopic correction of VUR.

VUR is currently graded on a system of severity from I–V (Fig. 3). As the grade of VUR increases, the chances of spontaneous resolution decrease and the likelihood of congenital renal dysplasia increases *(27)*. Severe VUR has also been shown to be an independent risk factor for urinary tract infection as well as pyelonephritis *(28)*.

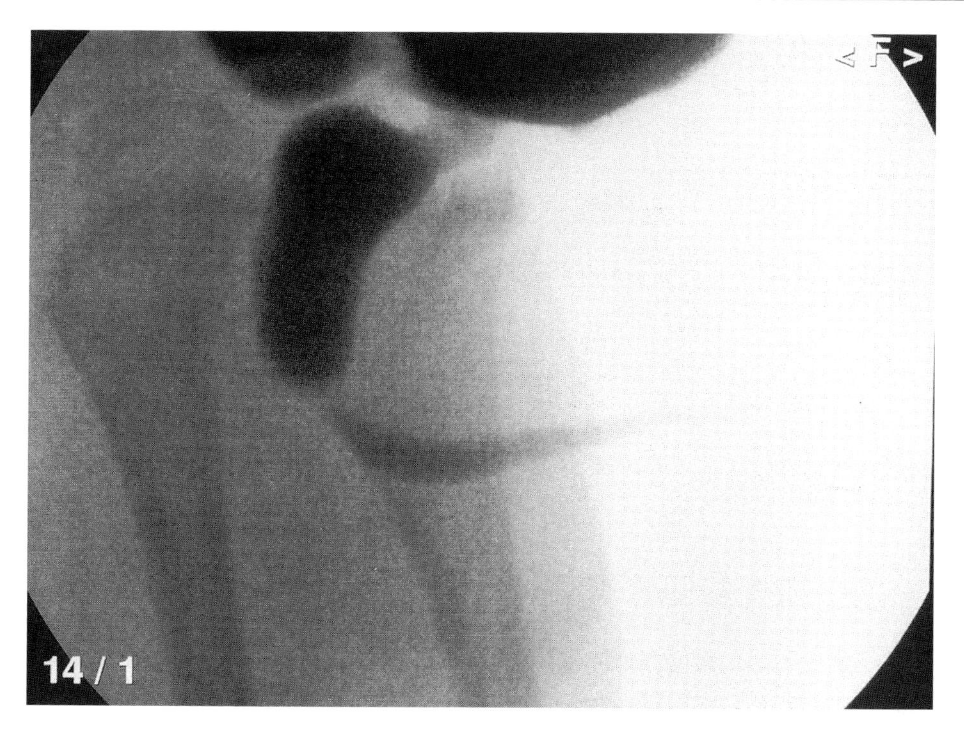

Fig. 4. A voiding cystouretrogram of a 3-wk-old boy with posterior urethral valves. Note marked discrepancy between the diameter of the posterior and anterior urethra.

Foreskin

Neonatal circumcision provides significant protection against UTI in male infants *(29)*. Clinical research has demonstrated a 12-fold increased risk for UTI among uncircumcised boys in the first 6 mo of life *(30)*. Other researchers have confirmed these observations in population-based cohort studies *(31,32)*. This increased risk appears to be a time-limited phenomenon. The increased risk of UTI associated with lack of circumcision is felt to be highest during the first year of life although some recently published data reported a fivefold increased risk of UTI associated with uncircumcised males in the first 5 yr of life, independent of age *(33)*. From a pathophysiologic perspective, the periurethral area of uncircumcised male infants is significantly more colonized with Gram-negative uropathogens than in circumcised males *(29)*.

Obstructive Uropathies

Children with obstructive uropathies may present with UTI. These conditions include posterior urethral valves (Fig. 4), obstruction of the urinary tract at the ureteropelvic junction or ureterovesical junction (obstructed megaureter; Fig. 5), and other congenital and acquired strictures of the ureter and urethra. Historically, children with these conditions presented with pain or UTI. With the advent of routine antenatal imaging studies, many of these anomalies are detected in utero and corrected soon after birth when indicated. However, children with a febrile UTI should be evaluated for an obstructive abnormality because one of these conditions may have gone previously undetected or

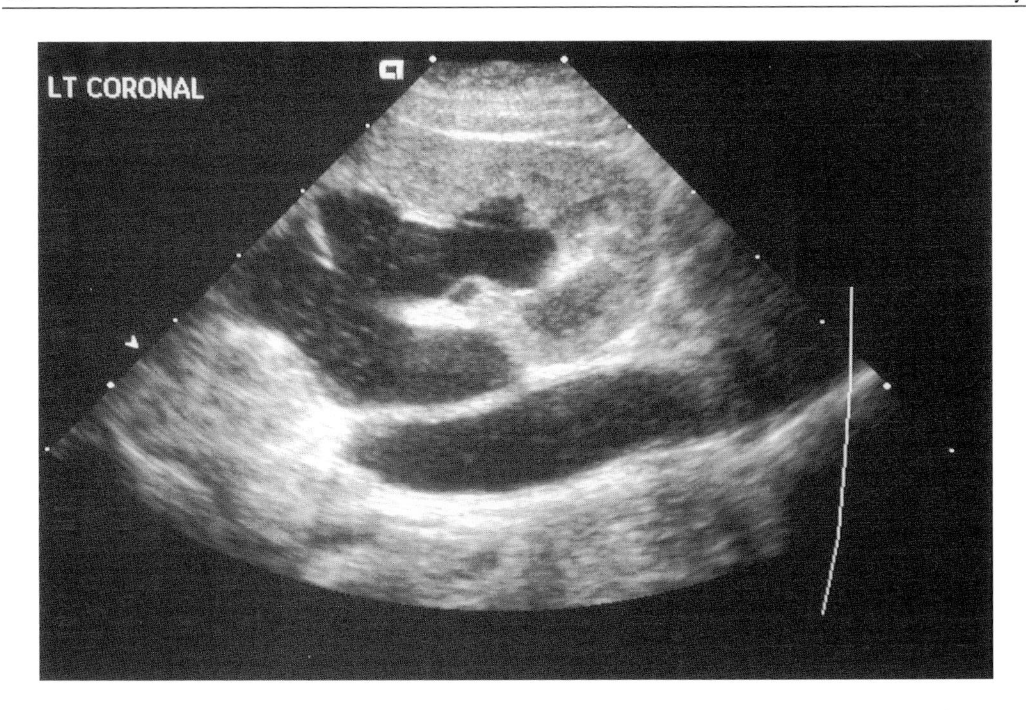

Fig. 5. A renal sonogram of a 2-mo-old girl with hydronephrosis and ureterectasis.

unrecognized. Ultrasonography serves as an excellent initial imaging modality for these conditions.

When detected by ultrasound, obstructive abnormalities are typically also evaluated by radioisotope diuretic renography and/or intravenous pyelography to access the degree of obstruction and function. Many of these lesions can be repaired surgically with reasonable rates of success.

Disorders of Elimination (Voiding Dysfunction and Constipation)

Children with voiding dysfunction are believed to be at higher risk of UTI because abnormal voiding can cause turbulent voiding, allowing the backwash of bacteria from the periurethral area into the bladder. In practice, an infrequent or inefficient voiding pattern is commonly associated with daytime urinary incontinence and UTI *(34,35)*. The underlying pathophysiology of voiding dysfunction remains incompletely understood. Clinically, children with voiding dysfunction will void infrequently. Parents note that these children are particularly adept at holding their urine for prolonged periods of time but will exhibit significant urinary urgency when they ultimately need to urinate. Imaging studies typically demonstrate a bladder capacity larger than predicted for age. Voiding studies may reveal a "spinning top" urethral configuration. This indicates that these children void with an incompletely relaxed external urinary sphincter. This causes a turbulent rather than laminar flow of urine that promotes vaginal filling during voiding and retrograde flow of urine into the bladder *(4)*. These children also often demonstrate incomplete voiding with high postvoid residual urine volumes. This is felt to be incomplete sphincter relaxation during detrusor contraction, a phenomenon that may also be recognized by the presence of staccato voiding or high-pressure voiding.

Currently, constipation is also felt to aggravate voiding dysfunction and, subsequently, contribute to an increased risk of UTI. Several investigators have shown that successful control of constipation improves daytime urinary incontinence and decreases the incidence of recurrent UTI *(36,37)*. Medical management for incontinence and UTI may remain unsuccessful until constipation is recognized and treated. Although some forms of constipation are readily apparent by history, other forms may be subtler. Some children may have fecal retention despite the regular passage of stool. In these cases, a plain radiograph may be the only method to effectively diagnose these children *(4)*.

When voiding dysfunction is identified, treatment is first directed at behavioral modification, including a timed voiding program and pelvic floor relaxation techniques. For those children who manifest partial urinary emptying with high postvoid residual volumes, biofeedback training can be particularly helpful. In contrast, children who experience detrusor instability with satisfactory bladder emptying may benefit from anticholinergic therapy. Several agents are available, including oxybutynin hydrochloride, tolterodine, and hyoscyamine. Of note, the Food and Drug Administration has approved none of these medications for use in children. This is also true of the majority of medications used in pediatrics.

Constipation may be treated by stool-softening agents followed by stool-bulking agents. Changes in diet, including the increased consumption of water and other fluids, are also important. A follow-up abdominal radiograph study may be necessary to assess the effect of treatment for some children.

LONG-TERM CONSEQUENCES OF UTIS FOR CHILDREN

The consequences of UTI in children include renal scarring and the sequelae of hypertension and renal insufficiency. Because children are at increased risk of renal scarring and recurrent UTI compared to adults, much attention has focused on reducing the risk of further infection in the pediatric population. Several recent studies have explored the long-term consequences of UTIs in childhood, and in particular, pyelonephritis.

Wennerstrom and co-workers *(38)* prospectively followed a group of 1221 patients after their first UTI. They specifically examined the data from patients with renal scarring after their first UTI. As part of this long-term study, they evaluated patients in this series with documented scarring by urography 16 to 26 yr after their first UTI and compared this group to an age-matched control group with no evidence of scarring after a UTI. On follow-up investigation, both groups underwent DMSA scans to assess scarring and 51Cr-EDTA investigation to measure glomerular filtration rate (GFR). Median GFR between these two groups was equivalent. However, patients with bilateral renal scarring demonstrated a significant drop in GFR on follow-up evaluation. The GFR of scarred kidneys also declined on follow-up investigation *(38)*. Wennerstrom also evaluated this same group for hypertension and found no difference between patients with renal scarring and those without renal scarring. Plasma renin levels, aldosterone, and angiotensin II levels were similarly unaffected, although atrial natriuretic peptide was significantly elevated in patients with renal scars *(38)*.These studies demonstrated that although global renal function remained intact for patients with renal scarring after UTI, the effects of renal scarring adversely affect involved kidneys over time.

The authors also examined gender-specific differences in renal scarring in this same group of patients in a different study. Of 652 children with a febrile UTI and no evidence of urinary obstruction, 74 developed scarring. Primary renal defects in boys occurred more often in the presence of VUR (67%), especially high-grade or dilated VUR. The parenchymal loss was global in many of the boys. In contrast, girls with renal scarring demonstrated focal scarring and only had VUR in 23% of the cases. Furthermore, acquired renal scarring only occurred in the setting of recurrent febrile UTI *(39)*. These findings support the concepts that high-grade VUR is associated with developmental renal abnormalities that occur during embryogenesis and that VUR in the absence of UTI does not damage kidneys. The data also highlight the danger of recurrent febrile UTI in childhood.

The link between end-stage renal disease (ESRD) in children and recurrent UTI in the setting of VUR has been termed reflux nephropathy. Some debate exists to the degree that recurrent infections play a role in ESRD in this condition. Craig et al. *(33)* retrospectively reviewed the dialysis and transplant registry in Australia and New Zealand between 1971 and 1998. They found no change in the incidence of reflux nephropathy as a cause of ESRD during this time when comparing subjects 25–34 yr of age, 15–24 yr of age, and 5–14 yr of age. The authors conclude that treatment to prevent UTI in the setting of VUR has not been accompanied by the expected decrease in ESRD because of reflux nephropathy. They suggest that ESRD caused by reflux nephropathy may represent congenital dysplasia/hypoplasia not amenable to postnatal intervention. In contrast, Hansson and colleagues reviewed the results of a quality assurance project in Sweden. This study suggests that the long-standing interest in Sweden in the early detection of UTI in children has led to a high diagnostic rate for UTI, which appears to have led to a decrease in the long-term consequences (scarring and reflux nephropathy associated ESRD) of UTI in that country *(40)*. Hansson's conclusions are supported by results from Nuutinen et al., who analyzed the data from children with acute UTI and compared it to data in the kidney transplant registry for England, Wales, and Finland *(41)*. Most believe that the aggressive medical treatment of UTI in children has reduced the incidence of reflux nephropathy-related ESRD.

SUMMARY

By recognizing the differences between adults and children in the treatment and evaluation of UTI, care providers can more effectively manage these infections in the pediatric populations they treat. Febrile UTI during childhood clearly can result in long-term damage to kidneys. Recognition of these long-term consequences should prompt a thorough evaluation into the potential risk factors for UTI that are more commonly found in children so that they may be appropriately treated.

REFERENCES

1. Dolan TJ, Meyers A. A survey of office management of urinary tract infections in childhood. Pediatrics 1973; 52: 21–24.
2. Roberts KB. A synopsis of the American Academy of Pediatrics' practice parameter on the diagnosis, treatment, and evaluation of the initial urinary tract infection in febrile infants and young children. Pediatr Rev 1999; 20: 344–347.
3. Naber K, Bergman B, Bishop, MC, Bjerlund-Johansen, TE, Botto H, Lobel B, Jimenez Cruz F, Selvaggi FP. EAU Guidelines for the management of urinary and male genital tract infections. Eur Urol 2001; 40: 576–588.
4. Strand W. Urinary infection in children: pathogenesis, bacterial virulence, and host resistance. In: Bauer S, Gonzales ET, ed. Pediatric Urology Practice. Lippincott, Williams, & Wilkins, Philadelphia, PA, 1999, pp. 433–461.

5. Dick P, Feldman W. Routine diagnostic imaging for childhood urinary tract infections: a systematic overview. J Pediatr 1996; 128 :15–22.
6. Larcombe J, Urinary tract infection in childhood. In: Barton S, ed. Clinical Evidence. British Medical Journal Publishing Group, London, England, 2000, pp. 239–245.
7. Bollgren I, Winberg J. The periurethral aerobic bacterial florain healthy boys and girls. Acta Pediatra Scand 1976; 65: 74–79.
8. Jodal U, the natural history of bacteriuria in childhood. Infect Dis Clin N Am 1987; 1: 713–718.
9. Winberg J, Andersen, HJ, Bergstrom T, Jacobsson B, Larson H, Lincoln K. Epidemiology of symptomatic urinary tract infection in childhood. Acta Pediatr Scand 1974; 252 (suppl): 3–15.
10. Stark H. Urinary tract infections in girls: the cost-effectiveness of currently recommended investigative routines. Pediatr Nephrol 1997; 11: 174–77.
11. Tullus K, Winberg J. Urinary tract infections in childhood. In: Brumfitt W, Hamilton-Miller J, Bailey R, ed. Urinary Tract Infections. Chapman & Hall Medical, London, England, 1998, pp. 175–197.
12. Goppert-Kattewitz F. Uber die eitrigen Erkrankungen der Harnwege im Kindersalter. Ergebinesse uber innern Medizin und Kinderheilkund 1908; 2: 30–73.
13. Lindblad B, Ekengren K. The long-term prognosis of non-obstructive urinary tract infection in infancy and childhood after the advent of sulphonamides. Acta Pediatrica Scandinavica 1969; 58: 25–32.
14. Hoberman A, et al. Oral versus initial intravenous therapy for urinary tract infections in young febrile children (*see* comments). Pediatrics 1999; 104(1 Pt 1): 79–86.
15. Moffatt M, Embree J, Grimm P, Law B. Short-course antibiotic therapy for urinary tract infections in children: a methodologic review of the literature. Am J Dis Child 1988; 142: 57–61.
16. Madrigel G, Odio, CM, MOhs E, Guevera J, McKracken, GH Jr. Single dose antibiotic therapy is not as effective as conventional regimens for management of acute urinary tract infections in children. Pediatr Infect Dis J 1988; 7: 316–319.
17. Lidefelt K, Bollgren I, Wiman A. Single-dosc treatment of cystitis in children. Acta Pediatrica Scandinavica 1991; 80: 648–653.
18. Bachur R. Nonresponders: prolonged fever among infants with urinary tract infections. Pediatrics 2000; 105: E59.
19. McDonald A, et al. Voiding cystourethrograms and urinary tract infections: how long to wait? Pediatrics 2000; 105: E50.
20. Goldraich N, Goldraich IH. Update on dimercapto-succinic acid scanning in children with urinary tract infection. Pediatric Nephrol 1995; 9: 211–226.
21. Rushton H, Majd M, Jantausch B, et al. Renal scarring following reflux and nonreflux pyelonephritis in children: evaluation with 99mTechnetium dimercaptosuccinic acid scintigraphy. J Urol 1992; 147: 1327–1332.
22. Majd M, Rushton HG, Jantausch B, Wiedermann BL. Relationship among vesicoureteral reflux, P-fimbriated Escherichia coli, and acute pyelonephritis in children with febrile urinary tract infection. J Pediatr 1991; 119: 578–585.
23. Hodson C, Maling TMJ, McManamon PJ, Lewis MG. The pathogenesis of reflux nephropathy (chronic atrophic pyelonephritis). Br J Radiol 1975; 13 (suppl): 1–26.
24. Ransley P, Risdon RA. Reflux and renal scarring. Br J Radiol 1978; 14 (suppl): 1–35.
25. Lenaghan D, Cass A, Cussen, LJ, Stephens, FD. Long-term effect of vesico-ureteral reflux on the upper urinary tract of dogs. J Urol 1972; 107: 758–761.
26. Group BRS. Prospective trial of operative vs. non-operative treatment of severe vesico-ureteral refluxin children: five years' observation. Br Med J 1987; 295: 237–241.
27. Risdon R, Yeung CK, Ransley PJ. Reflux nephropathy in children submitted to unilateral nephrectomy: a clinicopathologic study. Clin Nephrol 1993; 40: 308–314.
28. Jakobsson B, Jacobson SH, Hjalmas K, Vesico-ureteric reflux and other risk factors for renal damage: identification of high- and low-risk children. Acta Paediatr Suppl 1999; 88: 31–39.
29. Wiswell TE, The prepuce, urinary tract infections, and the consequences (comment). Pediatrics 2000; 105: 860–862.
30. Wiswell T, Hatchey WE. Urinary tract infections and the uncircumcised state: an update. Clin Pediatr 1993; 32: 130–134.

31. Canning DA. Cohort study on circumcision of newborn boys and subsequent risk of urinary-tract infection. J Urol 1999; 162: 1562.
32. Schoen EJ, Colby CJ, Ray GT. Newborn circumcision decreases incidence and costs of urinary tract infections during the first year of life (*see* comments). Pediatrics 2000; 105: 789–793.
33. Craig J, Knight JF, Sureshkumar P, Mantz E, Roy LP. Effect of circumcision on incidence of urinary tract infection in preschool boys. J Pediatr 1996; 128: 23–27.
34. Lapides J. Mechanisms of urinary tract infection. Urology 1979; 14: 2117–2225.
35. Koff S. Bladder-sphincter dysfunction in childhood. Urology 1982; 19: 457–463.
36. O'Reagan S, Yazbeck S, Shick E. Constipation, bladder instability, and urinary tract infection syndrome. Clin Nephrol 1985; 23: 152–158.
37. Loening-Baucke V. Urinary incontinence and urinary tract infection and their resolution with treatment of chronic constipation of childhood. Pediatrics 1997; 100: 228–235.
38. Wennerstrom M, Hansson S, Hedner T, Himmelmann A, Jodal U. Ambulatory blood pressure 16–26 years after the first urinary tract infection in childhood. J Hypertens 2000; 18: 485–491.
39. Wennerstrom M, Hansson S, Jodal U, Stokland E. Primary and acquired renal scarring in boys and girls with urinary tract infection. J Pediatr 2000; 136: 30–34.
40. Hansson S, Bollgren I, Esbjorner E, Jakobsson B, Marild S. Urinary tract infections in children below two years of age: a quality assurance project in Sweden. The Swedish Pediatric Nephrology Association. Acta Paediatr 1999; 88: 270–274.
41. Nuutinen M, Uhari M, Murphy MF, Hey K. Clinical guidelines and hospital discharges of children with acute urinary tract infections. Pediatr Nephrol 1999; 13: 45–49.

4 Screening and Early Detection for Genitourinary Cancer

Ian M. Thompson, MD
and Joseph Basler, MD

CONTENTS

INTRODUCTION

Genitourinary (GU) cancers constitute a significant fraction of all neoplastic disease. GU cancers include neoplasms of the prostate, bladder, kidney, testis, ureter, urethra, adrenal, penis, and testicular adnexae. Among the tumors represented, prostate cancer is the most common cancer in men and testicular cancer is the most common cancer in men between the ages of 15 and 30. Like most other tumors, survival of virtually all of these sites is directly related to stage at diagnosis. (In the case of testicular cancer, although survival is excellent even for advanced disease, the extent of therapy required for advanced disease is extremely more complicated and morbid than for disease localized to the testis.) It is for this reason that concerted early detection efforts for some of these tumors has been suggested.

To be a reasonable proposition for a specific organ-site, there are a number of requirements for early detection (or screening) that should be met. These include the following:

- The disease must have a high prevalence.
- Early detection tests must be available that have a high sensitivity and specificity.

From: *Essential Urology: A Guide to Clinical Practice*
Edited by: J. M. Potts © Humana Press Inc., Totowa, NJ

- Effective treatment for early stage disease must be available.
- Early detection tests must detect disease at a stage when treatment is effective.
- The cost of the early detection program must be acceptable.
- The morbidity associated with early detection must be acceptable.

Ideally, early detection for neoplastic disease should be proven to improve survival (as well as reduce mortality from the disease: two different outcomes) while preserving a high quality of life and while using an acceptable quality of health care resources. Unfortunately, no early detection test has been proven to meet all of these criteria. Even widely accepted early detection tests, such as screening mammography, continue to be the subject of debate regarding their efficacy *(1)*. In no GU site has screening been demonstrated to affect survival, mortality, or quality of life. For prostate cancer, two studies are currently underway to evaluate the impact of screening on survival. The Prostate, Lung, Colorectal, and Ovarian Cancer (PLCO) study in the United States and the European Randomized Study of Screening will address this issue late in the first decade of this century. For all other organ sites, no studies are currently ongoing, and all data must be extrapolated from clinical observations.

CONFOUNDS ASSOCIATED WITH SCREENING FOR GU MALIGNANCIES

A number of authors have pointed out many potential confounds associated with screening for malignancies in general. First among these is the issue of lead-time bias. This issue is graphically demonstrated in Fig. 1.

In this figure, it can be seen that in the upper case, a screening modality was used to identify a cancer early. Unfortunately, despite therapy, the disease recurred, metastasized, and ultimately led to the patient's demise. In the second case, the disease presented at a metastatic stage and the patient again ultimately died from the disease. The latter case presumes that the early detection effort was unable to affect the natural history of the disease. (A good example of this might be the use of chest x-ray for lung cancer when, by the time disease is diagnosed, it is beyond the ability of local excision to affect a cure.) In the former case, using early diagnosis, there is a perception that cancer survival is longer, whereas overall survival is actually unchanged.

Another confound with cancer screening is length-time bias. This concept reflects the propensity of screening tests that are generally administered on an infrequent basis to identify indolent, low-risk tumors. Figure 2 demonstrates this concept.

As can be seen in Fig. 2, there are three general types of tumors: those that grow quickly and rapidly lead to the demise of the individual (short and fat arrows), intermediate tumors, and tumors that develop and spread only over a long period of time (long, skinny arrows). If it is presumed that screening episodes are performed periodically, the results are those seen. The tumors that are most likely to be identified early, when cure is likely, are the long, skinny arrows—the most indolent of tumors. (In the case of the long, skinny arrows, all are detected while still curable. Unfortunately, of these, only half would have actually led to the demise of the patient.) However, none of the four rapidly growing tumors was detected sufficiently early to affect a cure and in all of these, the patient died of the disease. We have previously demonstrated that length-time bias is operational in patients screened with digital rectal examination for prostate cancer *(2)*. A concern of many authorities with respect to bladder cancer is the similar observation that the tumor that ultimately leads to the demise of the patient is

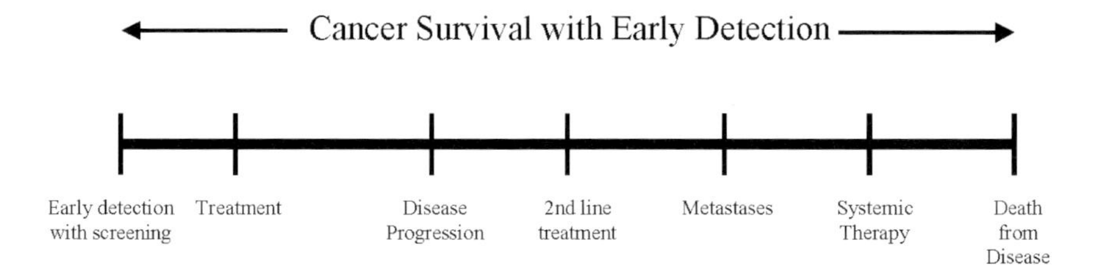

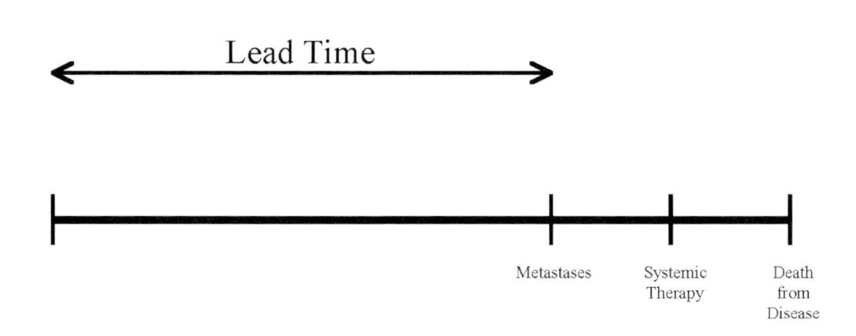

Fig. 1. Lead-time bias. Natural history of prostate cancer with and without early detection. If cancer is detected at the time of symptomatic metastases, short cancer survival is noted. If cancer is detected early with screening, much longer time (survival) is noted until death from cancer. However, no impact is noted on the actual length of the patient's life—just a longer time with the diagnosis of "cancer."

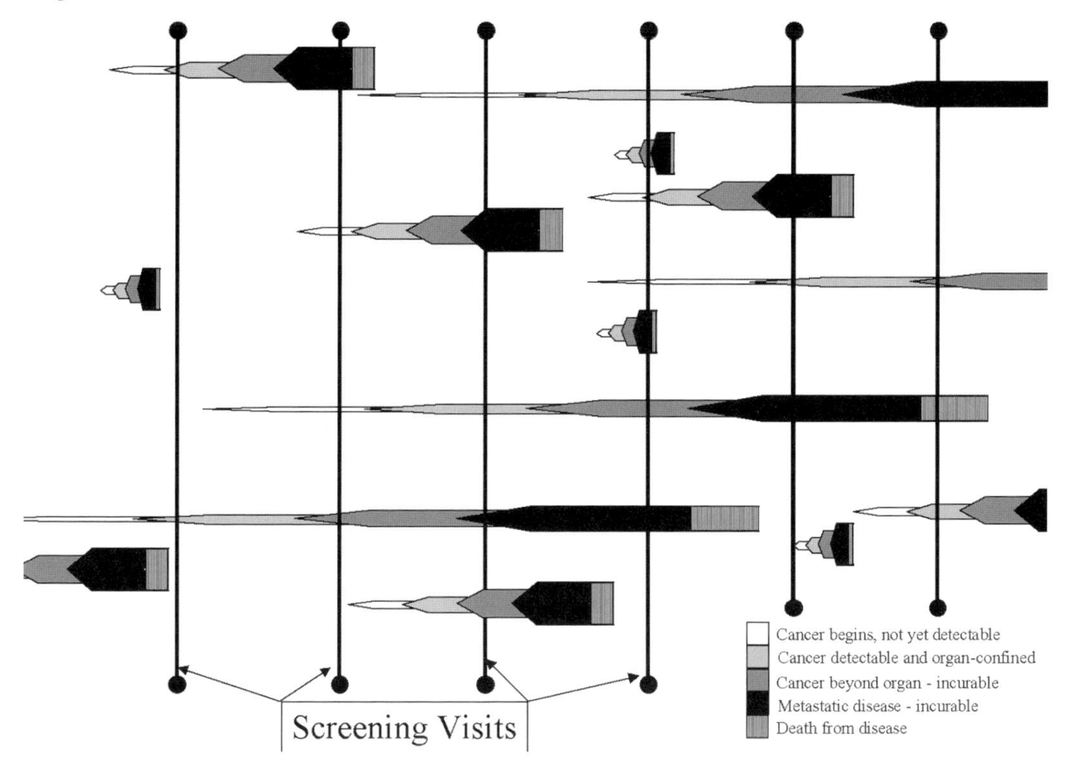

Fig. 2. Length-time bias. Regular screening visits are more likely to detect slow growth-rate rather than rapidly growing tumors while still curable. As a result, rapidly growing tumors, those that pose the greatest threat to a patient's life, are least likely to be found by screening.

rarely the one that develops after multiple superficial tumors; the lethal tumor generally presents with high-stage, advanced disease, suggesting a more rapid proliferation and development rate, much akin to the short, fat arrows in Fig. 2.

SCREENING FOR PROSTATE CANCER

Perhaps the most contentious of all screening modalities in medicine today, screening for prostate cancer is a fait accompli: it is widespread in the United States and, unless a major change occurs in the patterns of care or in information from clinical trials, it will probably continue for the foreseeable future. To provide the very best discussion, the format for this section will be that of a debate: the pros and cons of screening.

The Pros of Prostate Cancer Screening

Prostate Cancer Is a Public Health Problem

It is clear that prostate cancer represents a major public health concern. With almost 200,000 new cases annually and nearly 30,000 deaths each year, the human toll is substantial *(3)*. When one recognizes that approximately one man in four who undergoes prostate biopsy is found to have prostate cancer, then perhaps 800,000 prostate biopsies are being performed annually. If a man with prostate cancer lives, on average, 5–15 yr, then there are 1–3 million men in the United States with a diagnosis of prostate cancer and another 4–12 million who are at risk.

If Prostate Cancer Is Detected After It Is Symptomatic, Most Cases Are Metastatic

Localized prostate cancer is almost always devoid of symptoms. Although it is frequently recommended that men with obstructive voiding symptoms consider an evaluation for possible prostate cancer, this is an unusual presenting complaint. The reason: prostate cancer generally arises in the peripheral zone of the prostate and rarely will lead to urethral obstruction. It is only when metastases to bone (pain) or to regional lymph nodes (lower extremity lymphedema or deep vein thrombosis) or to the retroperitoneal lymph nodes (ureteral obstruction, flank pain, and uremia) occur that symptoms develop.

Once Prostate Cancer Has Metastasized, Most Men Will Die From the Disease

Despite advances in the management of advanced prostate cancer, the prognosis for a man with metastatic disease is quite poor. In a recent Phase III study of men with metastatic disease, median survival was only 30 mo *(4)*.

Tests Are Available That Allow for Early Diagnosis of Prostate Cancer

Since the advent of prostate-specific antigen (PSA) testing, in combination with digital rectal examination (DRE), prostate cancer diagnosis has been changed in a revolutionary manner. Approximately 10% of men tested with PSA will be found to have a value >4.0 ng/mL and between 3 and 10% will have an abnormal DRE. Of men undergoing biopsy, between 25 and 33% will be found to have prostate cancer *(5)*. With PSA screening, the more than 97% of prostate cancer cases diagnosed are clinically confined to the prostate *(6)*.

Table 1
Results of Cost Analysis of Screening for Prostate Cancer

Intervention	*Cost per quality-adjusted life-year saved*
Liver transplantation	$ 237,000
Screening mammography (<50)	$ 232,000
Worst case—prostate cancer screening	$ 145,600
CABG—two vessels with angina	$ 106,000
Captopril for hypertension	$ 82,600
Hydrochlorothiazide for hypertension	$ 23,500
Best case—prostate cancer screening	$ 8700
Physician "stop smoking" message	$ 1300

If Prostate Cancer Is Diagnosed Early, Treatments Are Generally Effective

Clearly, the outcome of treatment is related to the extent of disease. Although failures are greater if nodal disease, seminal vesicle involvement, or extracapsular disease is present, for tumors that are confined to the prostate, the progression-free probability at 10 yr exceeds 90% *(7)*.

Screening for Prostate Cancer Has Led to an Increase in the Rate of Localized Disease and a Fall in the Rate of Metastatic Disease

PSA screening in the United States began in earnest in the late 1980s. In association with this was a dramatic increase in the detection of disease. After a period of almost exponential rise in detection, the incidence rate fell to relatively stable rates. Beginning in 1991, and virtually every year since, a fall in the rate of metastatic disease has been seen *(8)*.

Screening for Prostate Cancer Has Preceded a Fall in Prostate Cancer Mortality

Since the early 1990s when the rate of metastatic disease began to fall, there has been a gradual decrease in prostate cancer mortality *(9)*. This was in the face of gradually increasing mortality rates in the late 1980s.

Screening for Prostate Cancer Is Cost Effective

In a decision analysis, using a range of efficacy rates of screening as well as actual charges for medical care, we previously demonstrated that quality-adjusted life-years gained from prostate cancer screening was in a range of commonly accepted preventive health measures *(10)*. Table 1 provides this data.

The Cons of Prostate Cancer Screening

Prostate Cancer Is Ubiquitous: We Don't Want to Find All of the Cases

A combination of autopsy data and national statistics suggest that although almost 70% of men will develop histological evidence of prostate cancer and 16% will be diagnosed, only 3–4% will die of the disease *(11)*. Thus, if we were able to detect disease in all men who had it, we would treat 20 men to prevent one death. (Of course, we diagnose nowhere close to that rate of the disease.) What fraction of the 16% of men diagnosed during their lifetime who are treated unnecessarily is unknown.

Screening Tests Are Ineffective

Despite the fact that the combination of regular PSA and DRE testing significantly reduces the stage of prostate cancer at diagnosis, they are not perfect. In those men in the Washington University series who were diagnosed with prostate cancer at the time of their initial PSA, 37% had clinically or pathologically advanced disease. Among those with serial PSA measurements, 29% still had advanced disease *(12)*. These observations suggest that, with time, even those men who are screened repetitively with PSA will be at risk for treatment failure and demise from their disease.

Treatment Is Not Always Successful

With prolonged follow-up after extirpative surgery (radical prostatectomy) even in men with organ-confined disease, there is a continued risk for disease recurrence (measured by development of a detectable level of PSA; ref. *13*). This risk of recurrence appears to increase over time *(14)*.

Treatment Carries With It Significant Risks and Complications

Treatment options for localized prostate cancer includes, generally, radiotherapy with external beam, brachytherapy, and surgery (radical prostatectomy). Each of these carries with it a unique spectrum of complications, including erectile dysfunction, urinary incontinence, urinary obstruction, radiation injury to the rectum or bladder, urethral strictures, and need for secondary therapies.

Screening Is Costly

We have demonstrated that the annual cost for screening for prostate cancer is in the range of $10–25 billion annually in the United States *(15)*.

There Is No Evidence That Screening Leads to an Improvement in Survival

To date, no appropriately powered and controlled clinical trials have demonstrated that screening neither improves survival of the general population nor enhances quality of life. Both the PLCO trial in the United States and the European trial should have results addressing these issues within the decade. Population observations regarding changes in mortality are subject to numerous confounds and do not clearly demonstrate an effect of screening or treatment.

SCREENING FOR KIDNEY CANCER

No studies have been conducted to evaluate the potential benefit of screening for kidney cancer. Nevertheless, there are interesting possibilities for investigation. Kidney cancer affects approx 30,000 individuals each year and causes about 11,000 deaths each year in the United States *(16)*. Like most other GU cancers, the outcome of the disease is distinctly related to its stage with 5-yr survivals for localized, regional, and distant disease of 88, 61, and 9%, respectively *(17)*.

High-Risk Groups

Clearly, the highest risk group for renal cell carcinoma (RCC) and the group in whom screening is standard-of-care are patients with Von Hippel-Lindau disease. In this patient population, although the incidence of renal cell carcinoma is between 25 and 50%, if a patient lives into his or her 70s, the risk of cystic or neoplastic disease is probably greater than 90% *(18–20)*. Certainly, in this population and in family members in whom the mutation has been identified (on 3p25), periodic surveillance of the kidneys is required. The age at which screening should begin has been disputed but certainly should have begun at or before age 20 *(21)*.

Other at-risk groups have been identified but not for RCC but for Wilm's tumor. In patients with Beckwith–Wiedemann syndrome, abdominal ultrasonography is indicated for both Wilm's tumor as well as hepatoblastoma *(22)*. Similar screening has been recommended for patients with hemihypertrophy and aniridia *(23)*. Finally, although some authorities have suggested screening kidneys being considered for transplantation, the risk of a tumor present at the time of transplant or developing over a 7-yr followup was 0.27 and 0.145%, respectively *(24)*.

Rationale for Screening

The primarily rationale for screening for RCC arises from repeated observations from the serendipitous detection of renal tumors through abdominal imagine performed for other reasons. Multiple authors have explored this concept and have repeatedly reached the following conclusions:

- With the increased use of abdominal imaging (for conditions such as cholelithiasis or evaluation of nonspecific complaints), the rate of serendipitous detection of renal tumors has increased dramatically.
- Tumors detected serendipitously:
  - Are smaller. In the series of Masood and colleagues *(25)*, the average size of serendipitously detected tumors was 5.9 cm compared with 9.2 cm for symptomatic tumors.
  - Are of a lower T-stage. In the series of Tsui and colleagues *(26)*, Stage I tumors constituted 62% of serendipitous tumors compared with 23% of tumors detected by virtue of symptoms.
  - Are more likely to be organ-confined *(26)*.
  - Are less likely to be metastatic *(25)*.
  - Have a dramatically improved survival *(27)*.

As a result of these observations, a number of authors have suggested that early detection of RCC should be considered. One large series has attempted to use abdominal ultrasonography to screen for abdominal disease processes *(28)*. In this remarkable report, the authors summarize the results of screening of 219,640 individuals over a period of 13 yr. A total of 192 RCCs were detected (0.09% of examinees) during this time and of these, 189 were organ-confined. Survival for cases was 97% at 5 yr and 95% at 10 yr.

In addition to the relatively low prevalence of RCC, another obstacle to widespread screening is the prevalence of cystic or complex renal masses that could be identified with imaging studies. These lesions are of such a complex issue that a system for their classification has been developed—the so-called Bosniak classification system.

Nonsolid lesions are grouped into four categories: group I are simple cysts, group II are mildly complicated but clearly benign cysts, group III are more complicated cysts that require histological confirmation for diagnosis, and group IV are overt cystic neoplasms *(29)*. Obviously, if the prevalence of RCC is as low as was seen in the Japanese experience and if there is a measurable rate of Bosniak III lesions in the general population, screening for RCC could not be considered.

At this time, early detection of RCC by routine screening of any group of patients other than the high-risk populations described above cannot be supported by data. However, the intriguing repeated observations relative to serendipitously detected tumors of a dramatic improvement in survival in "screen-detected" tumors strongly supports calls for prospective studies to evaluate this hypothesis.

SCREENING FOR BLADDER CANCER

Bladder cancer is the second most common GU cancer with 54,300 new cases annually and 12,100 deaths from the disease *(30)*. Almost all of these tumors arise from the bladder urothelium and are known as transitional cell (urothelial) carcinoma. The concept of early detection is well-supported by the substantial decrease in survival in advanced disease. Five-year survival rates for localized, regional, and distant disease for the period 1989–1996 were 93, 49, and 6%, respectively *(31)*.

In addition to the rationale for screening is the repeated observation that rarely is there a clinical progression from symptoms to local disease to regional and then advanced disease in most patients. Indeed, more than 90% of patients with advanced disease, present for the first time with symptoms at an advanced stage *(32)*. A final rationale for early diagnosis of bladder cancer is that treatment for superficial, noninvasive bladder cancer is generally considerably less morbid than that for more advanced disease. For tumors confined to the urothelium, simple transurethral resection is curative. For more deeply invasive tumors, partial or radical cystectomy is required with its attendant complications and impact on quality of life. The likelihood that tumors of no clinical significance would be identified in a screening program is extremely low as most studies have documented that tumors almost never are detected in patients without a history of bladder cancer at the time of autopsy *(33)*.

High-Risk Groups

Bladder cancer incidence increases with age and the primary risk factor for the disease is cigarette smoking. Other etiologies include exposure to various chemical agents. Screening programs have been conducted for employees exposed to these chemical agents and have confirmed that, for these very high-risk groups, early detection is a reasonable option *(34)*. A relatively unique population of patients at high risk for both urothelial and squamous cell carcinoma are spinal cord injury patients who often have indwelling Foley catheters. This group of individuals may have a 2–10% risk of bladder cancer over their lifetimes *(35)*.

Methods of Screening

Cystoscopy

No studies to date, with the exception of studies of spinal cord injured patients (in whom screening cystoscopy may influence survival through early detection in this very high-risk cohort), have used screening cystoscopy for detection of bladder cancer in otherwise-asymptomatic individuals. Cystoscopy is routinely used for follow-up of patients with a previous diagnosis of bladder cancer in whom there is a 25% risk of disease recurrence.

Hematuria Screening

Two retrospective studies have suggested that screening for bladder cancer using urinalysis on a single occasion for hematuria detection is ineffective *(36,37)*. In our own series, we found in 2000 men undergoing hematuria screening, we found a low rate of bladder cancer detection and no evidence of any improvement in population mortality or survival *(38)*.

Messing and colleagues *(39–41)* conducted a prospective study of 2431 men with repeated home hematuria evaluations using the Ames Hemastix test *(39–41)*. The population chosen was older males without a history of urological malignancies. Of those who were invited, only about half opted to participate. Just over 1% of participating men were found to have bladder cancer, yet more than 90% of men with hematuria did not have bladder cancer. An optimistic finding was that all but one tumor detected was muscle invasive. The population outcomes of this study are hard to evaluate, given that long-term follow up is not available. A major difficulty in a nonrandomized trial of this type is the inability of the investigators to determine whether the tumors detected were those with an invasive phenotype that would have otherwise developed invasive disease before symptoms. Thus, we do not know whether the hematuria screening merely added to the lead time without affecting the ultimate outcome.

Urine Cytology

One of the oldest forms of bladder cancer screening uses cytological examination of the urinary sediment for evidence of neoplastic cells. In general, cytology is a poor method to diagnose low-grade tumors but benefits from a relatively high sensitivity for higher grade tumors. In one nonpopulation-based study, the sensitivity of cytology for grade I, II, and III bladder tumors was 22, 38, and 83%, respectively *(42)*. Cytology has been tested in groups of occupationally exposed workers and has been suggested to be a reasonable method to identify individuals with a high risk of disease *(43)*.

Tumor Markers

A proliferation of bladder tumor markers has occurred over the past several years. One group of tests uses chromosomal variations at a number of loci where genetic loss or amplification has been identified. Exfoliated cells with these characteristics can then been identified with fluorescent *in situ* hybridization. Other genetic variations, microsatellite deletions, repeating regions that are deleted during the process of DNA repair and compared with genomic DNA, show promise for bladder cancer detection *(44,45)*. Several commercially available urinary tests are available for the detection of tumor markers associated with bladder cancer. In general, these tests are currently used for the detection of recurrent bladder cancer in patients with a previous history of bladder cancer. In these patients, traditionally, surveillance cystoscopy is performed on a regular basis. Advocates for these urinary tests suggest that their use can allow the reduction of the frequency of such cystoscopic examinations. No prospective studies have been conducted in at-risk populations who do not have a history of bladder cancer previously. It is, however, instructive to examine the performance characteristics of these tests within this very high-risk population. (The reader must realize that the recurrent-bladder-tumor population has a 25% or greater risk of bladder cancer compared to a 1% or less overall population risk. Such prevalence statistics provide little support for population-wide screening for bladder cancer.) In a recent study of 250 patients, 174 with a previous history of bladder cancer, 66 with newly diagnosed bladder cancer, and another 64 with microscopic hematuria, the authors assessed the performance of the NMP22, BTA stat, and UBC antigen tests *(46)*. The sensitivity for new tumors for these tests was 65, 75, and 60%, respectively. The specificity for disease recurrence was 64, 54, 72%, respectively. Interestingly, the sensitivity and specificity of cytology for new tumors was 41 and 94%, respectively.

Obviously, with sensitivity rates in the 60–70% range and specificity rates in the 50–70% range, none of these tumor markers would be acceptable for any program of mass screening. Whether the higher sensitivity of cytology for the very high-risk, grade III tumor is a potential advantage of this specific test remains to be determined. It would only be through properly powered, prospective, and randomized clinical trials that the efficacy of any of these tests for mass screening could be validated.

SCREENING FOR TESTICULAR CANCER

Testicular cancer, most commonly of germ-cell origin, is the most common neoplasm in young men. Approximately 7500 cases will be diagnosed in the United States each year and is the most common tumor in men 15 to 35 years of age *(47)*. About 400 men each year lose their lives from this disease. The current 5-yr survival in patients with testicular cancer is 95%. The extraordinary impact of platinum-based chemotherapy is evident in the extremely high survival rate of testicular carcinoma in every stage. The American Cancer Society has estimated that the 5-yr survival of localized, regional, and advanced testicular cancer is 99, 97, and 75%, respectively *(48)*.The attractive nature of early detection of testicular cancer is illustrated by the following observations:

1. Testicular examination is simple and convenient. Most testicular tumors will present with a solid mass within the testis that alters the testicular contour. The mass is generally painless.
2. If testicular cancer is detected early while confined to the testis, orchiectomy alone is a treatment option and will be curative for as many as 75% of patients with testicular cancer *(49)*.
3. If testicular cancer is detected when metastatic disease is present, not only does the potential for cure decrease, but the treatment also can be extensive, costly, and can have a major impact on quality of life. Treatments include first-line and salvage chemotherapy (side effects include renal toxicity, peripheral neuropathy, and infertility) as well as salvage surgery with its attendant risks.

Many organizations have recommended early detection for testicular cancer with periodic self-examination. Although a physician examination may be distinctly superior in quality to self-examination, the very low incidence rate of testicular cancer as well as its relatively rapid growth rate (which would make annual examinations insufficiently frequent), it is obviously not an appropriate choice. Despite this, no data have been published supporting the notion that regular self-examination will decrease mortality from the disease.

High-Risk Groups

An ideal approach to early detection of any tumor would be the implementation of early detection strategies in high-risk groups. For testicular cancer, some high-risk groups could be identified. Men with a history of cryptorchidism may have as much as a 20-fold increased risk of germ-cell cancer. Similarly, men with Klinefelter's syndrome and gonadal dysgenesis have a higher risk of disease *(50)*. Conversely, testicular cancer is uncommon among African-American men *(51)*. Finally, men with a history of testicular cancer have a higher risk of disease in the contralateral testis.

Considerable controversy has developed over the subject of infertility and testicular neoplasms *(52)*. At this point, because of the tremendous difference in rates of infertility in the population and that of testicular cancer, no recommendations can be made.

Method of Screening

Self-examination is the most commonly recommended screening modality. The potential for ultrasound screening has been suggested but carries with it serious problems. The risks of microlithiasis (suggested by some to be a potentially sign of malignancy) or of a hypoechoic lesion that is not testicular carcinoma are great *(53,54)*. For these reasons, ultrasound screening would be a poor choice for generalized use.

Recommendation

A program of mass screening for testicular cancer would be unlikely to reduce mortality or improve survival because of the excellent cure rates of even regional nodal and metastatic disease. Nevertheless, the potential reduction in morbidity of therapy if an increased fraction of tumors were diagnosed while localized to the testis, would be a laudable goal. For this reason, it is a reasonable approach to include a recommendation for periodic self-examination for young men. Certainly, removing the stigma for a young man to request an examination by a family physician or school nurse might lead to earlier diagnosis of some tumors in this emotionally sensitive organ site.

CONCLUSIONS

At this time, evidence is not clear-cut that mass screening for any GU malignancy will significantly reduce mortality and improve survival of the population. Of all organ sites, prostate cancer screening has the most mature data and is the most promising. Current screening trials should provide considerable evidence as to the efficacy within the next decade. The second most promising site is testicular cancer simply as screening can take the form of periodic public health messages regarding self-examination. Both bladder and kidney cancer, although having several potential screening modalities, do not appear to have sufficient evidence to warrant any use of screening at this time. Nevertheless, the data are developing that justify the development of clinical trials to employ existing tests. The ideal companion advance for all screening protocols will be the ability to identify high- and low-risk individuals who should be screened and need not be screened, respectively. Such pretesting will enrich disease prevalence in the screening group and will ultimately improve the performance characteristics of screening tests.

REFERENCES

1. Bomalaski JJ. Tabano M. Hooper L. Fiorica J. Mammography. Curr OpinObstet Gynecol 2001; 13: 15–23.
2. Gerber GS, Thompson IM, Thisted R, Chodak GW. Disease-specific survival following routine prostate cancer screening by digital rectal examination. JAMA 1993;;269:61–64.
3. Greenlee RT, Hill-Harmon MB, Murray T, et al. Cancer statistics 2001. CA Cancer J Clin 2001; 5: 15–36.
4. Eisenberger MA, Blumenstein BA, Crawford ED, Miller G, McLeod DG, Loehrer PJ, et al. Bilateral orchiectomy with or without flutamide for metastatic prostate cancer. N Engl J Med 1998; 339: 1036–1042.
5. Smith DS. Humphrey PA. Catalona WJ. The early detection of prostate carcinoma with prostate specific antigen: the Washington University experience. Cancer 1997; 80: 1852–1856.
6. Smith DS. Catalona WJ. The nature of prostate cancer detected through prostate specific antigen based screening. J Urol 1994; 152: 1732–1736.
7. Hull GW. Rabbani F. Abbas F. Wheeler TM. Kattan MW. Scardino PT. Cancer control with radical prostatectomy alone in 1,000 consecutive patients. J Urol 2002; 167: 528–534.
8. Hankey BF, Feuer EJ, Clegg LX, et al. cancer surveillance series: interpreting trends in prostate cancer—Part I: evidence of the effects of screening in recent prostate cancer incidence, mortality, and survival rates. J Natl Cancer Inst 1999; 91: 1017–1024.
9. Potosky AL, Feuer EJ, Levin DL. Impact of screening on incidence and mortality of prostate cancer in the United States. Epidemiol Rev 2001; 23: 181–186.
10. Thompson IM, Optenberg SA. An overview cost-utility analysis of prostate cancer screening. Oncology (Huntington). 1995; 9 (11 suppl): 141–145.
11. Merrill RM, Weed DL, Feuer EJ. The lifetime risk of developing prostate cancer in white and black men. Cancer Epidemiol Biomarkers Prev 1997; 6: 763–768.
12. Catalona WJ, Smith DS, Ratliff TL, Basler JW. Detection of organ-confined prostate cancer is increased through prostate-specific antigen-based screening. JAMA 1993; 270: 948–954.
13. Trapasso JG, deKernion JB, Smith RB, Dorey F. The incidence and significance of detectable levels of serum prostate specific antigen after radical prostatectomy. J Urol 1994; 152: 1821–1825.
14. Amling CL,. Blute ML, Bergstralh EJ, Seay TM, Slezak J, Zincke H. Long-term hazard of progression after radical prostatectomy for clinically localized prostate cancer: continued risk of biochemical failure after 5 years. J Urol 2000; 164: 101–105.
15. Lubke WL, Optenberg SA, Thompson IM. Analysis of the first-year cost of a prostate cancer screening and treatment program in the United States. J Natl Cancer Inst 199; 86: 1790–1792.
16. Jernal A, Thomas A, Murray T, Thun M. Cancer Statistics, 2002. CA Ca J Clin 2002; 52: 23–47.
17. American Cancer Society. Cancer Facts and Figures 2001. American Cancer Society, Atlanta, GA, p. 16.
18. Goldfarb DA. Nephron-sparing surgery and renal transplantation in patients with renal cell carcinoma and von Hippel-Lindau disease. J Intern Med 1998; 243: 563.
19. Chauveau D, Duvic C, Chretien Y, et al. Renal involvement in von Hippel-Lindau disease. Kidney Int 1996; 50: 944.
20. Latiff F, Tory K, Gnarra J, et al. Identification of the von Hippel-Lindau disease tumor supressor gene. Science 1993; 260: 1317.
21. Harries RW. A rational approach to radiological screening in von Hippel-Lindau disease. J Med Screening 1994; 1: 88–95.
22. McNeil DE, Brown M, Ching A, DeBaun MR. Screening for Wilms tumor and hepatoblastoma in children with Beckwith-Wiedemann syndromes: a cost-effective model. Med Pediatr Oncol 2001; 37: 349–356.
23. Craft AW, Parker L, Stiller C, Cole M. Screening for Wilms' tumour in patients with aniridia, Beckwith syndrome, or hemihypertrophy. Med Pediatr Oncol 1995; 24: 231–234.
24. Wunderlich H, Wilhelm S, Reichelt O, et al. Renal cell carcinoma in renal graft recipients and donors: incidence and consequence. Urol Int 2001; 67: 24–7.
25. Masood J, lane T, Koye B, et al. Renal cell carcinoma: incidental detection during routine ultrasonography in men presenting with lower urinary tract symptoms. BJU Int 2001; 88: 671–674.

26. Tsui KH, Shvarts O, Smith RB, et al. Renal cell carcinoma: prognostic significance of incidentally detected tumors. J Urol 2000; 163: 426–430.
27. Thompson IM, Peek M. Improvement in survival of patients with renal cell carcinoma—the role of the serendipitously detected tumor. J Urol 1988; 140: 487–490.
28. Mihara S, Kuroda K, Yoshioka R, Koyama W. Early detection of renal cell carcinoma by ultrasonographic screening—based on the results of 13 years screening in Japan. Ultrasound Med Biol 1999; 25: 1033–1039.
29. Bosniak MA. The current radiological approach to renal cysts. Radiology 1986; 158: 1.
30. American Cancer Society. Cancer Facts and Figures 2001. American Cancer Society, Atlanta, GA, p. 5.
31. American Cancer Society. Cancer Facts and Figures 2001. American Cancer Society, Atlanta, GA, p. 16.
32. Kaye KW, Lange PH. Mode of presentation of invasive bladder cancer: reassessment of the problem. J Urol 1992; 128: 31–33.
33. VF Marshall, Current clinical problems regarding bladder tumors. Cancer 1956; 3: 543–550.
34. Hemstreet GP, Yin S, Ma Z, et al. Biomarker risk assessment and bladder cancer detection in a cohort exposed to benzidine. J Natl Cancer Inst 2001; 93: 427–436.
35. Bejany DE, Lockhart JL, Rhamy RK. Malignant vesical tumors following spinal cord injury. J Urol, 1987; 138: 1390.
36. Mohr DN, Offord KP, Owen RA, et al. Asymptomatic microhematuria and urologic disease. A population-based study. JAMA 1986; 256: 224–229.
37. Hitt RA, Ordonez JD. Dipstick urinalysis screening, asymptomatic microhematuria, and subsequent urological cancers in a population-based sample. Cancer Epidemiol Biomarkers Prev 1994; 3: 439–442.
38. Thompson IM. The evaluation of microscopic hematuria: a population-based study. J Urol 1987; 138: 1189–1190.
39. Messing EM, Young TB, Hunt VB, et al. Hematuria home screening: repeat testing results. J Urol 1995; 154: 57–61.
40. Messing EM, Young TB, Hunt VB, et al. The significance of asymptomatic microhematuria in men 50 or more years old: findings of a home screening study using urinary dipsticks. J Urol 1987; 137: 919–922.
41. Messing EM, Young TB, Hunt VB, et al. Comparison of bladder cancer outcomes in men undergoing hematuria home screening versus those with standard clinical presentations. Urology 1995; 45: 387–397.
42. Ramakumar S, Bhuiyan J, Besse JA, Roberts SG, Wollan PC, Blute ML, O'Kane DJ. Comparison of screening methods in the detection of bladder cancer. J Urol 1999; 161: 388–394.
43. Bi W, Rao JY, Hemstreet GP, Fang P, Asal NR, Zang M, Min KW, Ma Z, Lee E, Li G. Field molecular epidemiology. Feasibility of monitoring for the malignant bladder cell phenotype in a benzidine-exposed occupational cohort. J Occup Med 1993; 35: 20–27.
44. Utting M, Werner W, Dahse R, et al. Microsatellite analysis of free tumor DNA in urine, serum, and plasma of patients: a minimally invasive method for the detection of bladder cancer. ClinCancer Res 2002; 8: 35–40.
45. Seripa D, Parrella P, Gallucci M, Gravina C, Papa S, Fortunato P, Alcini A, Flammia G, Lazzari M, Fazio VM. Sensitive detection of transitional cell carcinoma of the bladder by microsatellite analysis of cells exfoliated in urine. Int J Cancer 2001; 95: 364–369.
46. Boman H, Hedelin H, Holmang S. Four bladder tumor markers have a disappointingly low sensitivity for small size and low grade recurrence. J Urol 2002; 167: 80–83.
47. Jernal A, Thomas A, Murray T, Thun M. Cancer Statistics, 2002. Ca J Clin 2002; 52: 23–47.
48. American Cancer Society. Cancer Facts and Figures 2001. American Cancer Society, Atlanta, GA, p. 18
49. Sogani PC, Perrotti M, Herr HW, Fair WR, Thaler HT, Bosl G. Clinical stage I testis cancer: long-term outcome of patients on surveillance. J Urol 11998; 59:855–858.
50. Henderson BE, Benton B, Jing J, et al. Risk factors for cancer of the testis in young men. Int J Cancer 1979; 23: 598–602.

51. Moul JW, Schanne FJ, Thompson IM, Frazier HA, Peretsman SA, Wettlaufer JN, Rozanski TA, Stack RS, Kreder KJ, Hoffman KJ. Testicular cancer in blacks. A multicenter experience. Cancer 1994; 73: 388–393.
52. Giwercman A, Petersen PM. Cancer and male infertility. Best Practice Res Clin Endocrinol Metab 2000; 14: 453–471.
53. Peterson AC, Bauman JM, Light DE, et al. The prevalence of testicular microlithiasis in an asymptomatic population of men 18 to 35 years old. J Urol 2001; 166: 2061–2064.
54. Corrie D. Mueller EJ. Thompson IM. Management of ultrasonically detected nonpalpable testis masses. Urology 1991; 38: 429–431.

5 Basic Imaging in Urology

Martin B. Richman, MD *and Martin I. Resnick,* MD

CONTENTS

INTRODUCTION

Radiology, like most other fields of medicine and science, has seen substantial advancement and change with the continuing growth of technology. The first 75 years of urological imaging were performed with plain-film radiography and the 1970s, 1980s, and 1990s saw the introduction and then widespread usage of sonography (ultrasound), computed tomography (CT), magnetic resonance imaging (MRI), and radionuclide imaging. Urological imaging has benefited from these advances with a more precise ability to diagnose and evaluate genitourinary disorders without surgical exploration.

PLAIN-FILM IMAGING (RADIOGRAPHY)

Plain-film imaging of the urinary tract has been recognized since the end of the 19th century when Swain reported visualization of renal calculi on a glass abdominal flat plate *(1)*. Radiography uses x-rays to develop an image on a piece of film based on the amount of energy that passes through the object between the source and the film plate. Tissues of the body and foreign or organic materials that may be found within the body absorb different amounts of the radiation to create a readable image.

From: *Essential Urology: A Guide to Clinical Practice*
Edited by: J. M. Potts © Humana Press Inc., Totowa, NJ

Contrast Media

More precise evaluation of the upper urinary tracts became possible in the 1920s with cystoscopic-guided retrograde injection of Collargol, a colloidal silver suspension. Several years later, in 1930, Moses Swick reported on Uroselectan, the first relatively safe intravenous contrast agent *(2)*.

Since the 1950s and 1960s, sodium and meglumine salts of the fully substituted tri-iodinated benzoic acid compounds have been used as intravenous contrast agents. These ionic agents, also known as high-osmolality contrast media, dissociate in solution into the radiopaque anions and cations. These agents often exceed the osmolality of serum by five- to sevenfold, leading to many of their adverse effects. More recently, nonionic, low-osmolality contrast media have been developed. These agents are also tri-iodinated benzoic acid compounds but have hydrophilic hydroxyl groups instead of cations. Elimination of cations reduces the adverse effects of these contrast agents.

Toxicity of contrast media is caused by both the biochemical effects of injecting the agent into the bloodstream and to the possible hypersensitivity reaction that can occur. Chemotoxicity occurs with ionic contrast media that both disrupts the electrolyte balance of the serum and extracellular fluids and is three to four times more hypertonic than serum. This leads to disruption of endothelial surfaces and alters the conductivity of bodily fluids. Renal damage may occur from the subsequent decrease in renal perfusion and direct glomerular and renal tubular injury. Patients with a history of renal insufficiency or diabetes mellitus are at a higher risk for chemotoxicity and a transient increase in serum creatinine may occur in up to 10% of these patients.

Hypersensitivity or a systemic allergic reaction can also occur with injection of contrast media. These reactions can range in severity from nausea, vertigo, fevers, and rash to anaphylaxis and possible death. The overall incidence of adverse reactions to contrast media is between 0.5 and 5%, and the risk of mortality is between 0.9 and 2 per 100,000 patients. Patients with known previous reactions to contrast media or allergies to iodine or shellfish can be pretreated with corticosteroids and antihistamines (both H1 and H2). Nonionic contrast media generally have fewer adverse effects than conventional ionic media and are frequently used in patients with previous reactions to ionic contrast media. Treatment of adverse reactions includes supportive measures and the administration of antihistamines, epinephrine, corticosteroids, vascular volume expanders, and other appropriate measures.

PLAIN FILM OF THE ABDOMEN (KUB)

The kidneys–ureters–bladder (KUB) is often the first imaging study performed to visualize the abdomen and urinary tract (Fig. 1). The film is taken with the patient supine and should include the entire abdomen from the base of the sternum to the pubic symphysis.

The KUB can show bony abnormalities as well as calcifications and large soft tissue masses. The kidneys can usually be visualized because of the perirenal fatty tissue within Gerota's fascia. This study can provide information regarding the number of kidneys and their position relative to the bony structures and the shadows of the psoas muscles. Radiodense renal, ureteral, and bladder calculi can be seen on a KUB, and this study can be used to plan treatment or to assess for clearance of calculi after treatment (Figs. 2 and 3).

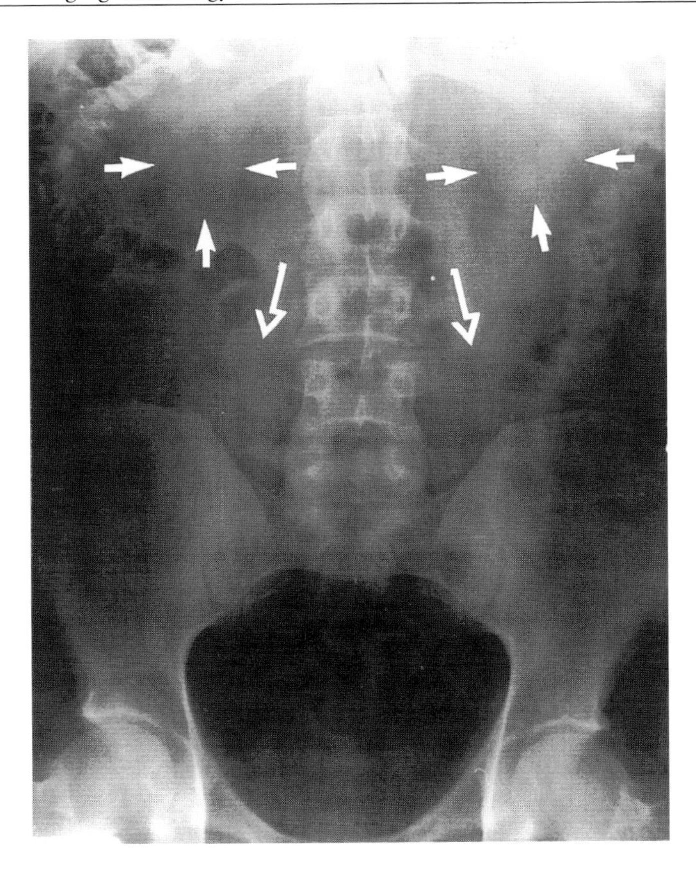

Fig. 1. Normal plain-film KUB showing the renal shadows (white arrows) caused by perinephric fatty tissue, and psoas shadows (open arrows). (From ref. *3*.)

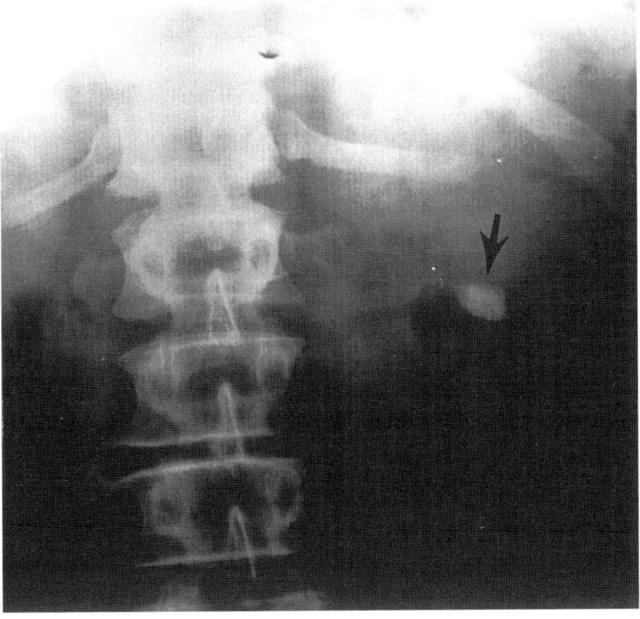

Fig. 2. Plain-film KUB showing a round density (arrow) overlying the left renal shadow indicative of a left renal calculus. (From ref. *3*.)

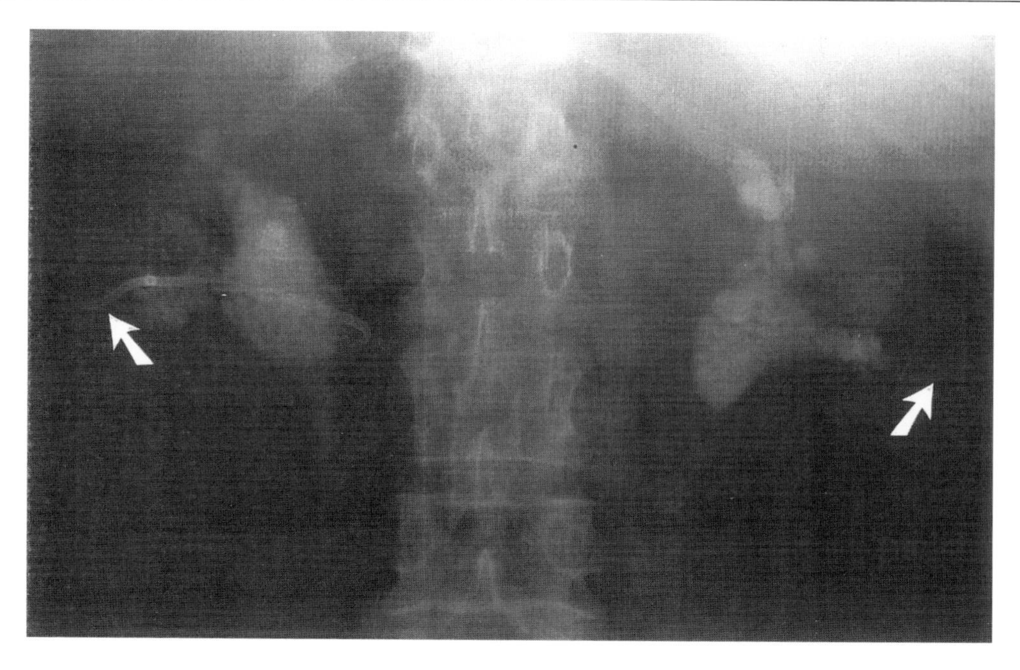

Fig. 3. Plain-film KUB showing calcific densities overlying bilateral pelvicalyceal systems indicative of "staghorn" calculi. Bilateral percutaneous nephrostomy tubes (white arrows) are seen. (From ref. *3*.)

UROGRAPHY

Urography involves injection or instillation of contrast material to better visualize the collecting or lumenal structures of the kidneys, ureters, bladder, and urethra. This can be done after intravenous injection or direct instillation into the urinary tract.

Intravenous Urography

The intravenous urogram (IVU), also called the intravenous pyelogram, is the classical modality for imaging the entire urothelial tract from the pyelocalyceal system through the ureters to the bladder. Although newer imaging modalities are frequently used in place of the IVU, the IVU is an excellent study for identifying small urothelial lesions as well as the severity of obstruction from calculi. This study provides anatomical and qualitative functional information about the kidneys (Figs. 4 and 5).

The IVU is performed after a gentle bowel catharsis to reduce interference from air or stool in the intestines. A preliminary KUB is taken. This film is used to demonstrate calculi or other abnormal calcifications that may be obscured by the contrast. Radiographic contrast is then injected, usually as a bolus, and a second image is obtained. This first contrast image is the nephrogram phase and shows enhancement of the renal shadows as the kidneys are perfused with contrast. Additional images are taken at timed intervals to display excretion into the collecting system, and drainage through the ureters. Filling of the bladder with contrast can demonstrate mucosal lesions or foreign bodies, which are represented as filling defects (Fig. 6). Nephrotomograms are frequently obtained to better visualize the more posterior upper and anterior lower renal poles. Tomograms can also be used to eliminate interference from overlying bowel gas.

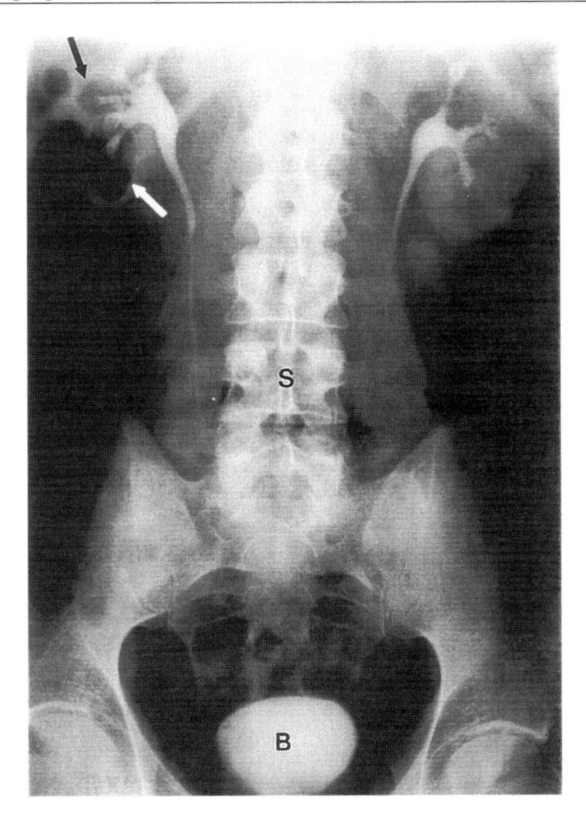

Fig. 4. Normal excretion phase of an intravenous urogram. The kidneys, collecting systems, ureters, and bladder appear normal. Bowel catharsis before the study is to prevent obscuring bowel gas (arrows). S, spine; B, bladder. (From ref. *3*.)

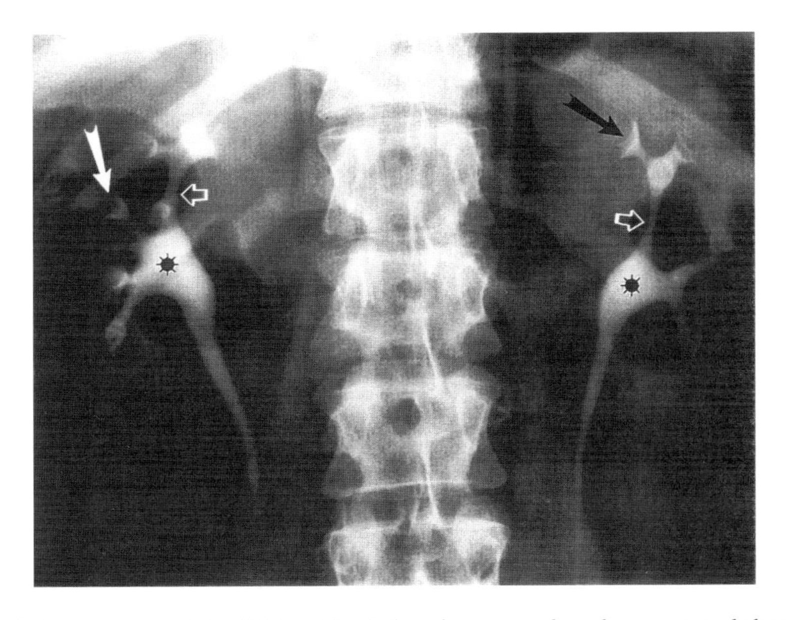

Fig. 5. Coned-down image of the IVU in Fig. 2 showing normal nephrogram and sharply defined calyces (solid arrows), which drain to the renal pelvis (symbols) by way of the infundibula (open arrows). The ureteropelvic junctions and proximal ureters are normal. (From ref. *3*.)

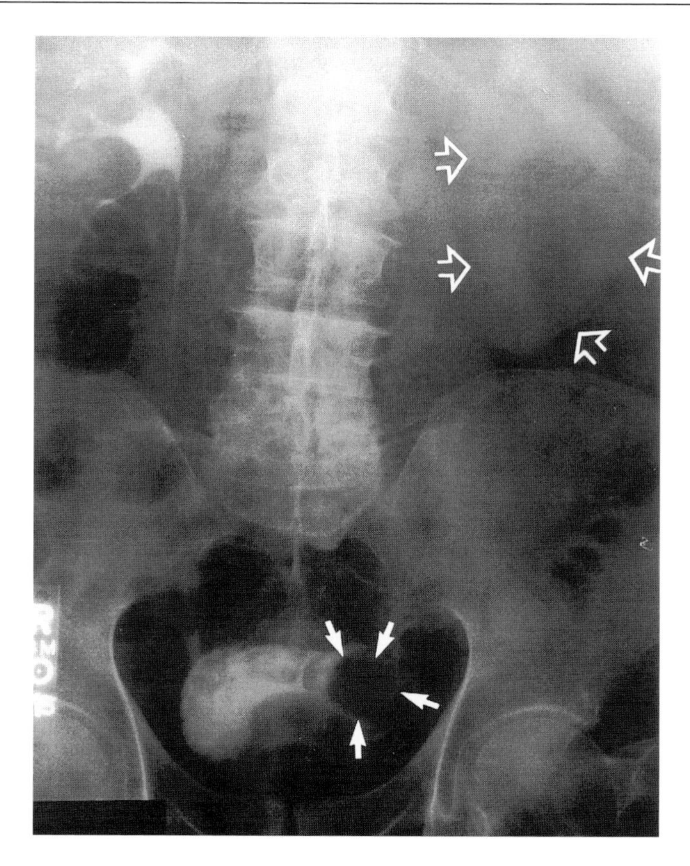

Fig. 6. IVU of a patient showing a large filling defect in the left side of the bladder from an invasive carcinoma (white arrows). The left kidney is not functioning (there is no contrast excretion) because of a distal ureteral obstruction from the bladder tumor (open arrows). The right kidney appears normal. (From ref. *3*.)

The study is usually continued for 45 min or until the right and left collecting systems and ureters are adequately seen. Delayed views are often needed in obstructed systems. A postvoid image is also taken to show bladder residual volume and to allow further drainage of the upper tracts. The postvoid film can sometimes reveal small urothelial lesions of the bladder that were previously obscured when full of contrast containing urine.

Cystography

Cystography permits imaging of an opacified urinary bladder after retrograde instillation of contrast media through a urethral or suprapubic catheter. Imaging is usually performed with fluoroscopy to allow real-time imaging. This study is most often used to demonstrate a suspected urine leak, either from traumatic bladder rupture or after bladder surgery. Cystography can also be used to demonstrate the presence of a fistula between the bladder and the vagina or the bowel and to identify and characterize bladder diverticuli.

Cystography is performed by first obtaining a plain film before instillation of contrast media. As with the IVU, this shows the underlying anatomy of the area to be opacified.

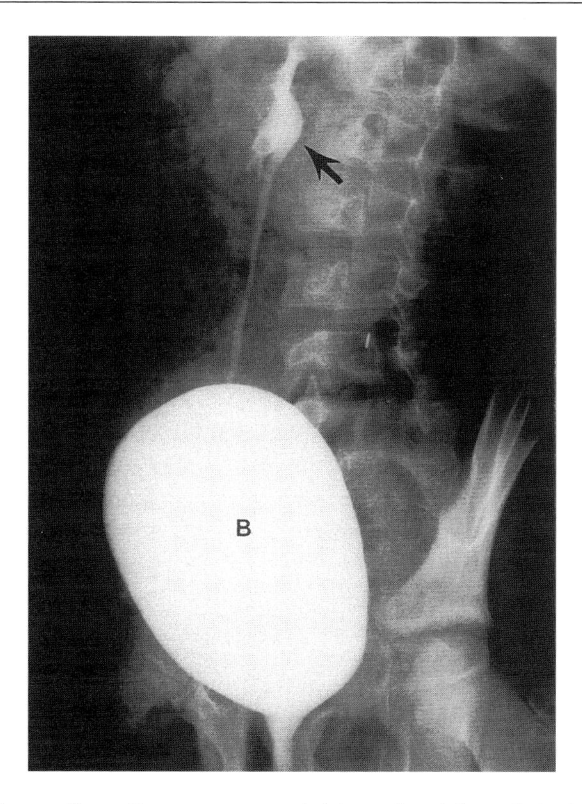

Fig. 7. VCUG showing reflux of contrast material into the right pelvicalyceal system without hydroureteronephrosis (grade II). B, bladder. (From ref. *3*.)

Contrast material is then instilled into the bladder through the urethral or suprapubic catheter until the bladder is distended. Images may be taken in various planes to fully evaluate the bladder. The bladder is drained, and a postdrainage film is taken to evaluate for abnormalities previously obscured by the distended bladder. Bladder rupture can be extra or intraperitoneal. Extraperitoneal extravasation forms an irregular shape, and intraperitoneal extravasation follows the contour of the bowel and other visceral organs. Fistulas can be identified when adjacent, nonurinary organs are opacified with contrast.

Voiding Cystourethrography

Voiding cystourethrography (VCUG) can be used to evaluate for abnormal anatomy and function of the lower urinary tract in both children and adults. This study is started similar to the cystogram with instillation of contrast material into the bladder through a urethral catheter. After full distension of the bladder, the patient is instructed to void either after removing the catheter or around the catheter.

Abnormal findings include vesicoureteral reflux (VUR), ureterocele, posterior urethral valves, or strictures in males and urethral diverticula and bladder or urethral hypermobility in females. VUR (Fig. 7) predisposes the patient to upper-urinary tract infections and subsequent renal damage. There is an international grading system for VUR with a range of I to V. Grade I is the reflux of urine into the ureter without reaching the renal pelvis. Grade II reflux extends to the renal pelvis without abnormal dilation. Grade III reflux has dilation of the renal pelvis and ureter, and grades IV and V reflux describe increasing severity of dilation from blunting of the renal calyces to complete renal distortion and intrarenal reflux.

Retrograde Urethrography

Complete evaluation of the urethra includes both antegrade and retrograde urethrography. The antegrade urethrogram is part of the VCUG as described above. The retrograde urethrogram allows visualization of the anterior male urethra. This is used for evaluating a suspected traumatic urethral injury or urethral stricture. It can also be useful for diagnosis of a urethral diverticulum in females.

The procedure involves placing a catheter in the fossa navicularis and occlusion of the urethral meatus with 1 to 2 mL of water in the catheter balloon. Contrast is gently instilled and images are obtained of the anterior urethra. For female retrograde urethrography, a double balloon catheter (Trattner type) with one balloon at each end of the urethra can be used to fully distend and evaluate the urethra.

ULTRASONOGRAPHY

Sonography uses ultrasound frequencies to image organs of the body. Images are produced by using a transducer that emits ultrasonic waves into the tissues, and then detects those that are reflected back to the transducer. Medical sonography uses frequencies that are between 3.5 and 10 Mhz, which is beyond the range of human hearing, hence the term ultrasound. Lower frequencies have better tissue penetration and are better for imaging deeper structures, whereas more superficial structures are better imaged with higher frequency ultrasound.

Ultrasound transducers are piezoelectric crystals that use the pulse-echo principle, transforming electrical energy into ultrasonic waves and generating an electric energy potential when struck by reflected waves. This energy potential is digitized and displayed on the monitor screen as an image. When the burst of ultrasound waves from the transducer encounter an interface between tissues of different density or stiffness, echoes are produced. This difference in tissues is referred to as acoustic impedence, and if the difference is small, few of the sound waves are reflected to the transducer. When the acoustic impedence is large, many of the pulsed waves are reflected to the transducer. The differing impedence of various tissues relative to surrounding tissues results in the image seen on the monitor screen. Real-time ultrasonography, which is most commonly used, is the continuous, live-image generation that occurs as the transducer is moved from one area to another. This permits dynamic imaging of the function of a single organ or the relationship between adjacent organs or structures.

Doppler sonography detects a moving object, such as blood flow, moving toward or away from the transducer. The Doppler effect is the change in frequency of the sound pulse when it is reflected from a moving object. This can be used to detect the presence and degree of blood from within an artery or a vein. Color Doppler imaging takes the Doppler information from real-time gray scale imaging and converts it to color-coded imaging to facilitate differentiation between flow toward and away from the transducer. Power Doppler ultrasound has increased sensitivity for detecting blood flow in smaller vessels by displaying the integrated power of the Doppler signal. This modality does not, however, show the direction or velocity of flow.

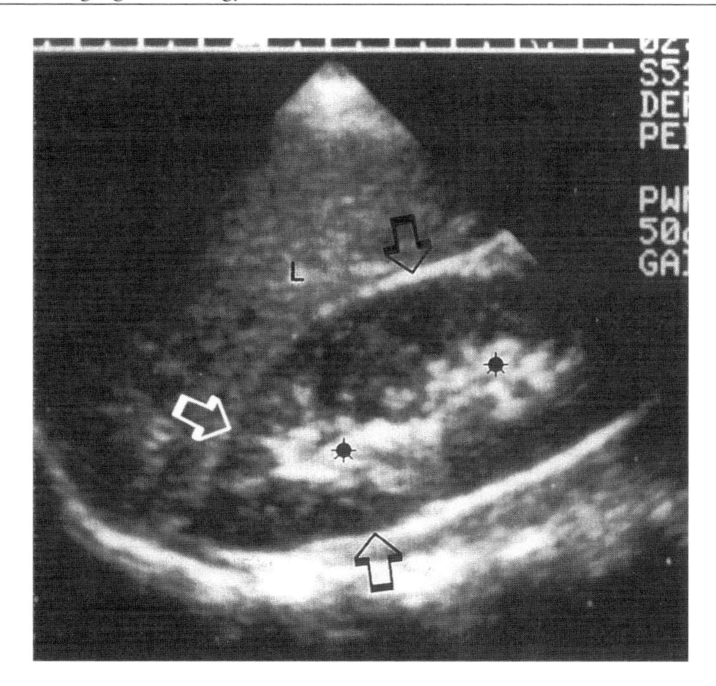

Fig. 8. Sagittal sonogram of a normal right kidney. The renal parenchyma (open arrows) is less echogenic than the adjacent liver (L). The bright central sinus (symbol) is very echogenic because of the presence of fat. (From ref. *3*.)

Ultrasound is widely used for diagnostic purposes in urology. It serves as a portable, non- or minimally invasive technique that does not produce ionizing radiation, and with a skilled operator, can produce accurate, high-quality imaging studies. It is commonly used for imaging the kidneys, ureters, bladder, prostate, testis, and scrotum.

Kidney

Sonography can be used to evaluate the renal parenchyma as well as the pyelocalyceal system. Ultrasound of the parenchyma can show lesions, such as cysts and tumors, and differentiate between the two. It can also be used to evaluate the thickness and echogenicity of the parenchyma. Increased echogenicity of the cortex is often an indicator of medical renal diseases.

The normal appearance of the kidney on ultrasound is a low-echogenic, bean-shaped organ with increased echogenicity of fat within the central renal sinus (Fig. 8). The central echo complex normally has no significant lucent areas, and the presence of a hypoechoic lucency indicates hydronephrosis. The renal cortex is typically slightly less echogenic than the adjacent liver. The normal adult sonographic length of the kidney is typically between 9.5 and 13 cm.

Renal cortical lesions can usually be differentiated with sonography alone or in combination with other imaging modalities. Ultrasound is very effective for differentiating benign cortical cysts from suspicious solid lesions. Cysts appear as anechoic structures with very thin walls and enhanced posterior acoustic transmission. Cystic masses may be hypoechoic or anechoic, with thickened walls, septa, and decreased or absent poste-

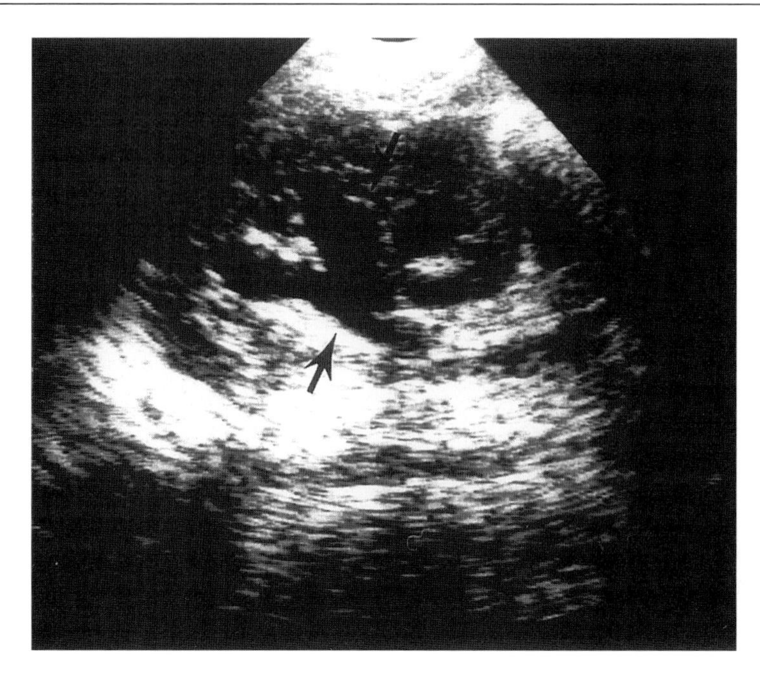

Fig. 9. Longitudinal sonogram of a right kidney with hydronephrosis. There is dilation of the renal calyces and separation of the central sinus by nonechogenic urine (arrow). (From ref. *3*.)

rior acoustic transmission. Solid renal masses are variably echogenic, may have calcifications, and have decreased through transmission. Calcifications are hyperechoic and produce acoustic shadows that block through transmission.

Although sonography has very high sensitivity for detection of renal masses, staging of parenchymal and urothelial tumors is not as sensitive as computed tomography or magnetic resonance imaging in regard to detection of lymphadenopathy, capsular invasion, and invasion of adjacent structures. Ultrasound is useful for detecting tumor thrombus extension into the inferior vena cava.

Hydronephrosis is seen on sonography as an anechoic space within the bright echoes of the central renal sinus (Fig. 9). This anechoic space will include the ureter with hydroureteronephrosis. When infected urine with debris or hematuria with clots is present in the hydronephrotic renal pelvis, the sonographic appearance will be more hypoechoic than anechoic, and the debris can give variable echogenic shadows. Calculi, like parenchymal calcifications are hyperechoic and block through transmission, creating acoustic shadows.

Ureter

The normal, nondilated ureter cannot be adequately evaluated by sonography. The ureteropelvic and ureterovesical junction can be visualized when abnormalities result in dilation of the structure. Calculi and ureteroceles, when present, can be seen with ultrasound. Calculi in the distal ureter, like those in the renal pelvis and calyces are hyperechoic with posterior shadowing. A ureterocele appears as a round, anechoic, intravesical structure, adjacent to a dilated distal ureter. The ureterocele may contain a calculus that would appear as described above.

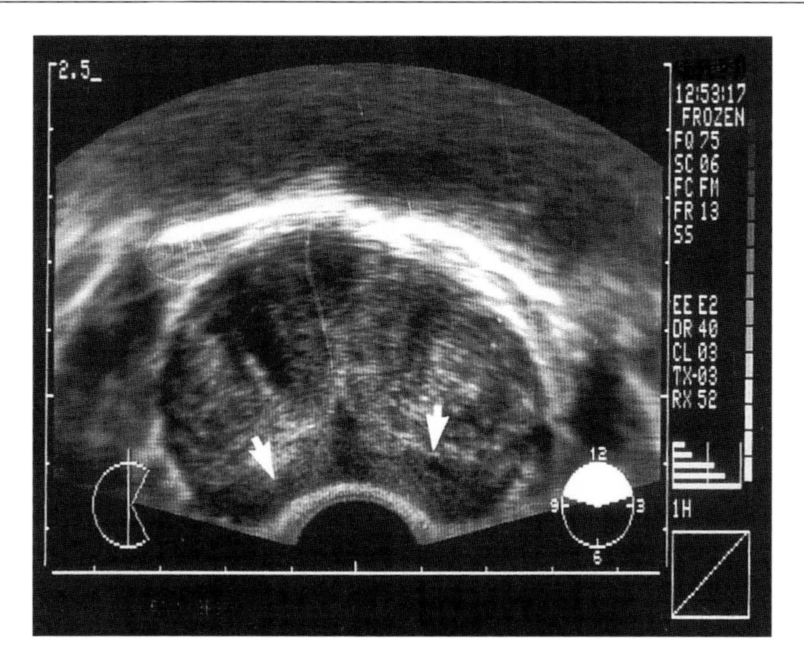

Fig. 10. Transverse view of a transrectal sonogram of the prostate gland showing benign prostatic hyperplasia. The white arrows show the border between the more hypoechoic anterior transition zone and the surrounding peripheral zone. (From ref. *3*.)

Bladder

Transabdominal bladder sonography is commonly performed and can be used to assess bladder volume or postvoid residual volume, bladder wall thickness, and the presence of intraluminal disorders such as tumors or calculi. Transurethral bladder ultrasound can be used at the time of cystoscopy for staging bladder neoplasms, however this practice is not commonly used.

Prostate

Sonography of the prostate gland is commonly used for guidance during transrectal or transperineal core needle biopsy of the prostate. The prostate gland is examined sonographically with an endolumenal probe at a frequency of 5 to 7 Mhz using a transrectal approach. The normal gland is a symmetric, triangular, or ellipsoid organ surrounded by periprostatic fat that has a bright echogenic appearance. It normally has a sonographically measured volume of 10 to 25 cm^3. Benign prostatic hyperplasia on ultrasound has a mixed heterogeneous transition zone that is usually somewhat hypoechoic compared with the homogeneous surrounding peripheral zone (Fig. 10). Prostate cancer usually appears as a hypoechoic lesion in the peripheral gland (Fig. 11). Advanced lesions can produce an irregular asymmetrical appearance of the prostatic capsule with possible invasion into surrounding structures.

Testis and Scrotum

Sonography is an important modality for imaging testicular and scrotal disorders. Because of the superficial position of these structures, high-frequency 5- to 10-Mhz

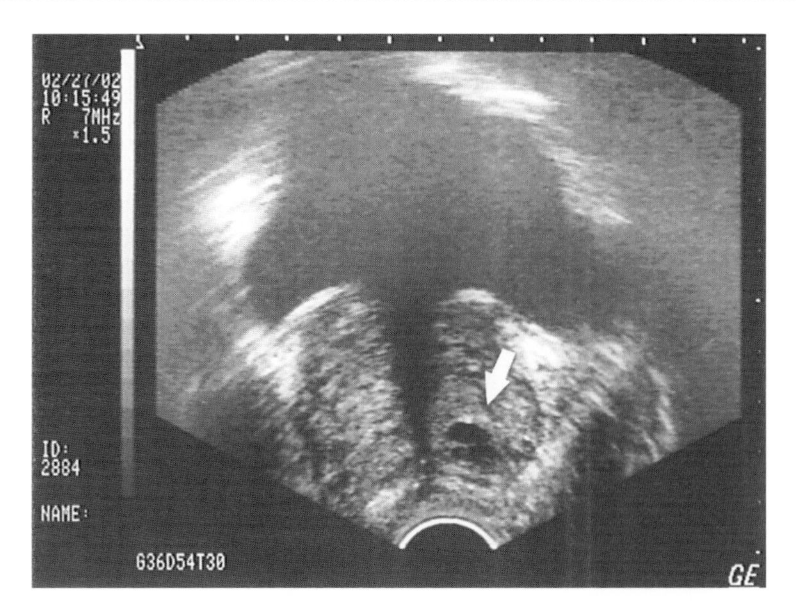

Fig. 11. Transverse view of transrectal sonogram of the prostate showing hypoechoic lesions in the left peripheral zone with distortion of the capsule (white arrow), suspicious for carcinoma. (Picture courtesy of Dr. Elizabeth Anoia.)

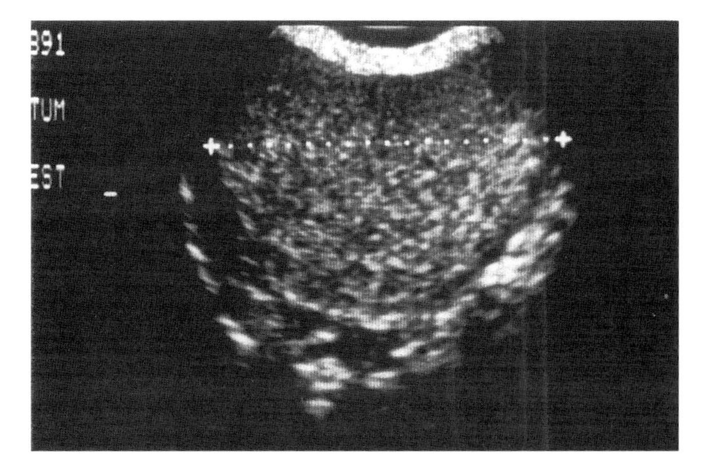

Fig. 12. Sonogram of a normal testis (From ref. *3*.)

transducers are used. The sonogram of a normal testis shows homogeneous echogenicity and a smooth contour (Fig. 12). There should be no distinct hypo- or hyperechoic areas within the tunica albuginea. The epididymis is observed as a separate structure and has similar echogenicity as the testis.

Color Doppler sonography can characterize blood flow to the testes and can be used to identify the etiology of acute scrotal pain. Ischemic pain, as would present with testicular torsion, can be separated from hyperemic pain, associated with inflammation or infection. Traumatic injury to the scrotum can be assessed sonographically. Findings can include hematoma, hydrocele, hematocele, and testicular fracture.

Sonographic findings can triage the testicular symptoms as a surgical emergency or as best managed with medical treatment. Ultrasound can also be used as the initial study to evaluate a male with a nonpalpable testis and can identify cryptorchid testes distal to the internal inguinal ring. Intraabdominal testes are better identified on CT or MRI.

Testicular sonography is very accurate for the differentiation of intratesticular vs extratesticular disease when a scrotal mass is palpated. Extratesticular masses are usually benign processes, such as cysts of the epididymis or dilation of the rete testis. Varicoceles, which are dilation of the pampiniform venous plexus, can be seen with ultrasound, and although moderate-sized and large varicoceles are palpable, sonography can be useful in identifying a subclinical, nonpalpable varicocele.

Testicular malignancies usually appear as hypoechoic intratesticular masses that frequently have a heterogeneous appearance and may invade the tunica albuginea and scrotal wall. The sonographic appearance of an testicular neoplasm can sometimes predict the histology of the tumor but is generally nonspecific, and there is a fairly significant overlap in appearance depending on the stage of the tumor.

COMPUTED TOMOGRAPHY

CT scanning produces high-definition images of a patient's anatomy by passing a thin collimated beam of x-rays through the patient from multiple sources, which are then absorbed by a linear array of detectors. These x-ray images are assembled by a computer, generating cross-sectional views of the patient on a monitor. The images can then be stored digitally or printed on radiographic film for review and storage. Spiral CT rotates continuously using sliding contacts or brushes while the table moves at a constant speed through the x-ray beam. This allows rapid acquisition of image data during a single breath-hold by the patient, limiting overlapping images and motion artifact.

Hounsfield units (HU) are numerical representations of the relative density of imaged tissues. They are based on water density, which is assigned the number zero, with a range of –1000 to +1000. Structures with greater density than water have positive HU numbers and those less dense than water have negative HU numbers. Unenhanced tissue density is approx +30 HU or greater, and fatty tissues are –50 or less.

Patients are usually supine for CT imaging. Scans can be with or without contrast. Oral contrast is given to outline the gastrointestinal tract and to differentiate loops of bowel from adjacent normal and abnormal structures. Intravenous contrast media is similar to that used for IVU and the same patient screening must be instituted before usage. Patients must have normal renal function and no previous history of hypersensitivity to contrast material. In high-risk patients, nonionic contrast media should be considered to minimize the risk of adverse reactions. CT scans with intravenous contrast material are used to evaluate perfusion and function of normal organs and abnormal masses. Scans without intravenous contrast are used to identify radiodense lesions, such as calculi, that may be obscured by intravenous contrast that is excreted into the renal collecting system. Comprehensive imaging without and with intravenous contrast is frequently used to differentiate active bleeding from urinary extravasation, and to assess for contrast enhancement of suspected malignant lesions.

Kidney

CT can be used for evaluation of many types of renal disorders (Fig. 13). A complete renal evaluation with CT involves imaging in three phases, noncontrast imaging, imme-

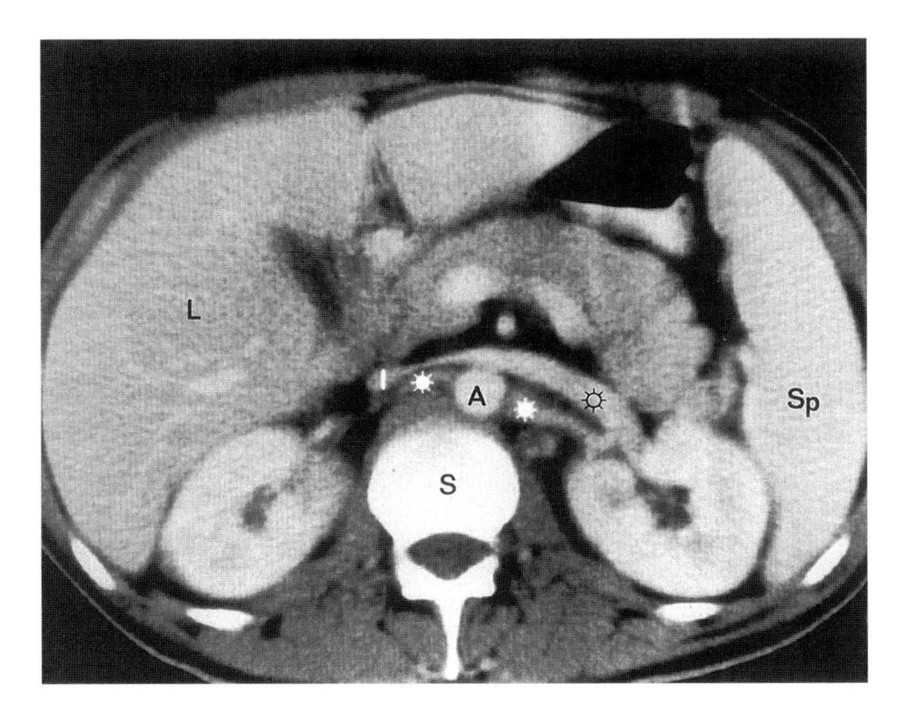

Fig. 13. Axial CT scan of normal kidneys. Right and left renal arteries are identified (solid symbols) as is the left renal vein (open symbol). Other adjacent structures identified include the aorta (A), inferior vena cava (I), liver (L), spleen (Sp), and spine (S). (From ref. *3*.)

diate post-contrast bolus imaging, and delayed postcontrast bolus imaging, to evaluate the excretion phase of the urinary tract. As already mentioned, plain, nonenhanced CT imaging alone is very sensitive for renal and ureteral calculi in a patient with renal colic. This study can be performed in minutes compared with nearly an hour for an IVU. Nonenhanced CT scans are also useful for evaluating acute hemorrhage around the kidney or in the retroperitoneum. Acute bleeding produces a hyperdense collection, whereas old blood, urine, and ascites are relatively hypodense.

Contrast media, as with IVU is taken up by the kidneys, enhancing the parenchyma, and is excreted into the collecting system, opacifying the hollow structures of the urinary tract. Renal parenchymal masses can be differentiated by comparing non-contrast with contrast CT images. Cysts, unless complicated by hemorrhage or infection, do not enhance with intravenous contrast (Fig. 14) Solid renal masses that enhance with contrast are considered to represent renal cell carcinoma until proven otherwise (Fig. 15). CT scan can also be effectively used to stage renal malignancies (Figs. 16 and 17). It can provide information regarding the relationship between the renal mass and adjacent structures, and the presence or absence of lymphadenopathy. CT can also be used for postoperative surveillance for tumor recurrence after partial nephrectomy.

Renal cysts are graded for their malignant potential based on a classification system proposed by Bosniak. Category I cysts are simple cysts that are universally considered benign. These are usually round and smooth in a well-defined plane from the normal renal parenchyma. Category II lesions are also considered benign but are more complex from previous hemorrhage or infection. These cysts may have one or two delicate,

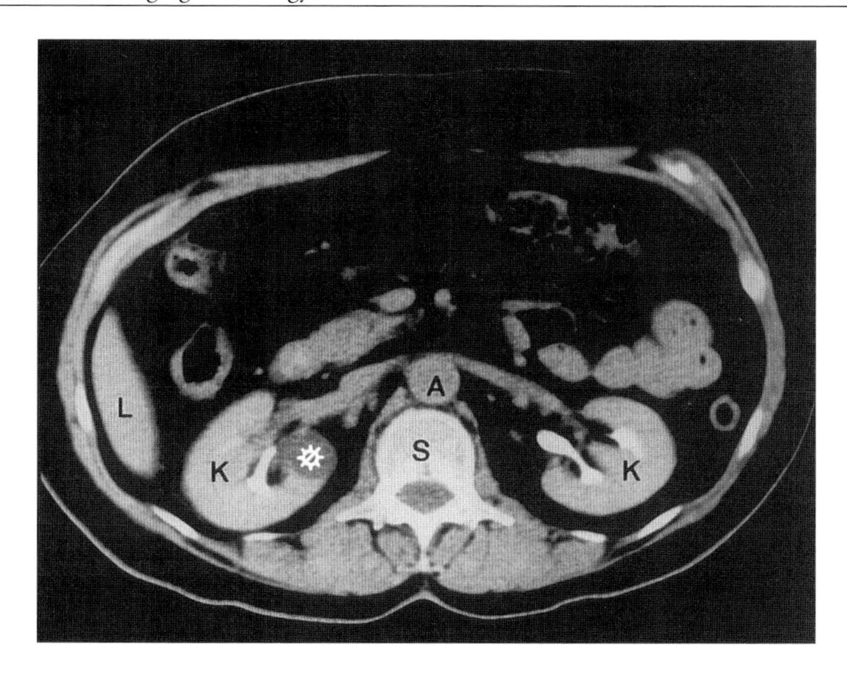

Fig. 14. Contrast-enhanced axial CT of the mid-abdomen demonstrates a simple cyst in the right kidney (symbol). This lesion has a smooth border and did not enhance with contrast compared to noncontrasted images of the same lesion. A, aorta; K, kidney; L, liver; and S, spine. (From ref. *3*.)

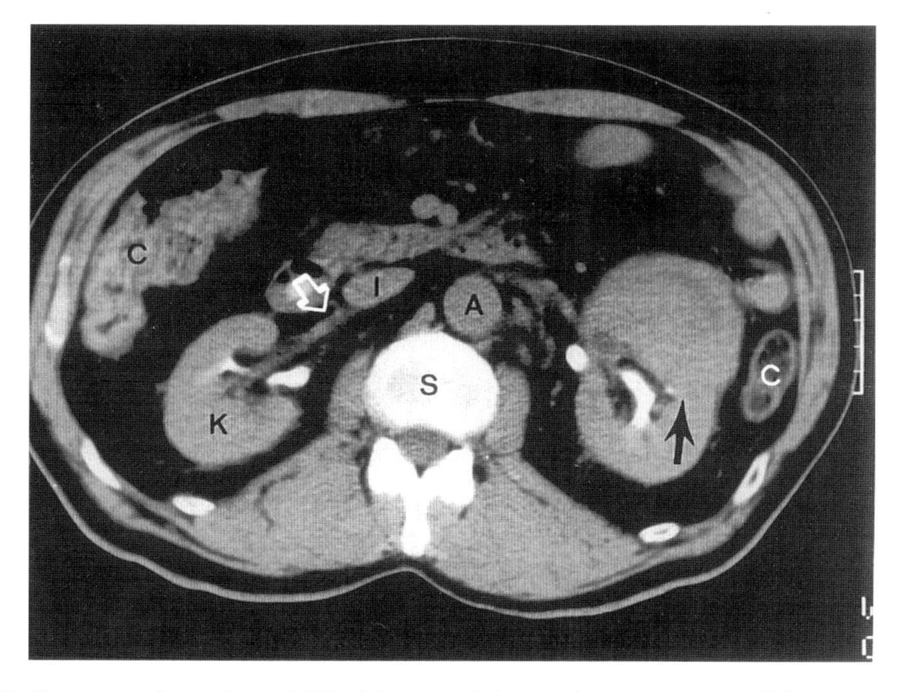

Fig. 15. Contrast-enhanced axial CT of the mid-abdomen demonstrates a solid enhancing anterior mass of the left kidney (solid arrow) consistent with renal cell carcinoma. Contrast is seen in the renal pelvis and proximal ureter. Other structures include the aorta (A), inferior vena cava (I), right kidney (K), right renal vein (open arrow), and colon (C). (From ref. *3*.)

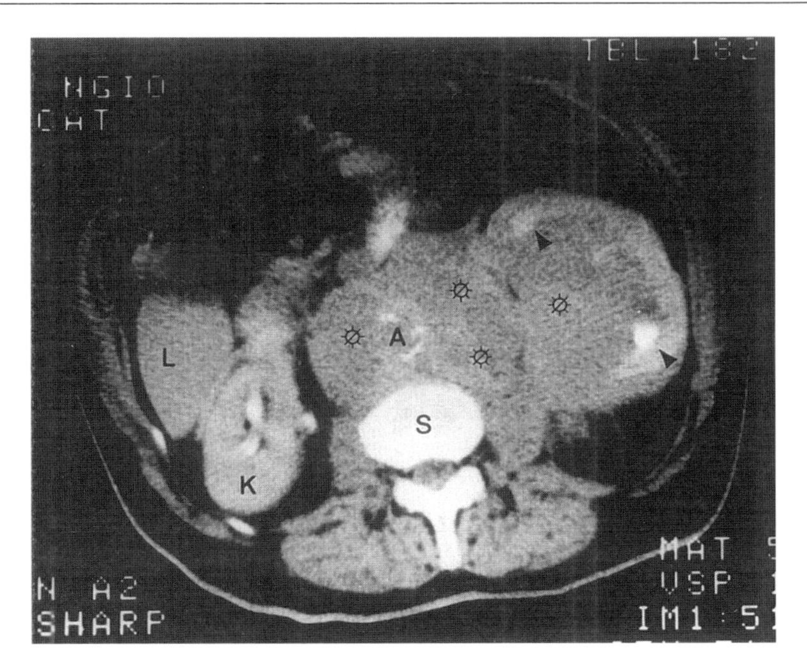

Fig. 16. Contrast-enhanced axial CT of the mid-abdomen demonstrates a large heterogeneous left renal cell carcinoma (symbols) with local extension to the retroperitoneum, surrounding the aorta (A) anterior to the spine (S). The left kidney demonstrates function with contrast excretion into the collecting system (arrowheads). The right kidney (K) and adjacent portion of the liver (L) are normal. (From ref. *3*.)

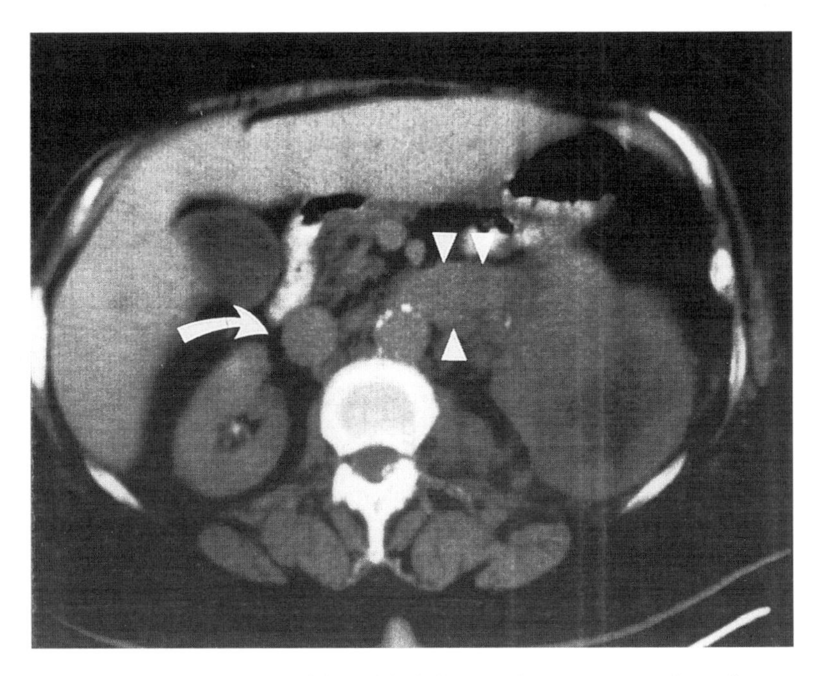

Fig. 17. Contrast-enhanced axial CT of the mid-abdomen demonstrates a large heterogeneous left renal cell carcinoma with tumor thrombus in the left renal vein (white arrowheads) and in the inferior vena cava (white arrow). The vena cava is normally flat (*see* Fig. 13) and a round, full appearance indicates thrombus. (From ref. *3*.)

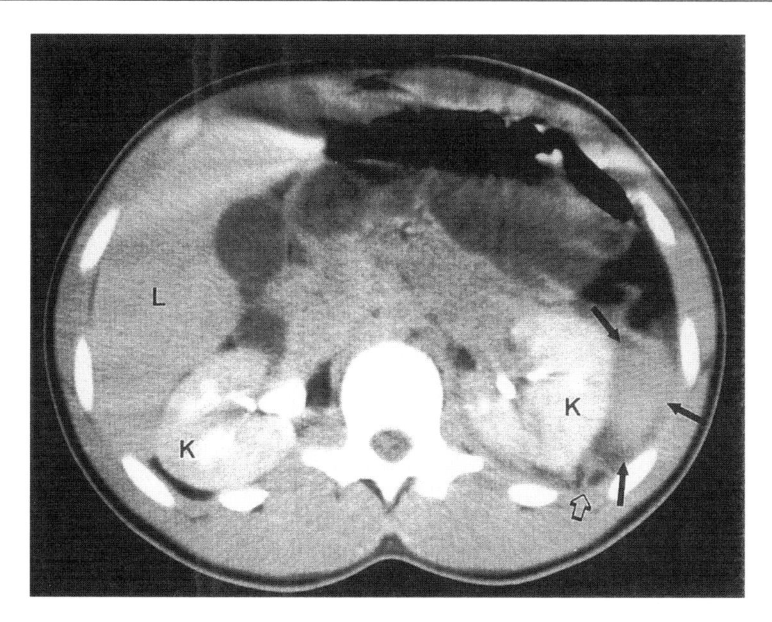

Fig. 18. Contrast-enhanced axial CT of the mid-abdomen identifies left renal contusion (K) from blunt abdominal trauma. Demonstrated is a perirenal hematoma (black arrows) that contains old (darker) blood and evidence of active bleeding (lighter blush in middle of hematoma). There is also some edema of the left perirenal fat (open arrow). L, liver. (From ref. *3*.)

nonenhancing internal septa, linear delicate calcifications in the wall or septa, or may be hyperdense because of blood, protein, or colloid content. Category IIF was created for category II cysts presenting with any degree of certainty of malignant potential. These lesions should be followed with interval CT scans to ensure that the lesion is stable. Category III lesions are cystic masses. These lesions may have thick, irregular calcification in the wall or septa, irregular borders, wall thickening, or small, nonenhancing nodules. These lesions may be malignant because they have the same radiographic appearance as cystic renal cell carcinoma and must be excised for treatment and pathological evaluation. Category IV lesions are malignant lesions. Their cystic appearance results from necrosis or liquefaction of a solid tumor. These lesions have irregular, thickened walls and may have enhancing nodules. Surgical excision is indicated for category IV lesions.

Upper urinary-tract infections can also be evaluated by CT. Acute pyelonephritis appears as one or multiple patchy wedge-shaped perfusion defects that can appear similar to segmental infarction. Relevant clinical history can be helpful in differentiating these disease processes when interpreting the CT. With pyelonephritis, there is also a stranding appearance of the perinephric fat from edema. Renal abscesses appear as hypodense lesions in the parenchyma surrounded by a hyperdense wall, the pseudocapsule. Emphysematous pyelonephritis is very evident with CT scanning and has the appearance of gas or air pockets within the renal parenchyma.

CT is the primary imaging modality for evaluating renal trauma (Fig. 18) Contusions, lacerations, and fractures of the renal parenchyma and injuries to the collecting system are readily visualized. Acute bleeding is best evaluated with noncontrast CT, while extravasation of urine from the collecting system can be seen during the excretion phase of a contrasted study.

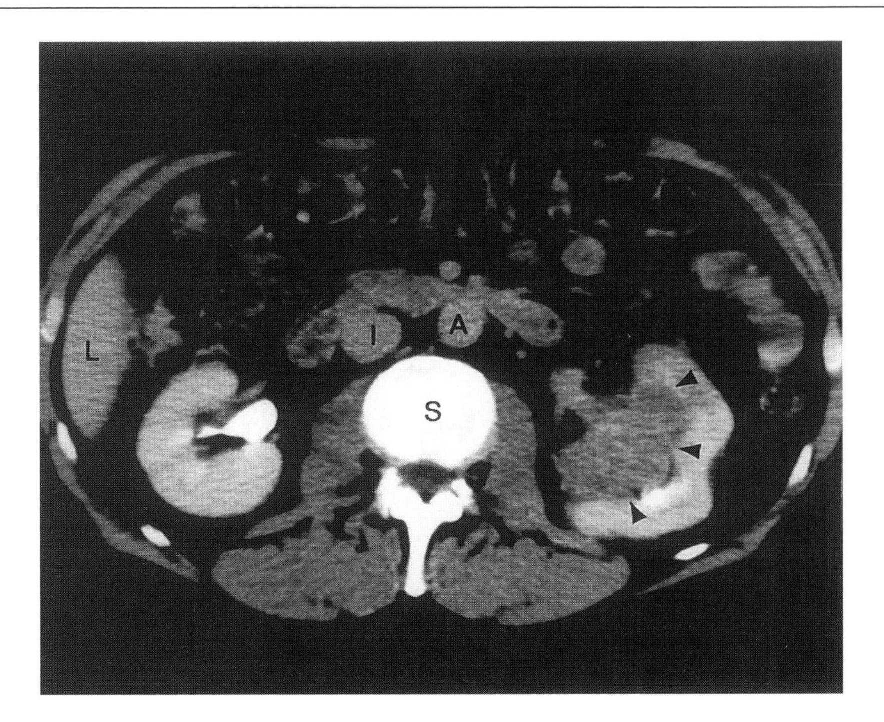

Fig. 19. Contrast-enhanced axial CT of the mid-abdomen demonstrates a large mass in the collecting system of the left kidney (arrowheads). This lesion is a transitional cell carcinoma of the renal pelvis urothelium. S, spine; L, liver; I, inferior vena cava; A aorta. (From ref. *3*.)

Renal Pelvis, Ureters, and Bladder

Urothelial tumors appear as filling defects seen during the excretion phase of a contrast-enhanced CT scan (Figs. 19 and 20). Bladder tumors may appear as thickened areas of the bladder wall or as filling defects within the contrast filled bladder on delayed images (Figs. 21 and 22). CT is primarily used for staging of urothelial tumors. Lymphadenopathy from advanced bladder and prostate cancers can be detected with a CT scan of the pelvis (Fig. 23). CT cystogram can be performed with retrograde injection of contrast through a urethral catheter and is very sensitive for diagnosing bladder tumors and bladder rupture from trauma.

Adrenal

The adrenal glands are readily imaged with CT for benign and malignant disorders. (Fig. 24) Adrenal cysts appear as large, hypodense, lobulated masses that can have calcification of the walls. Acute adrenal hemorrhage, like other etiologies of active bleeding, appears as hyperdense collections. Adrenal adenomas are small, well-defined, homogeneous masses, whereas adrenal carcinomas appear as large, heterogeneous masses with calcifications and central necrosis. Pheochromocytoma on CT appears as large hypodense mass with central necrosis and occasional small calcifications. These lesions enhance significantly with intravenous contrast. Differentiation of adrenal cortical carcinoma from pheochromocytoma is based on biochemical and clinical studies, as they appear similar on CT.

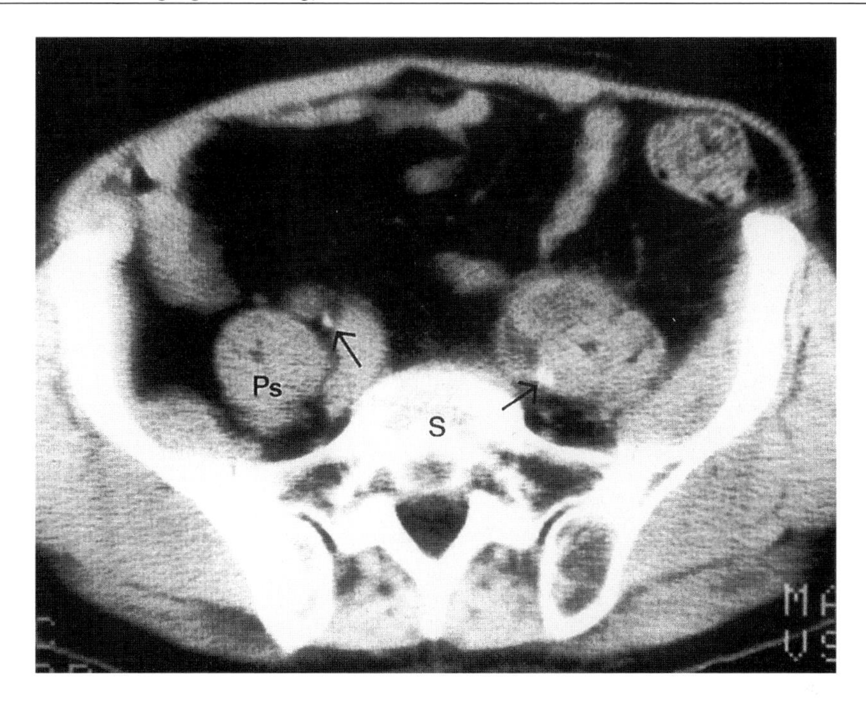

Fig. 20. Contrast-enhanced axial CT of the pelvis demonstrates a mass in the left ureter with local extension into the psoas muscle. This is a transitional cell carcinoma of the urothelium in the ureter. Contrast can be seen in both ureters (arrows), as this lesion is not causing left ureteral obstruction. S, spine, Ps, psoas muscle. (From ref. *3*.)

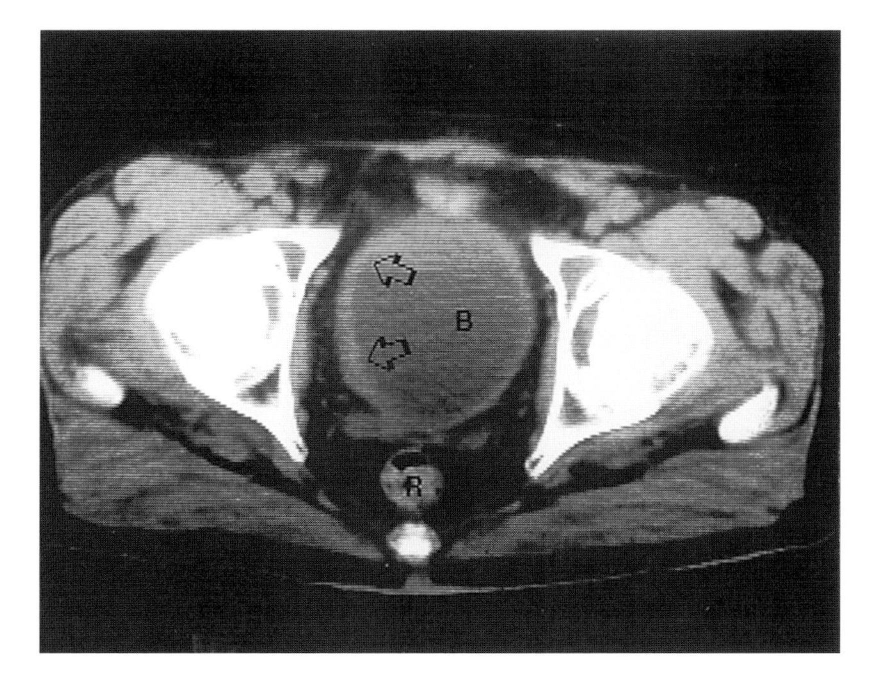

Fig. 21. Axial CT of the pelvis demonstrates diffuse bladder wall thickening, worse on the right (open arrows). Asymmetric bladder wall thickening usually indicates a tumor but could be the consequence of longstanding bladder outlet obstruction with detrusor hypertrophy. R, rectum; B, bladder. (From ref. *3*.)

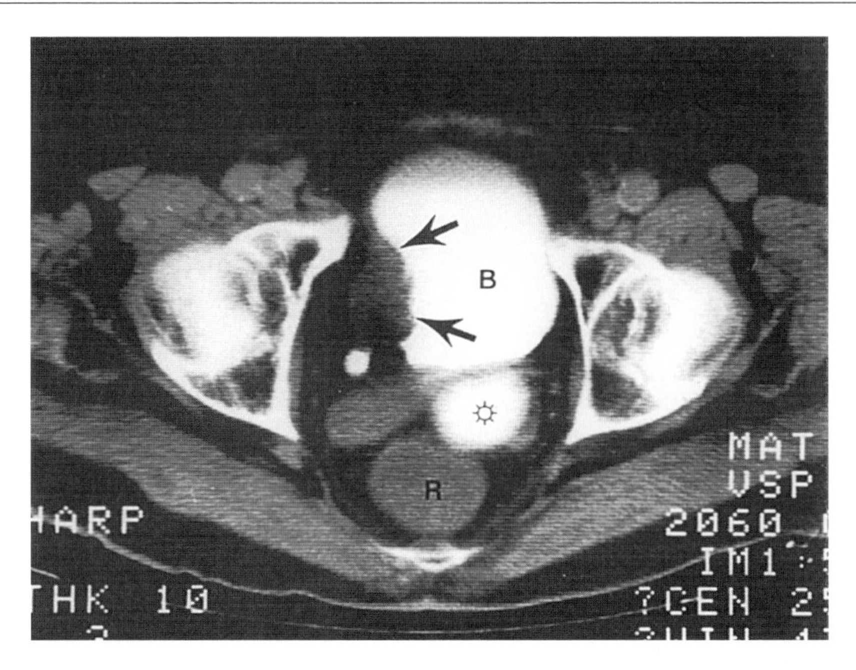

Fig. 22. Contrast-enhanced axial CT of the pelvis demonstrates a contrast-filled bladder with a large filling defect along the right bladder wall. This soft tissue density lesion is a sessile bladder tumor (arrows). This patient also has a posterior bladder diverticulum (symbol), just anterior to the rectum (R). B, bladder. (From ref. *3*.)

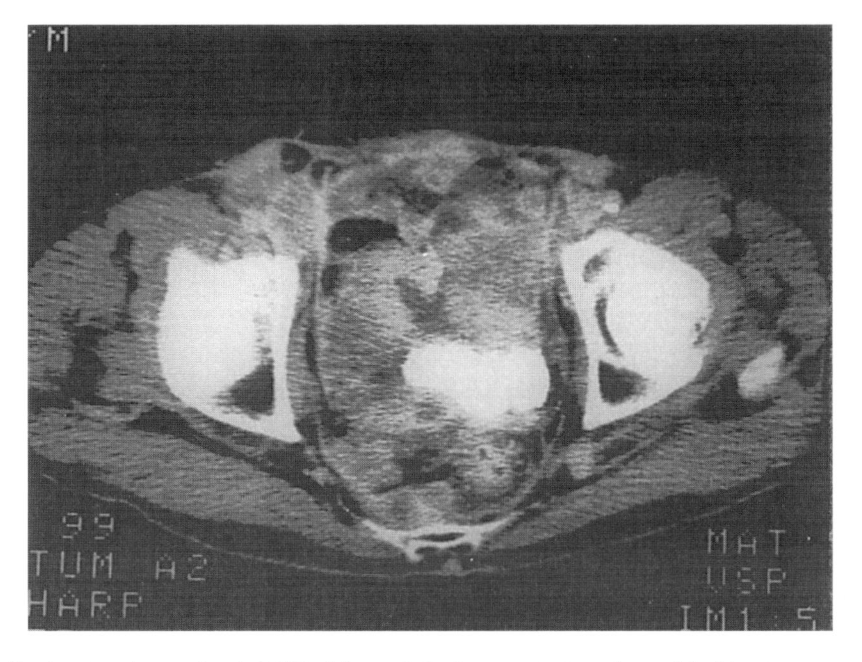

Fig. 23. Contrast-enhanced axial CT of the pelvis demonstrates a large bladder tumor anterior to the contrast filled bladder lumen. Bilateral pelvic lymphadenopathy is present indicating spread of the carcinoma. Similar pelvic lymphadenopathy can be seen with advanced carcinoma of the prostate. (From ref. *3*.)

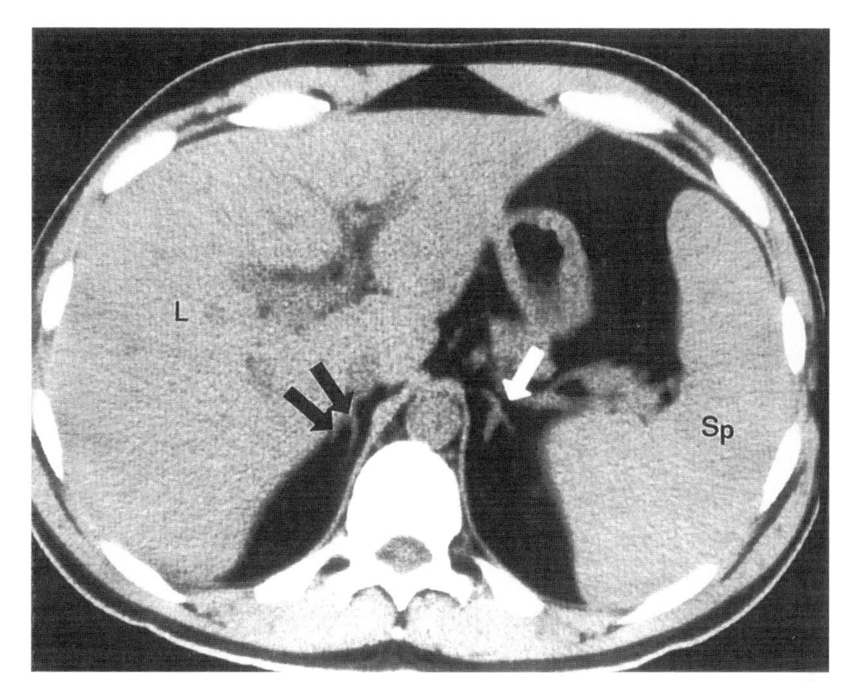

Fig. 24. Axial CT scan of the upper abdomen shows normal right and left adrenal glands (arrows). L, liver; Sp, spleen. (From ref. *3*.)

Retroperitoneum

CT is routinely used for staging of urological malignancies and other retroperitoneal tumors. Pelvic and para-aortic lymphadenopathy from bladder, prostate, testicular, and renal carcinomas can be readily assessed (Fig. 25) This evaluation is best performed with intravenous contrast injection. Lymph nodes greater than 1 cm in the pelvis and 1.5 cm in the para-aortic region are considered significant.

Retroperitoneal fibrosis, often an idiopathic process that can lead to vascular and ureteral obstruction has a distinct appearance on CT. It has a symmetric distribution, and results in medial deviation of the ureters with loss of distinct tissue planes between the great vessel and surrounding structures.

MAGNETIC RESONANCE IMAGING

MRI uses the behavior of atomic nuclei with odd numbers of nucleons when exposed to a magnetic field. The most abundant atom with an odd number of nucleons within the human body is hydrogen, and normally the spin axes of the hydrogen nuclei are randomly oriented. However, when nonionizing radiofrequency pulses of energy are used to induce a brief excitement of the protons of the hydrogen atoms, they invert their orientation to a higher energy state. After the pulse terminates, the hydrogen nucleus returns to its original state, called relaxation. Relaxation times are then measured in longitudinal (T1) and transverse (T2) planes. Images are generated based on the amount and orientation of hydrogen in different tissues. Different tissues have inherent T1 and T2 relaxation time constants, and the image can be manipulated by changing the excitation and relaxation time. MRI produces better soft-tissue differentiation than

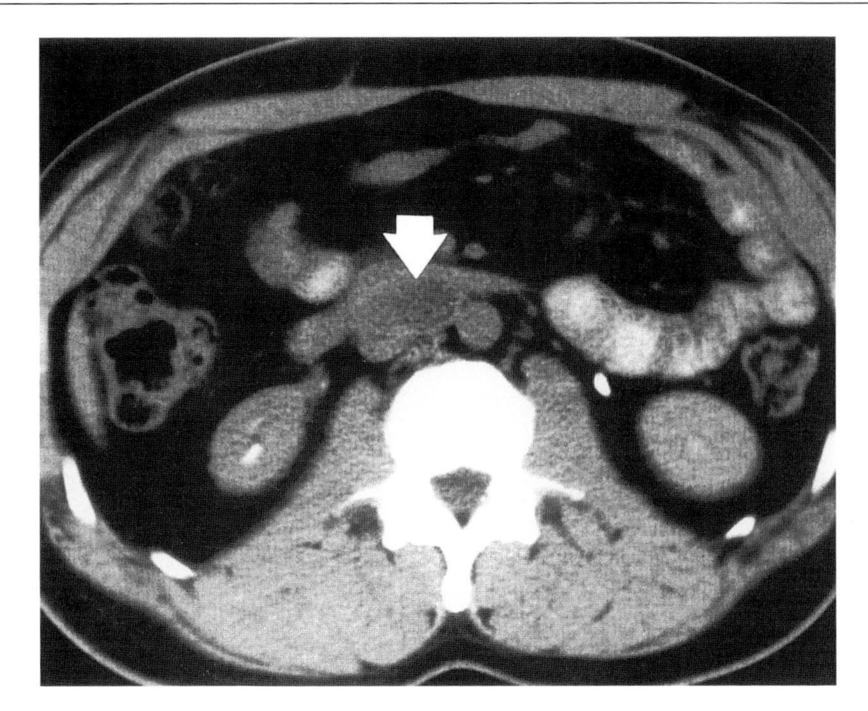

Fig. 25. Contrast-enhanced axial CT of the mid-abdomen demonstrates retroperitoneal lymphadenopathy (white arrow) from metastatic testicular carcinoma. (From ref. *3*.)

CT and generates image reconstructions in multiple perspectives, such as cross-sectional, sagittal, coronal, and oblique, as well as three-dimensional orientations. MRI is performed in large, uniform magnetic field, and classically this required a narrow, enclosed imaging tube. Newer machines are available with open configurations that allow patients who could not tolerate classic scanners to be imaged. The open machines also permit imaging a patient who is not supine to allow imaging in normal physiological positions.

Intravenous contrast in MRI uses compounds with paramagnetic properties that cause deflection in the magnetic field, changing the T1 and T2 relaxation constants of certain tissues. Gadolinium-diethylenetriaminepentaacetic acid (DTPA) is the most commonly used contrast agent with MRI. The enhancing effects of gadolinium on MRI tissue signal intensity depends on its concentration. Gadolinium is not nephrotoxic and it can be used for MRI in patients with pre-existing renal insufficiency.

Contraindications to MRI include pacemakers, ferromagnetic intracranial aneurysm clips, cochlear implants, and metallic pieces in vital locations of the body. Titanium is not ferromagnetic and therefore is not affected by MRI. Patient claustrophobia can prevent adequate imaging from a standard MRI. These patients can be imaged in an open MRI, or if standard MRI is needed, they may need to be sedated.

Kidney

With MRI of the normal kidney, the medulla is lighter than the cortex on T1-weighted imaging (Fig. 26), and the same density as the medulla on T2-weighted imaging. Fat is bright on both T1- and T2-weighted images unless fat suppression is used. Urine and

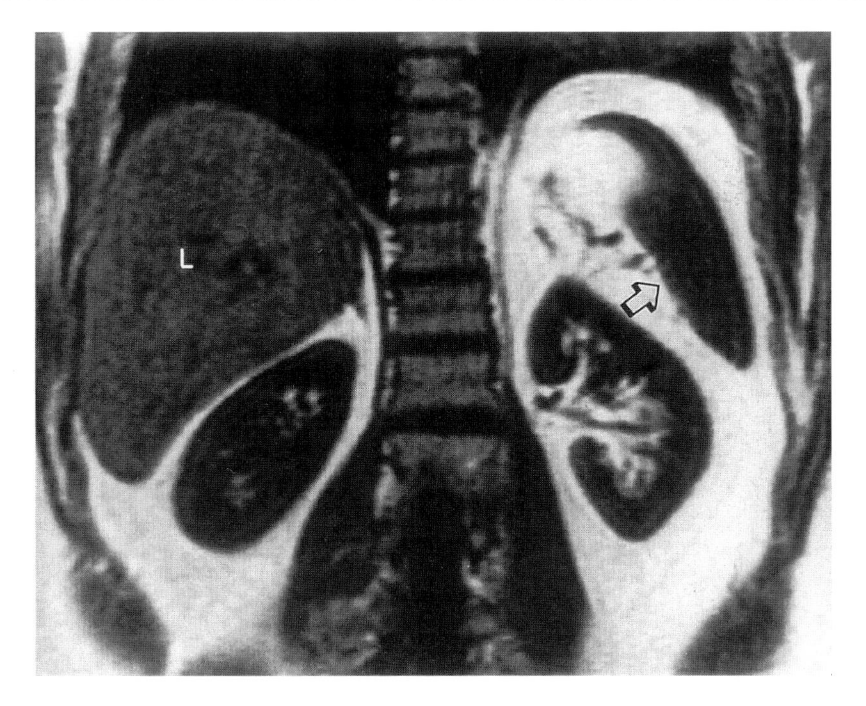

Fig. 26. Coronal T1-weighted MRI showing normal right and left kidneys. Retroperitoneal fat appears bright. The liver (L) and spleen (open arrow) are also seen. (From ref. *3*.)

most renal cysts and tumors are dark on T1- and light on T2-weighted images. For this reason, differentiation between cysts and solid tumors may be difficult. MRI imaging of the kidneys is most useful to demonstrate contrast enhancement of suspicious renal lesions in a patient who cannot receive iodinated contrast media for CT scanning. MRI is also useful for staging of renal tumors as anatomic differentiation between the kidneys and surrounding organs is superior to that seen with CT. MRI can reveal local invasion of tumor into perinephric fat, as well as the presence or absence of tumor thrombus in the renal vein and inferior vena cava. MRI can also be used to perform magnetic resonance angiography to evaluate the renal arteries for stenoses, aneurysms, thrombosis, and arteriovenous fistulas.

Ureters and Retroperitoneum

MRI is no better than CT for imaging the ureters and retroperitoneum for normal and abnormal anatomy. An exception to this is the evaluation for lymphadenopathy in a metastatic workup of renal, bladder, prostate, and testicular cancer or when lymphoma or metastatic cancer from other sites impinges on the urinary tract. MRI is not limited by the presence of artifacts, such as metallic clips or prostheses, and does not require the injection of intravenous contrast to distinguish lymph nodes from adjacent vessels. Like CT, MRI cannot distinguish benign from malignant lymphadenopathy.

Bladder and Prostate

Although MRI can be used to detect and evaluate carcinomas of the bladder and prostate (Figs. 27 and 28), it is infrequently used because ultrasonography with biopsy

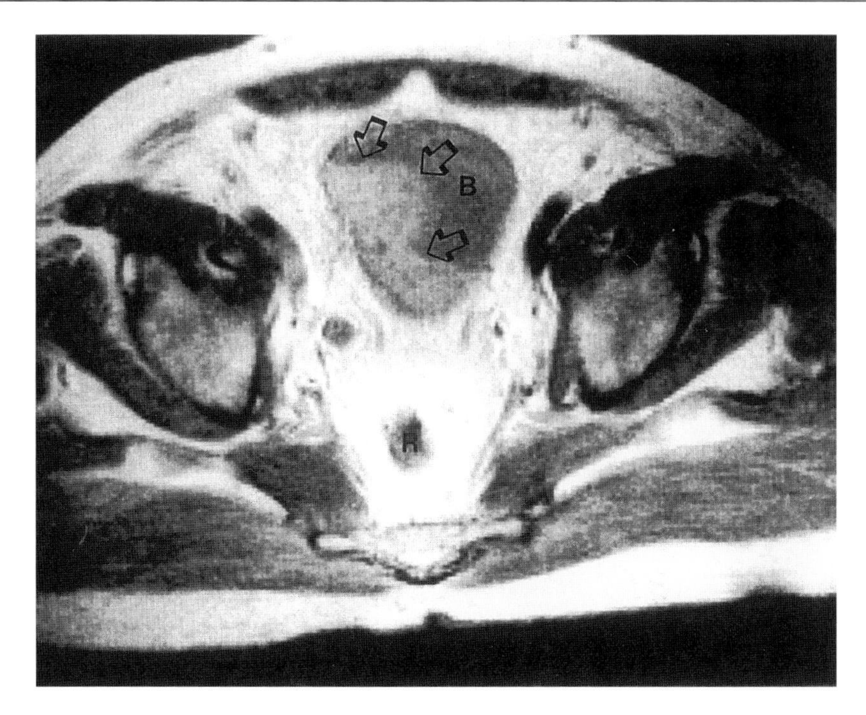

Fig. 27. Axial MRI through the pelvis demonstrates an irregular mass originating from the right-posterior bladder wall (open arrows) and extending into the bladder (B). R, rectum. (From ref. *3*.)

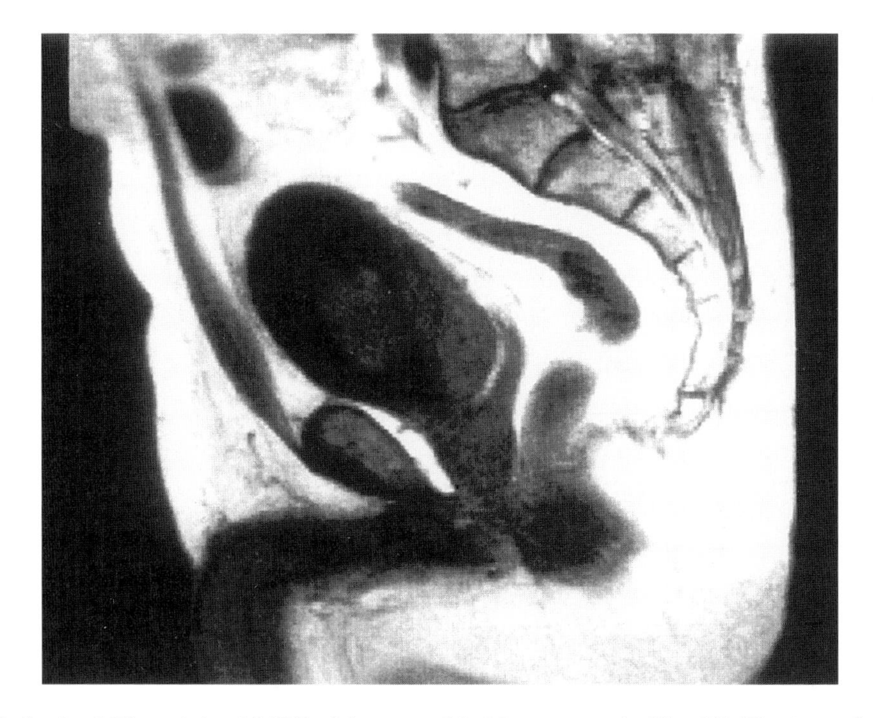

Fig. 28. Sagittal T1-weighted MRI of the same bladder as seen in Fig. 27. The irregular tumor can be seen originating from the posterior wall, extending into the bladder. (From ref. *3*.)

of the prostate and cystoscopy with biopsy of the bladder both give more accurate information about the grade and local stage of tumors, and MRI adds little additional information about the local disease. However, as previously mentioned, MRI is useful in the evaluation of metastatic lymphadenopathy, especially in patients who cannot receive iodinated contrast media with CT scanning.

Adrenal

Evaluation of the adrenal glands with MRI has become more common as this imaging modality is very accurate in differentiating benign adenomas from metastases. Opposed-phase chemical shift MR imaging takes advantage of the different resonance frequency peaks for the hydrogen atom in water and lipid molecules. Tissues containing lipids and water have a decreased signal intensity compared with tissues without lipids. This technique accurately differentiates lipid containing benign adenomas from metastases that are devoid of lipid. Adrenocortical carcinomas often have focal collections of macroscopic lipid, which can result in focal regions of signal intensity loss on opposed-phase chemical shift MRI. In contrast to adrenocortical lesions, pheochromocytomas typically are high-intensity adrenal masses on T2-weighted MRI.

Female Pelvis

MRI is used to accurately evaluate pelvic organ prolapse because it provides a multiplanar global view of the pelvis, including the pelvic floor musculature, the pelvic organs, and their relationship to the bony pelvis. This can be used to diagnose the presence of a cystocele, rectocele, enterocele, and prolapse of the vagina and uterus in a patient who presents with incontinence, urinary retention, pain, constipation, and defecatory dysfunction. To accurately assess prolapse, dynamic MRI must be employed using fast imaging techniques. Imaging is performed both before and during Valsalva maneuver to demonstrate pelvic floor dysfunction at rest and with straining. Imaging helps to delineate the degree of prolapse prior to surgical exploration and repair.

RADIONUCLIDE IMAGING

Radionuclide imaging uses radiophamaceuticals with specific properties that permit them to become integrated into normal physiologic and pathologic processes. This modality can provide anatomic and functional data about the genitourinary tract.

Once the radionuclide is instilled, usually by intravenous injection, it accumulates in the target organ by incorporation into normal physiologic pathways. The amount of radiotracer present within organ or system of interest can then be monitored externally with a scintillation camera. The camera has a crystal that releases visible-light photons on detection of incident photons from the radiolabeled organ. These visible-light photons are then processed by a photomultiplier, which is able to determine the spatial relationship of the original incident photons. This information can be analyzed by a computer, resulting in mapping of the data onto visual media such as film. The gamma camera can rotate around the patient to obtain a series of images from multiple angles, called single-photon emission computed tomography (SPECT). Computer analysis of the SPECT data can display graphs, images, and tables showing function of the imaged organ. For example, with SPECT imaging of the kidneys, total and differential split function of the right and left kidney can be determined.

Kidney

Nuclear imaging of the kidney provides important data about its anatomy and function. These studies are noninvasive and spare the patient the risk of iodinated contrast injection as with IVU and CT.

Renal cortical imaging is performed with radiopharmaceutical agents that bind to renal tubular cells and the most commonly used agent is technetium-99m labeled dimercaptosuccinic acid (DMSA). An intravenous dose of DMSA is administered and within 4 h, at least 50% is bound to the renal proximal tubular cells. Detailed renal parenchymal imaging is then performed with the gamma camera. DMSA renography is valuable for demonstrating parenchymal abnormalities, such as scarring from recurrent pyelonephritis. It can also demonstrate tumors and traumatic renal lesions.

Functional or excretory nuclear renal imaging must use an agent isotope that is rapidly excreted by the kidney to quantify glomerular or renal tubular function. Technetium-99m labeled DTPA shows glomerular filtration rate as it is freely filtered by the glomerulus and is minimally reabsorbed or secreted by the tubular or collecting duct cells. Technetium-99m labeled mercaptoacetyltriglycine (MAG3) estimates renal blood flow, as it is nearly all filtered by the glomerulus with one pass through the kidney. Imaging with either of these isotopes quantifies the amount of the isotope entering and leaving the collecting system, which allows for simultaneous dynamic, functional and anatomic imaging (Fig. 29).

Radionuclide renography can be used to evaluate the degree of obstruction and function when a hydronephrotic kidney is identified by other imaging techniques. The study should be performed in a well-hydrated patient, and bladder catheterization is recommended to prevent interference because of bladder outlet obstruction or VUR. After the isotope is injected intravenously, the amount of isotope uptake and excretion by the kidneys is analyzed over a standard time frame. These data are graphed as a washout time-activity curve. A hydronephrotic system inherently drains slower, and a diuretic, such as furosemide, is administered approx 15 min into the scan if the washout time-activity curve is still rising or becomes static. After injecting the diuretic, an obstructed system produce a static or rising time-activity curve, and a nonobstructed system will show a decreasing number of counts over the kidney as the isotope drains into the ureter.

Bladder

Radionuclide VCUG with DTPA can be performed in much the same way as a regular VCUG (Fig. 30). The isotope is instilled into the bladder through a urethral catheter, and then the patient voids during gamma camera imaging. Nuclear VCUG is highly sensitive for VUR and exposes the patient to minimal radiation. However, the degree of reflux cannot be accurately graded with nuclear VCUG because the resolution is relatively poor. This study is an excellent low-radiation means to evaluate a patient after ureteroneocystostomy or after expected spontaneous resolution of VUR.

Adrenal

The adrenal cortex and medulla can be assessed with radionuclide imaging. Adrenal cortical functioning tumors can be identified by intravenous injection of radiolabeled derivatives of cholesterol, such as 7-iodomethyl-19-norcholesterol, labeled with iodine-131. This agent is incorporated into steroids synthesized in the adrenal cortex and

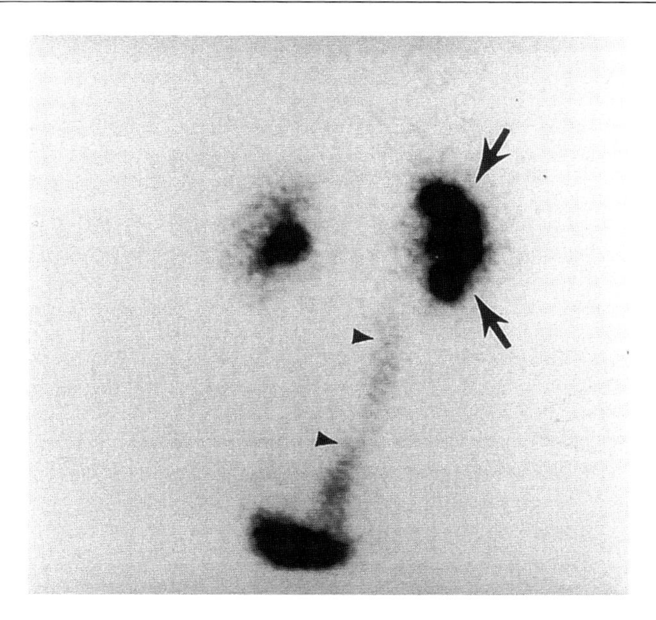

Fig. 29. DTPA renogram shows bilateral isotope uptake and excretion with pooling of excreted isotope in the right collecting system (arrows) and ureter (arrowheads). This patient has a right obstructing ureterovesical junction calculus. (From ref. *3*.)

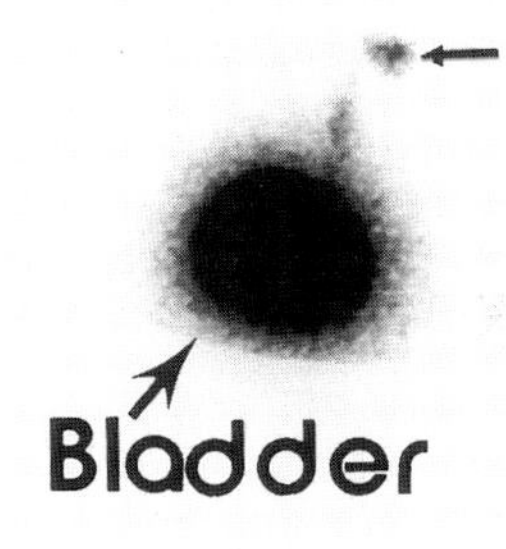

Fig. 30. Radionuclide VCUG with Tc-99 sulfur colloid shows right vesicoureteral reflux to the level of the renal pelvis (small arrow). (From ref. *3*.)

hyperproduction of cortical steroids by a functional tumor will be seen with gamma camera imaging.

Pheochromocytoma of the adrenal medulla can be evaluated after the injection of meta-iodobenzylguanidine (MIBG), which is taken up by adrenergic neurons. MIBG is also radiolabeled with iodine-131 for the gamma camera to image the adrenal medulla and any other endocrinologically active adrenergic tissues. This is especially useful when a patient has biochemical evidence of a pheochromocytoma, but no obvious adrenal mass on CT scan. MIBG scanning is very sensitive and specific for localizing intra-adrenal and extra-adrenal pheochromocytoma and neuroblastoma.

Prostate

Creating radiolabeled monoclonal antibodies (MAb) to tumor antigens allows cancer-specific radionuclide imaging. This is the mechanism of Prostascint imaging, which uses indium-111 labeled capromab pendetide. Capromab is a MAb against prostate-specific membrane antigen found only on the surface of prostate cells. After intravenous injection of the tracer, the patient is immediately imaged with the gamma camera. This is to assess blood pool distribution of the capromab. The patient is then reimaged 4 to 7 d, later revealing areas of the body with prostate tissue. This study is most useful when evaluating a patient with a rising prostate-specific antigen after radical prostatectomy. Tracer may be seen in the prostatic bed with local recurrence or in the pelvic lymph nodes or other metastatic sites with advanced disease.

Bone Scan

Radionuclide imaging of the skeletal system is important in staging known genitourinary malignancies, especially prostate cancer. Bone scintigraphy is performed with technetium-99m-labeled methylene diphosphonate. The tracer is taken up into bone crystals and the amount of tracer the bone takes up depends on how vascular the bone is. Bone involved with metastatic tumors or inflammation tends to be hyper-vascular and takes up more tracer. This produces "hot" areas when analyzed with the gamma camera.

CONCLUSIONS

For more than 75 yr, urological imaging consisted of plain-film radiography, first without, and then with, contrast enhancement. The last 25 yr have seen the development and widespread use of advanced imaging techniques, including ultrasonography, CT, MRI, and radionuclide imaging. These advances, along with the continued use of basic imaging techniques, have enabled the urologist to better identify genitourinary disease without early surgical exploration and to formulate early definitive treatment plans for the best-possible management of a patient's disease.

SUGGESTED READINGS

Amis Jr ES, Newhouse JH. Essentials of Uroradiology. Little, Brown and Company, Boston, MA, 1991.

Barbaric ZL. Principles of Genitourinary Radiology, 2nd Ed. Thieme Medical Publishers Inc., New York, NY, 1994.

Bechtold RE, Zagoria RJ. Imaging approach to staging of renal cell carcinoma. Urol Clin North Am 1997; 24: 507–522.

Bosniak MA. The current radiologic approach to renal cysts. Radiology 1986; 158: 1–10.

Chan DY, Soloman S, Kim FJ, Jarret TW. Image-guided therapy in urology. J Endourol 2001; 5: 105–110.

Cohan RH, Ellis JH. Iodinated contrast material in uroradiology: choice of agent and management of complications. Urol Clin North Am 1997; 24: 471–492.

Curry NS, Bissada NK. Radiologic evaluation of small and indeterminate renal masses. Urol Clin North Am 1997; 24: 493–506.

Davidson AL, Hartman DS. Radiology of the Kidney and Urinary Tract, 2nd Ed. W.B. Saunders Co., Philadelphia, PA, 1994.

Dohke M, Mitchell DG, Vasavada SP. Fast magnetic resonance imaging of pelvic organ prolapse. Tech Urol 2001; 7: 133–138.

Dunnick NR, McCallum RW, Sandler, CM. Textbook of Uroradiology, 2nd Ed. Williams & Wilkins, Baltimore, MD, 1997.

Friedland GW, Chang P. The role of imaging in prostate cancer. Radiol Clin North Am 1991; 29: 581–590.

Goldman SM, Sandler CM. Genitourinary imaging: the past 40 years. Radiology 2000; 215: 313–324.

Haaga JR, Alfidi RJ. Computed Tomography of the Abdomen. C.V. Mosby Company, St. Louis, MO, 1985.

Hartman DS, Aronson S, Frazer H. Current Status of Imaging Indeterminant Renal Masses. Radiol Clin North Am 1991; 29: 475–496.

Horstman WG. Scrotal Imaging. Urol Clin North Am 1997; 24: 653–672.

Hricak H, Okuno W. Radiology of the urinary tract. In: Tanagho EA, McAninch JW, eds. Smith's General Urology, 15th Ed. McGraw-Hill (Lange), New York, NY, 2000, pp. 65–119.

Koff SA, Thrall JH, Keyes JW Jr. Diuretic radionuclide urography: a non-invasive method for evaluating nephroureteral dilation. J Urol 1979; 122: 451–454.

Kogan BA, Hattner RS, Cooper JA. Radionuclide imaging. In: Tanagho EA, McAninch JW, eds. Smith's General Urology, 15th Ed. McGraw-Hill (Lange), New York, NY, 2000, pp. 183–195.

Korobkin M, Francis IR. Imaging of adrenal masses. Urol Clin North Am 1997; 24: 603–622.

McClennan BL, Stolberg HO. Intravascular contrast media: ionic vs. nonionic: current status. Radiol Clin North Am 1991; 29: 437–454.

Newhouse JH. Urinary tract imaging by nuclear magnetic resonance. Urol Radiol 1982; 4: 171–175.

Newhouse JH. Clinical use of urinary tract magnetic resonance imaging. Radiol Clin North Am 1991; 29: 455–474.

Papanicolaou, N. Urinary Tract imaging and intervention: basic principles. In: Walsh PC, Retik AB, Vaughan ED, Wein AJ, eds. Campbell's Urology, 7th Ed, W.B. Saunders Co., Philadelphia, PA, 1998, pp. 170–221 and 233–237.

Resnick MI. Prostatic Ultrasonography. B.C. Decker, Philadelphia, PA, 1990.

Resnick MI, Rifkin, MD. Ultrasound of the Urinary Tract, 3rd Ed. Williams & Wilkins, Baltimore, MD, 1991.

Rifkin MD. Ultrasound of the Prostate. Raven Press, New York, NY, 1988.

Sagel SS, Stanley RJ, Levitt RG, Geisse G. Computed tomography of the kidney. Radiology 1977; 124: 359–370.

Vasile M, Bellin MF, Helenon O, Mourey I, Cluzel P. Imaging evaluation of renal trauma. Abdom Imaging 2000; 25: 424–430.

REFERENCES

1. Swain J. The effect of the roentgen rays on calculi: with the report of a case of renal calculus in which the diagnosis was confirmed by skiagraphy. Bristol Med Chirurgical J 1897; 15: 1–13.
2. Swick M. Intravenous urography by means of the sodium salt of 5-IODO-2-pyridon-n-acetic acid. JAMA 1930; 95: 1403.
3. Hoffman D, Gazelle GS, Seftel AD, Haaga JR, Resnick MI. Atlas of Urologic Imaging. Williams & Wilkins, Baltimore, MD, 1995.

6 Hematuria

Mark J. Noble, MD

CONTENTS

INTRODUCTION

Gross hematuria (visible blood in the urine) can be one of the most frightening symptoms experienced by a patient. If encountered for the first time, a patient will not-uncommonly consider it to represent an emergency and will sometimes present to the hospital emergency room with this complaint. Many patients who see blood in their urine fear the presence of cancer, and they remain uneasy until they have completed an evaluation to rule out this type of problem. Even microscopic hematuria can be quite upsetting to a patient when he or she is informed of this finding by the physician or through work-related testing. It is important for the physician to be sensitive to such feelings and to proceed in an expeditious manner to find out the cause of the hematuria and to thus alleviate a patient's understandable anxiety. To begin this evaluation, a physician should start with a thorough history, perform an appropriate physical examination, and order tests pertinent to the clinical circumstances. These may include one or more of the following tests: urinalysis, urine cytology (including tests for cancer markers), intravenous pyelography (IVP), renal ultrasonography, computed tomography (CT), renal arteriography, magnetic resonance imaging (MRI), retrograde pyelography, and cystoscopy. The following will provide a guide for a better understanding

From: *Essential Urology: A Guide to Clinical Practice*
Edited by: J. M. Potts © Humana Press Inc., Totowa, NJ

of hematuria including its definitions and types, its common causes, its evaluation, some of the complications that may result from hematuria, and its proper treatment.

TAKING THE HISTORY (TYPES OF HEMATURIA)

Blood in the urine may be present in microscopic amounts (microhematuria) or it may be directly visible (gross hematuria). On occasion, a patient may complain of the finding of a spot of blood on the underwear. In male patients, this can actually be from bloody semen, not hematuria, whereas in females it might be caused by bleeding from a source within the vagina and not the urinary tract. Thus, spotting may or may not relate to hematuria but it should be noted as part of the history. If blood is present under the microscope, presumably the patient has been informed that a routine urinalysis showed microscopic bleeding (by chemical dipstick test, by the presence of red blood cells under the microscope, or both). It is especially important to find out if the patient has had previous reports of microhematuria or if this is the only occasion. If the hematuria is grossly visible, determination of the type of gross hematuria can be very helpful.

Because a male usually voids in the standing position, he can view his urination from start to finish. This permits the male who experiences gross hematuria to be questioned as to whether the blood was seen only at the beginning of micturition (initial hematuria), at the completion of micturition (terminal hematuria), or throughout the entire voiding process (total hematuria). Blood in the ejaculate (hematospermia) is not related to hematuria *per se*, and it will not be a significant part of this discussion.

Initial (gross) hematuria in the male indicates a urethral bleeding source. Terminal (gross) hematuria suggests a prostatic etiology, since the prostate constricts at the end of micturition (to eliminate small amounts of urine from the prostatic urethra). Total gross hematuria can be from any urinary tract source but commonly originates from the bladder or higher.

A female usually voids in the sitting position (or sometimes while squatting, as in a public restroom). A woman nearly always views her urine in the toilet bowel after voiding is completed. It is thus difficult to obtain a history from a female as to whether gross hematuria was initial, terminal, or total. However, a woman will often notice whether there was blood on the toilet tissue with wiping, or if the blood was merely seen in the toilet bowl before flushing.

Along with details regarding the hematuria, other information relating to voiding symptoms can be important in forming a differential diagnosis. Does the patient have dysuria, nocturia, frequency, urgency, incontinence, fever, chills, flank pain, hesitancy, or a history of previous genitourinary surgery or kidney stones? Is there any family history of genitourinary malignancy or nephrolithiasis? Was there any history of trauma, long-distance running, or extreme contact sports? What medication does the patient take? What other medical or surgical disorders does the patient have in his or her history?

In males, a sexual history should be obtained whenever possible. This should include the age virginity was lost, whether the hematuria has any relation to sexual activity, any previous sexually transmitted diseases, or any self-instrumentation or experimentation (not uncommon in younger males with spina bifida or other conditions that render the lower genitourinary tract insensate).

In females, a gynecologic history should be obtained. Details regarding menstruation should be obtained at the outset. Is the patient menstruating regularly? How many pads per day, how many days per menstrual cycle, and how many days between cycles? Is there a possibility of pregnancy? If the patient is a teenager, ask about age of menarche, regularity vs irregularity, frequency and severity of any accompanying pain, and type of pads used (internal vs external). Ask about previous pregnancies, live births, and miscarriages or abortions. Ask about the approximate date of the last Pap smear, whether or not it was normal, and if abnormal, what follow-up testing was performed. When feasible, obtain a sexual history, including age of loss of virginity, exposure to (or treatment for) sexually transmitted diseases, use of contraceptive devices or hormones, and other relevant information as befits the clinical circumstances. Sometimes simple inquiry into the correlation between sexual relations and the finding of hematuria can be very revealing, especially with microhematuria.

PHYSICAL EXAMINATION

In completing a general physical examination, attention should be focused on the genitourinary tract and signs should be sought that pertain to the hematuria complaint. Examine the flanks with inspection, palpation, and percussion. Is there ecchymosis that might indicate retroperitoneal bleeding (or that could indicate trauma)? Is the patient tender over one or both flanks? If so, it could indicate stone, infection, obstruction of a kidney, and/or inflammation. Is there a palpable mass (which could be a sign of cyst, tumor, severe hydronephrosis, or phlegmon)? The abdominal examination will be a continuation of the flank examination, but in addition to inspection, palpation, and percussion there should also be auscultation. A bruit could indicate a vascular process relating to the bleeding (i.e., aneurism or arteriovenous malformation). Changes in bowel sounds may be nonspecific clues relating to an inflammatory process causing an ileus (or a mass causing bowel obstruction). A lower, midline abdominal (supra-pubic) mass that is dull to percussion suggests a distended bladder.

The male genital examination should include retraction of the foreskin in uncircumcised patients, gentle spreading of the urethral meatus (to look for polyp or condyloma), palpation of the penis and urethra, examination of the testicles for mass, hernia, swelling, tenderness, varicocele, or other pathology, and a digital rectal examination to check the prostate and rectum for abnormalities. Tenderness and bogginess of the prostate might relate to acute prostatitis, whereas a hard, irregular prostate could indicate prostate cancer.

The female genital examination should include a complete pelvic examination. Inspect the external genitalia for lesions. Lacerations could indicate sexual assault. The urethral meatus might contain a caruncle or tumor. Use a speculum to examine the cervix and vaginal canal. Palpate the uterus and bladder and feel for any pelvic masses or tenderness during bimanual examination. A rectal examination should be performed as well, because sometimes a pelvic mass is better felt during this part of the exam, especially if it involves the posterior cervix or uterus. Rectal examination might also reveal retroperitoneal tumor forming a "shelf-like" mass that is palpable in the anterior wall of the proximal rectum (in proximity to the peritoneal reflection).

DIAGNOSTIC TESTING

Urinalysis

In many cases, patients who give a history of gross hematuria experience the bleeding only intermittently. It is important to do a thorough urinalysis and to be certain regarding the method of urine collection. This latter can't be over-emphasized. If the patient is an uncircumcised male, or an obese female (or a female who is menstruating), the urinalysis can reflect bleeding from areas outside rather than inside the urinary tract. To avoid such confusion, it may be necessary to obtain a catheterized urine specimen. Although the insertion of a catheter can sometimes itself cause hematuria, especially if traumatic, it provides a rapid method to bypass external genital factors that can sometimes mislead the physician. Furthermore, in cases of factitious bleeding (i.e., Munchausen's syndrome), catheterization may prevent the patient from putting blood in the specimen cup containing his or her urine.

The urinalysis is an extremely important tool for evaluation and screening of patients with hematuria. A standard dipstick includes a test of urine pH and also tests for protein, glucose, ketones, and blood. A comprehensive dipstick usually includes these tests and in addition has tests for white blood cells (WBC) by detection of leukocyte esterase, uropathogenic bacteria by nitrite measurement, bilirubin and/or urobilinogen, and specific gravity. The microscopic examination of the urine is usually performed on the resuspended pellet after centrifugation of a 5- to 15-mL aliquot (and discarding most of the supernatant). The microscopic examination includes a count of the number of WBCs per high-powered microscopic field (HPF), the number and appearance of red blood cells (RBCs) per HPF, an estimate of the amount of bacteria (none, few, moderate, many), numbers of epithelial cells per HPF, presence or absence of casts (and what type of casts, if present), presence or absence of crystals (and type), and sometimes a comment if other cells are present, such as spermatozoa and trichomonas. There are some who believe that the appearance of the RBCs can relate to their origin, either bladder or kidney, on the theory that cells from the kidney are older and thus appear less round, even crenated. RBCs from the renal tubule may also be paler than if they originate from the bladder or renal collecting system. Others do not fully accept these as reliable indicators of RBC origin.

A nephrology consultation should be considered (to evaluate for nephritis or other primary medical disorders of the kidneys) when one finds significant protein or one or more red blood cell casts in the urine or when there is persistence of microhematuria despite completely normal x-rays and normal lower urinary tract endoscopy (*see* section on cystoscopy). For example, there exists a condition termed "benign, idiopathic, microhematuria" which is a diagnosis of exclusion. In other words, all surgical and medical causes for microscopic hematuria should be ruled out (with appropriate tests) before this diagnosis is entertained. Benign, idiopathic, microhematuria is characterized by the unchanged finding of small numbers of red blood cells in the urine (more than three per microscopic HPF but usually fewer than 10, depending on the concentration of the urine) over a period of years, with at least two separate anatomic evaluations of the urinary tract yielding no definable cause. The patient may or may not have a family history of this disorder. It is thought to be caused by the slight leakage of RBCs past the glomerular basement membrane during filtration. It is benign because it is not associated with any malignancy and there is no evidence of renal damage over time or any harm to the patient. The defect in the glomerular basement membrane is thought to have little chance of progression and is not associated with any other illness or organ dysfunction elsewhere in the body; hence its benign character.

Cytology

A urine cytology has value in screening for urothelial cancer, the most common malignancy found in patients with microscopic hematuria. Cytological testing of the urine consists of a microscopic examination of Pap or equivalently stained cells obtained by centrifugation of an aliquot of urine, usually at least 10 mL. Cytology results usually are reported in three categories as noted in the following:

1. Negative for malignant cells.
2. Atypical cells, cannot rule out transitional cell carcinoma (TCC).
3. Positive for cells consistent with TCC.

It is important when listing the source of the urine specimen to indicate whether it is clean voided urine or one obtained by instrumentation (catheterization or after placing a cystoscope). Typically, an instrumented cytology will contain clumps of cells rubbed off by the catheter or cystoscope, and these may somewhat resemble clusters of cells seen in the urine from a patient with known TCC. Therefore, an other-wise negative instrumented cytology specimen that is not so-labeled will often be reported as containing atypical cells, and this can create confusion for the physician and fear for the patient. Because of a large number of specimens historically reported as category 2 (atypical cells), cytology lacks high sensitivity and specificity as a test for screening for the presence of TCC. That is, patients with known TCC display only a 30% positive rate with standard urine cytology, although patients with more aggressive TCC (high-grade or invasive cancers) will have a higher rate of positive cytology approaching 65–75%, and these are the more life-threatening cancers. Still, the cytology test is not as accurate as one would like, and attempts have been made to improve these results by looking at biologic markers (cell surface or genetic) within urine cells. Such tests as NMP-22 and BTA-STAT have shown promise, but the most promising to date (and Food and Drug Administration-approved for detection of recurrent bladder cancer in a patient with prior bladder malignancy) is the "FISH" test (fluorescent *in situ* hybridization analysis for chromosomal alterations). The FISH test is performed in conjunction with regular cytology, but stains are used to identify up to four genetic markers that correlate highly with neoplastic transformation of epithelial cells. It has a specificity and sensitivity (lack of false-positives and false-negatives) in the 85–90% range, and multicenter studies with FISH suggest it is such an accurate test that a positive FISH in the absence of cystoscopic evidence of bladder cancer nearly always implies that a patient will develop bladder cancer within 1 yr of the positive test.

Plain Abdominal Film (Kidneys, Ureters, and Bladder, or KUB)

For evaluation of hematuria, the plain abdominal film is often of little help by itself. It is sometimes useful if a kidney or ureteral calculus is suspected (up to 85% of symptomatic urinary calculi can be seen on a KUB alone, although sometimes other calcifications such as pelvic phleboliths can be confused with ureteral calculi). Occasionally, a large renal mass lesion is visible on a KUB. In the pediatric population, a KUB often shows more structures than in the adult, chiefly due to the lower amount of fat in children. But a KUB does not really show much detailed anatomy with respect to the upper urinary tract (kidneys and ureters). It is, however, important to obtain this film as part of most other x-ray series (IVP, CT, arteriogram, retrograde pyelogram), because the KUB or "scout" film enables comparison of structures before and after contrast administration, as will be seen later in this chapter (clinical case 2).

Intravenous Pyelography

Traditionally, the IVP has been the method of choice for evaluating the upper urinary tract (kidneys and ureters). It is also called excretory urography. The best way to prepare (prep) the patient for urography is to order clear liquids beginning the evening before the study and nothing by mouth for 6 h before the study. Laxatives are rarely needed. An IVP is performed by injecting radiographic contrast intravenously into the patient and then performing a series of x-rays as noted below. The usual film sequence for IVP is as follows:

1. Plain film: the KUB must be visualized to evaluate calcifications and bony structures.
2 One minute: the nephrogram visualizes the renal parenchyma.
3. Five minutes: early visualization of the upper collecting system (calices, pelvis, upper ureter).
4. Tomograms: performed to assess renal outlines and fine calcifications. Routine on patients over 40 yr old and used selectively below age 40.
5. Fifteen to twenty minutes: late visualization should include the lower ureters and bladder.

Certain "tricks" during the study are used to improve the diagnostic yield:

1. Delayed films: to assess the level of obstruction in hydronephrotic kidneys.
2. Plain tomograms: before contrast, these are used to assess renal calcifications.
3. Ureteral compression: a compression band surrounding the lower abdomen helps to fill the upper ureters better.
4. Prone films: demonstrate better visualization of the pelvic portion of the ureters.
5. Oblique films: help to visualize abnormalities in three dimensions.
6. Post void film: provides a better assessment of bladder pathology and residual urine.

The plain film helps to assess bony structures and to discern any calcifications. The nephrogram enables gross assessment of renal function (normal, delayed, or not visualized). Tomograms permit improved viewing of the renal outlines and may demonstrate the presence of a mass or small calcifications within the kidney not otherwise seen. Early films can depict hydronephrosis, filling defects, distorted calices, malposition, mass, and/or renovascular disease. Late films may reveal filling defects, dilation, or constriction of the ureter. The bladder should be assessed for size, filling defects, mucosal pattern (thickened, trabeculated), and shape (teardrop: pelvic lipomatosis; Christmas tree: neurogenic bladder).

In general, an IVP is unable to differentiate cyst from solid mass or tumor, and it is not particularly sensitive for masses smaller than 3 cm in diameter. An IVP is also of little or no value if a patient has a serum creatinine above 2.0 because the visualization of the kidneys will be poor and little or no visualization of the ureters will be obtained. Patients should be warned of the risks of having an IVP (allergic reaction and renal toxicity); this is usually performed by the radiologist. Certain disorders increase the risk of toxicity. They include diabetic nephropathy, multiple myeloma, hyperuricosuria, amyloidosis, pre-existing chronic renal failure, and other conditions producing severe proteinuria. Patients with a previous history of contrast reaction, asthma, or other severe allergies are at increased risk of allergic reaction during an IVP and most radiologists recommend a special "prep" before administering intravenous contrast in such cases. This prep can vary from institution to institution but often includes several doses of Benadryl and Prednisone (antihistamine and corticosteroid) before the study. If a patient has a previous history of anaphylaxis to intravenous contrast, one might consider alternative testing such as retrograde pyelography to view the ureters. Ordinarily, when contrast is instilled retrograde into the ureters using a cystoscope inserted into the bladder, the contrast does not enter the bloodstream and therefore does not cause allergic reaction or toxicity. Renal ultrasound, noncontrast CT, or MRI can be used to examine the renal parenchyma.

Renal Ultrasonography

Renal ultrasound imaging can be very helpful for evaluating the kidneys and is especially useful for differentiating a solid mass from a cyst. Renal ultrasonography has the advantage of being totally noninvasive (no radiation that might injure a fetus if a female is pregnant, no contrast and thus, no chance of toxicity or contrast allergy) and relatively inexpensive. Ultrasound units have become fairly compact and many medical offices have them, so an ultrasound is readily available (compared to a CT scanner, which is less available and which may be scheduled 2–3 wk in advance for nonemergent tests). It is not a very comprehensive test for evaluating the anatomy of the kidneys and ureters with respect to causes of hematuria, but a sonogram can exclude biologically significant renal masses (those greater than 2–3 cm), hydronephrosis, or medium-to-large renal calculi (those likely to become lodged in the ureter, 5 mm or larger). With Doppler imaging, a measurement of renal blood flow can be obtained and compared (left vs right). Renal ultrasound might not demonstrate a urothelial malignancy such as a TCC of the renal collecting system, unless it is large or causing segmental renal obstruction (with hydrocalyx). A renal sonogram also has difficulty resolving small renal calculi (4 mm or less), and it is not useful for examination of a nondilated ureter. If a cyst is not perfectly smooth-walled, or if it is multiloculated, or if a cyst has some internal echo characteristics that are not typical of water density, then a CT scan is usually recommended for further evaluation to rule out a tumor within a cyst.

Computed Tomography

CT has proven revolutionary in the evaluation of patients for a variety of ailments and has only recently been supplanted by MRI for certain areas of the body. But for imaging the kidneys, ureters, and bladder, MRI offers little additional information in the great majority of cases. MRI also typically costs approximately twice as much as an abdominal CT scan. A fine-cut CT scan of the abdomen without contrast ("renal stone protocol") has been found to be the most sensitive test (96–98%) for determining the presence or absence of a renal or ureteral calculus (significantly more accurate than an IVP, which is 70–80% sensitive). A noncontrast CT scan can also detect pathology in organs adjacent to the urinary tract ("incidental" findings), such as gallstones, pancreatic mass or pseudocyst, uterine or ovarian mass, aortic aneurism, and other lesions that may or may not relate to hematuria but that can be clinically significant. A CT scan with intravenous contrast (it usually includes oral contrast as well) is extremely sensitive for detecting renal malignancies and often can demonstrate lesions within the ureters or the bladder. An IVP may demonstrate a "bulge" in the renal outline, which could be a mass, a cyst, or a dromedary hump. A CT scan will almost always differentiate between these. The CT scan is far more expensive than an IVP or ultrasound, and it does expose the patient to significant amounts of radiation (which could be detrimental to the fetus in a pregnant patient). A CT with intravenous contrast has the same toxicity and allergy risks as an IVP, and intravenous contrast is usually not administered if the serum creatinine is greater than 2.0, just as with IVP. Finally, CT scans can, on rare occasions, show a false mass, or pseudotumor. This nonexistent renal mass can be the result of the phenomenon of "volume-averaging" that was more a problem with older CT scanners but which still can occur. In this circumstance, a CT image shows what appears to be a mass within or extending from the capsule of a kidney when in fact no actual mass is present. Although exceedingly rare, such has resulted in nephrectomy in a few instances. Newer techniques, such as a "triple-phase CT" have all but eliminated this type of false image phenomenon. One of the newest techniques, a three-dimensional CT scan, can demonstrate the number of main renal arteries and veins, the precise relationship of a renal lesion or mass to the rest of the kidney, and the relationship to other organs adjacent to the kidney. The clarity is striking and almost resembles that seen in an anatomic model (i.e., "The Visible Man"). It has proven quite helpful for surgery designed to remove or ablate a portion of a kidney while preserving the remainder.

Renal Arteriography

Until the advent of CT scanners in the mid- to late 1970s, a renal arteriogram or "angiogram" was the definitive test to evaluate a possible renal mass seen on IVP. Most malignant renal tumors are hypervascular, and the tumor vessels have a characteristic appearance that differs from that of normal renal vasculature. Furthermore, tumor vessels usually lack smooth muscle in their walls, so it was possible to administer epinephrine in the contrast injected into a renal artery, which would constrict the normal renal vessels but not the vessels within a renal cell carcinoma, thus enhancing the appearance of the tumor. A renal arteriogram is still the best test for demonstrating the anatomy of the renal vasculature and can demonstrate the presence of an arteriovenous malformation, renal artery aneurysm, or other vascular lesion that may be a source of hematuria. If a patient's kidney has multiple renal arteries (approx 30% of patients have a kidney with more than one artery) and one needs to surgically remove part or all of the kidney because of disease within it, it is helpful to know the precise number and course of the arteries to that organ. Until the advent of three-dimensional CT or MRI angiography, renal arteriography was the only method available for imaging the renal vasculature. Angiography is not as sensitive as CT for demonstration of renal masses, and it is significantly more invasive as it requires femoral arterial puncture with its attendant risks and complications. Even with digital subtraction techniques (to enhance the clarity of images and lower the amount of radiation exposure), there is still likely to be more radiation exposure than with other imaging techniques. Administration of radiographical contrast directly into a renal artery also carries increased risk of nephrotoxicity compared with intravenous contrast, and an interventional radiologist is usually required to perform the procedure. However, angiography has an important place in circumstances where other tests are equivocal, and by the very fact that it is invasive, it can be used therapeutically to treat certain lesions (i.e., embolization of an arteriovenous malformation).

Magnetic Resonance Imaging

This modality has been shown to demonstrate certain genitourinary lesions with far better clarity than other available radiographic imaging techniques. Tumor thrombus in the vena cava can be best staged with MRI, and certain adrenal lesions (such as pheochromocytoma) are more apparent than with CT scan. MRI can demonstrate the main renal vasculature with gadolinium enhancement. Furthermore, MRI is currently felt to be the most accurate test for demonstrating the anatomy of pelvic prolapse in the female and for depicting the presence of urethral diverticulum. With an endorectal coil, MRI can image the prostate with a great deal of detail. However, MRI offers no significant anatomic advantage over CT scan with respect to renal mass lesions, stone disease, or other abnormalities involving the upper genitourinary tract. Furthermore, it costs as much as twice the price of a CT scan. Because an MRI produces a very powerful magnetic field, it cannot be used with good clarity in patients with metallic objects (surgical clips) in the area of study, and it also cannot generally be used in patients with cardiac pacemakers.

Retrograde Pyelography

A retrograde pyelogram is performed by injecting radiographic contrast into a ureter through the ureteral orifice in the bladder. A cystoscopy is performed and a small catheter is gently inserted into the ureteral orifice of interest. In the adult, typically 10 mL of radiographic contrast solution is injected slowly, often under fluoroscopy, with appropriate "spot" or hard-copy x-rays taken as may be appropriate. If there is significant hydronephrosis, an amount of contrast greater than 10 mL may be needed to fully delineate the renal collecting system. The entire course of the ureter is observed from the bladder retrograde-fashion up to the kidney and its collecting system (renal pelvis, infundibula, and calyces). Before actual instillation of contrast, a plain abdominal x-ray is taken to enable comparison. Retrograde pyelography relies on undiluted or partly diluted contrast and depicts the ureters with far more detail than an IVP. Filling defects may be observed and can be due to calculus, blood clot, or tumor. Occasionally, an air bubble is injected with the contrast and this can create confusion as to presence or absence of a true filling defect. Many female patients can undergo retrograde pyelography under local anesthesia, but most male patients will require a regional or a general anesthetic, or at least a fair amount of sedation, as the discomfort appears to be significantly greater because of the significantly longer urethra and the need to negotiate more curves with the cystoscope (which usually needs to be a rigid type of instrument in order to do retrograde studies).

Cystoscopy

All of the above studies can be done (or ordered) by a primary care physician. Cystoscopy (bladder endoscopy), however, is the mainstay of the urologist and is the best test for evaluation of the bladder as a possible source of hematuria. (Nephrologists in a number of European countries perform diagnostic cystoscopy to evaluate the bladder for possible cancer, and gynecologists who specialize in female urology are sometimes trained to perform cystoscopy in conjunction with certain female incontinence surgery. But in the United States, nearly all patients with hematuria who require a cystoscopic evaluation are examined by urologists.) Cystoscopes are available as both rigid and flexible instruments. Patients find the flexible scope to be more comfortable than the rigid, especially male patients as previously mentioned, but females apparently also share this view. A flexible cystoscope is less useful if the bleeding is severe because the rate at which irrigant can be instilled (to clear the lens to see) is usually much faster with a rigid instrument. Rigid instruments, at least in adult sizes, usually have larger working channels (than flexible instruments), enabling a more effective cautery instrument to be introduced in order to stop bleeding. Also, it is much more difficult, for a variety of technical reasons, to thread a ureteral catheter through a flexible cystoscope and to direct it into a ureteral orifice in order to perform retrograde pyelography. But the flexible cystoscope can be deflected 180° at its tip and thus can be used to view the bladder neck from the inside, something that is virtually impossible to accomplish with a rigid cystoscope. Although tumors are rare in this location, they do occur from time to time.

Cystoscopy is performed after using local anesthetic jelly as a means to numb the urethra. Most rigid cystoscopy sets contain two telescopes, usually a 30° lens and a 70° lens. These give different views within the bladder. Only the rigid telescope with a 30° view is useful for examining the urethra, however. A cystoscopy can yield a lot of information about bladder anatomy and function in addition to providing a sensitive test for detection of an abnormal bladder lesion that might be a source of hematuria (tumor, bladder calculus, or other problem). For example, some patients with incontinence may be voiding under very high pressures because of a condition called detrussor-sphincter dyssyneria. In this neurological dysfunction of the bladder, the urinary sphincter is improperly coordinated with a bladder contraction and the sphincter fails to open (or relax), thus creating a degree of obstruction. A urodynamic (bladder nerve and voiding test) may be required for complete diagnosis of such a condition, but cystoscopy alone can provide evidence to strongly suggest a nerve imbalance simply by the finding of significant bladder trabeculation (thickening of the detrussor muscle). If a patient has this condition (common with a number of spinal cord lesions), it is not unusual to sometimes see some microhematuria on routine urinalysis. This is thought to be caused by abnomally high bladder pressures necessary for voiding, and correction of this condition will frequently rectify the condition of microhematuria.

SOME COMMENTS ON INITIAL AND SUBSEQUENT EVALUATION FOR HEMATURIA

In 2001, a report was issued by the Microscopic Hematuria Guidelines Committee under the auspices of the American Urological Association. This comprehensive text reports on the committee's findings with respect to gross and microscopic hematuria and provides recommendations for evaluating patients with either problem. It can be accessed using an Internet Web Browser at the following URL: https://shop.auanet.org/timssnet/products/guidelines/main_reports.cfm It can also be printed (and viewed more completely) by using a utility, such as Adobe Acrobat. This report sets forth a de facto standard for the evaluation of hematuria.

A simplified flow chart, modified with permission (from the above report) is presented in Fig. 1 to help the reader with methodical evaluation of hematuria. Clinicians are in general agreement that all patients with gross hematuria require evaluation. This may range from history, physical examination, urinalysis, and urine culture (to document an actual hemorrhagic urinary tract infection) in an otherwise healthy young adult female with "honeymoon cystitis" to more detailed work-up (for a patient who may have cancer) using some or all of the radiographic and urological procedures described here.

Note that patients with initial findings that strongly suggest a primary nephrologic basis for hematuria are referred for medical work-up to this end. Clues would be the finding of high amounts of protein in the urine, the presence of one or more RBC casts, a strong family history of medical-renal disease (African-American patients with a relative with sickle trait or disease would be included in this group), the presence of conditions that commonly result in renal parenchymal damage and that might cause hematuria (such as long-standing or poorly controlled diabetes), and possibly the presence of RBCs that have a suspicious appearance (consistent with origin in the glomerulus). A patient who is not initially felt to have hematuria relating to a medical cause, as well as one who has undergone medical evaluation with results that fail to support medical-renal disease as an etiologic factor for hematuria, should undergo a work-up

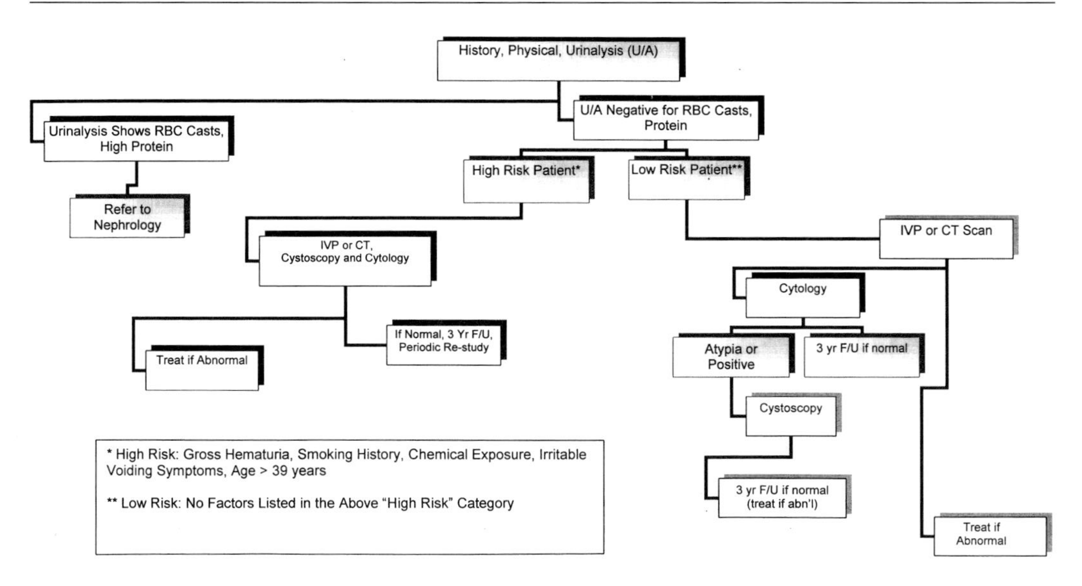

Fig. 1. Flow chart for management of hematuria (modified from ref. *17*, with permission).

with anatomic study of the urinary tract. It is recommended that an IVP or CT scan be obtained to image the upper urinary tract, and additional testing to evaluate the lower urinary tract for pathology should be obtained as noted in Fig. 1. Patients who have no gross hematuria and no "risk factors," such as age 40 or older, previous smoking, chemical exposure, or irritative voiding symptoms (frequency, dysuria, urgency) can be considered "low risk" for having bladder cancer, and such patients with otherwise negative evaluation may have a urine cytology and, if negative, deferral of an endoscopic procedure (cystoscopy with or without retrograde pyelography). The rationale is that patients with high-grade urothelial malignancies will have a finding of at least atypia if not frankly positive cytology and these are the life-threatening conditions involving the bladder that one would need to discover immediately. A patient with a low-grade TCC of the bladder or microscopic hematuria from benign prostate enlargement does not have an immediately life-threatening condition and will still be accurately diagnosed because of the persistence of the hematuria with follow-up (which would result in endoscopy at some point). When following a patient with microhematuria, most physicians would see the patient every 3–6 mo and perform repeat urinalysis and cytology (FISH augments the accuracy of cytology as noted earlier). A patient who has gross hematuria on anticoagulants still falls within the high-risk category even though some patients bleed from multiple sites, including the urinary tract (without the presence of a bladder tumor), when clotting is overly prolonged. That patient still needs full anatomic work-up and in fact, many bladder tumors present in just that fashion (of course, many patients on anticoagulants are patients with cardiovascular disease, which correlates with prior smoking, so they are "high risk" anyway). Whenever there is a question about which path to follow for a patient with hematuria, consultation with a urologist should be strongly considered.

COMPLICATIONS OF HEMATURIA

It is rare for patients to experience complications from microscopic hematuria itself. If the microscopic hematuria is severe (hundreds of RBCs per microscopic field on urinalysis) and prolonged, there may be some possibility that a patient will develop anemia, but more likely, the anemia will be the result of some other co-existing factor. For example, patients with medical renal disease generally experience diminished erythropoetin levels because of decreased secretion by the damaged kidney cells, and this is more important than loss of the equivalent of 3–5 mL of blood daily, which a normal person can easily handle. Many cancers cause systemic effects, including anemia (renal cell carcinoma frequently does this, even when the tumor is relatively small). A patient with recurrent or persistent gross hematuria, however, can easily become anemic just as can the patient with chronic gastrointestinal bleeding, and such patients may need treatment for this condition as part of their overall management.

A patient with severe, gross hematuria can experience urinary clot retention, as the clots may be too large to pass through the urethra. These clots require evacuation through a large Foley catheter or sometimes through a cystoscope under anesthesia, or bladder rupture could result. A patient with significant bleeding from a kidney may be able to pass clots through the urethra but may still experience clot "colic" similar to the pain felt with passing a ureteral calculus. Such discomfort can obviously be severe and often requires parenteral analgesics for management. Exsanguination is extremely rare but can occur in extreme cases of gross hematuria; for this reason any patient with hematuria along with clots (or significant gross hematuria in a patient on anticoagulants) requires rapid evaluation, possibly in an emergency room setting, to see if immediate or emergent treatment is needed.

SPECIAL SITUATIONS

Blood in the semen, termed hematospermia, has no direct relationship to microscopic or gross hematuria. It is thought to result from infection or inflammation in one or both seminal vesicles or sometimes the prostate. Furthermore, there is no known relationship between hematospermia and prostate cancer, yet hematospermia often frightens male patients to nearly the same degree as does the observation of gross hematuria. Sometimes a male may experience this when he awakens in the morning and finds a blood spot on his underwear, possibly relating to a nocturnal emission. It should not be difficult to differentiate this in the history from hematuria and also should be simple to differentiate this from a bloody urethral discharge, which may be from the prostate or from any lesion, infection, or inflammation within the urethra (intraurethral condyloma acuminata may present as bloody urethral discharge or spotting on the underwear and requires endoscopy for diagnosis). Of course, urethral bleeding, if severe enough, will also color the urine red but should be lighter or clearer as the bladder urine washes through the urethra.

Examples

Case 1

M.D. is a 40-yr-old female who presented with right flank pain and gross hematuria. Physical examination was noncontributory. Urinalysis showed grossly bloody urine. A urine sample was sent for cytology and showed atypia. IVP demonstrated a right ureteral filling defect (Fig. 2A–F). Cystoscopy did not reveal any bladder tumors, but two right ureteral orifices were observed. Retrograde pyelography was performed

Fig. 2. *(Opposite page)* IVP demonstrates poor visualization of the lower pole collecting system **(A–F)**.

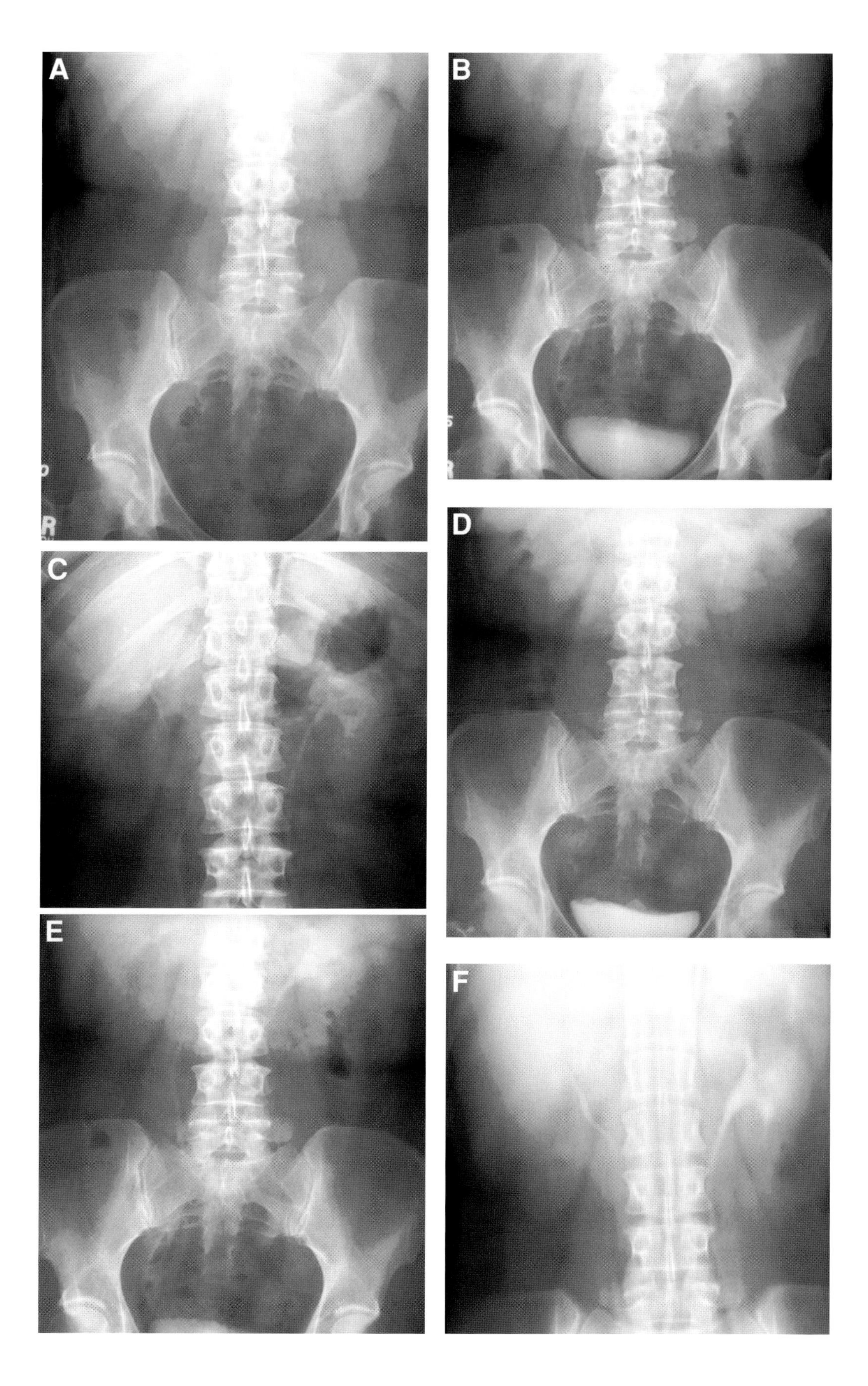
A
B
C
D
E
F

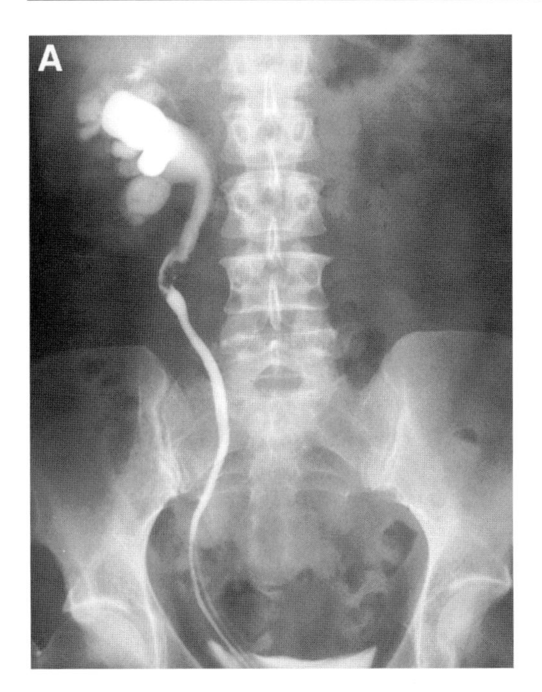

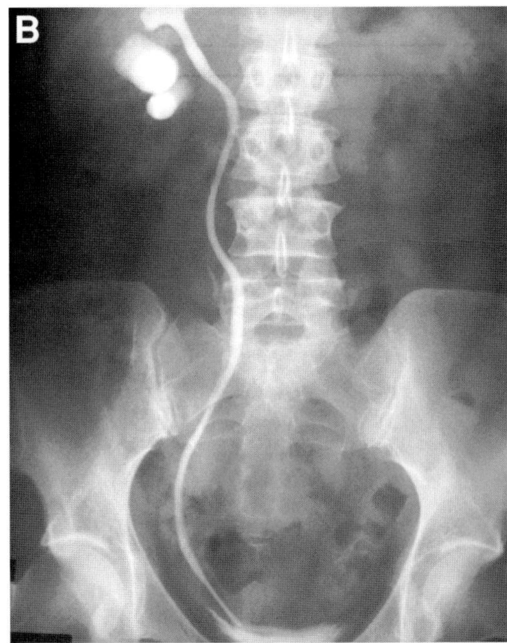

Fig. 3. The ureter to the right lower renal segment is seen to have a filling defect on retrograde pyelography **(A)**, whereas that to the upper renal segment is without any defects **(B)**.

and showed a nonmobile filling defect in the ureter to the right lower renal segment but no abnormality of the ureter to the right upper renal segment (Figs. 3A and B)—a complete ureteral duplication existed in this patient. CT scanning showed no evidence of a periureteral mass but demonstrated some obstructive changes, hydronephrosis, in the lower renal segmental collecting system as the result of a compromise of drainage from the ureteral lesion (Fig. 4A and B). The patient underwent surgical exploration and a segmental ureteral resection was performed along with fusion of the remaining proximal and distal segments into the second right ureter, essentially conjoining them. Pathology report showed a grade 2/3 TCC of the ureter. Postoperative IVP revealed an excellent surgical result with no recurrence, and a repeat urine cytology was normal.

Case 2

M.C. is a 49-yr-old female with a long history of recurrent urinary tract infections associated with positive cultures. She was followed for years with microhematuria but never had gross hematuria, and she was repeatedly treated with antibiotics for her infections. However, a recent urine culture was negative yet she still had microhematuria. A urine cytology was negative. An IVP showed a normal left kidney and a complex staghorn calculus in the right kidney (Fig. 5A and B). A renal scan showed the right kidney to have 34% (roughly one-third) of total renal function (Fig. 6). An open, anatrophic nephrolithotomy was performed with complete removal of the staghorn calculus and successful reconstruction of the kidney (Fig. 7A–E). The patient had a good, long-term result.

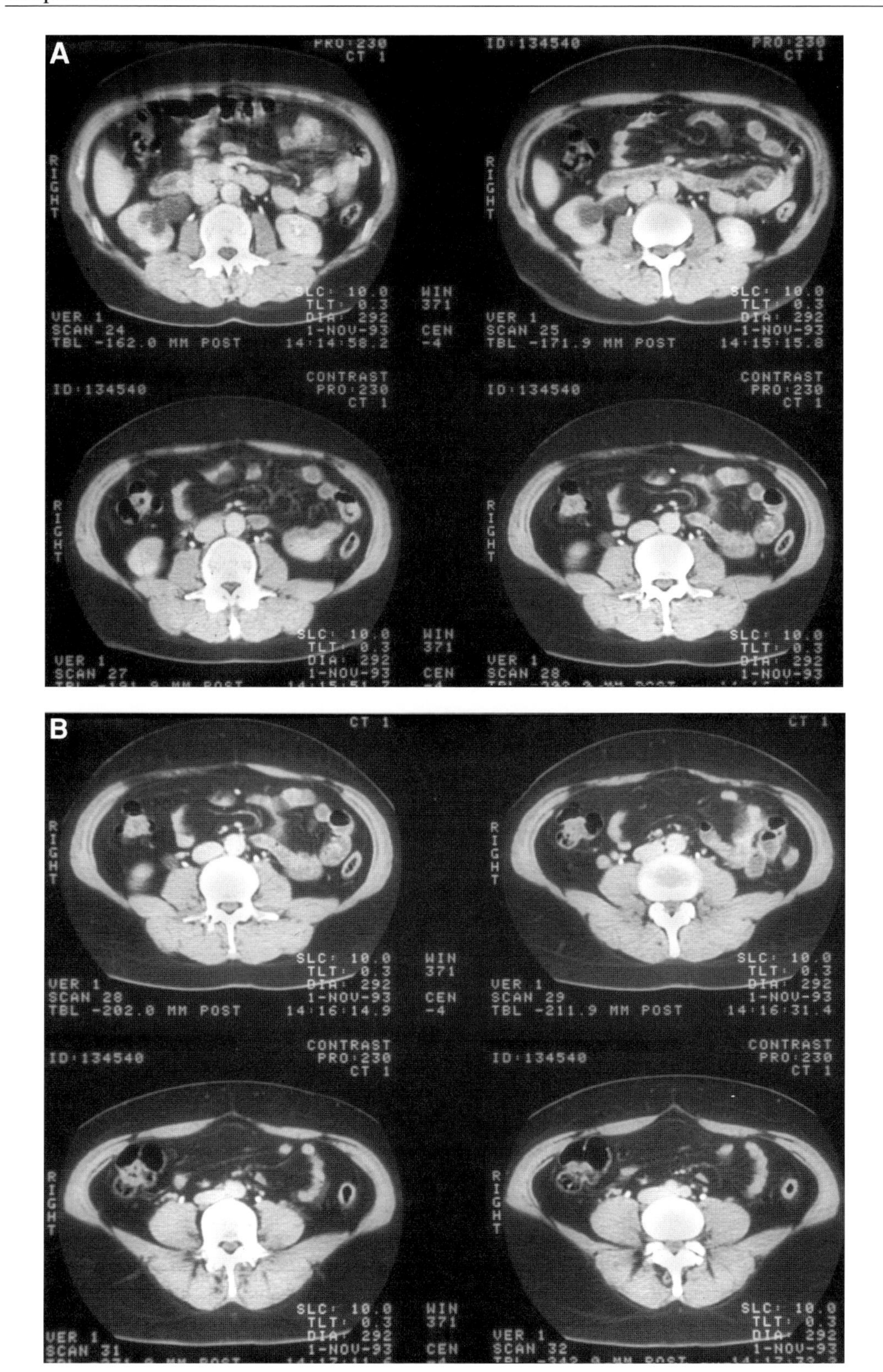

Fig. 4. CT reveals hydronephrosis of the right lower pole renal segment (**A** and **B**).

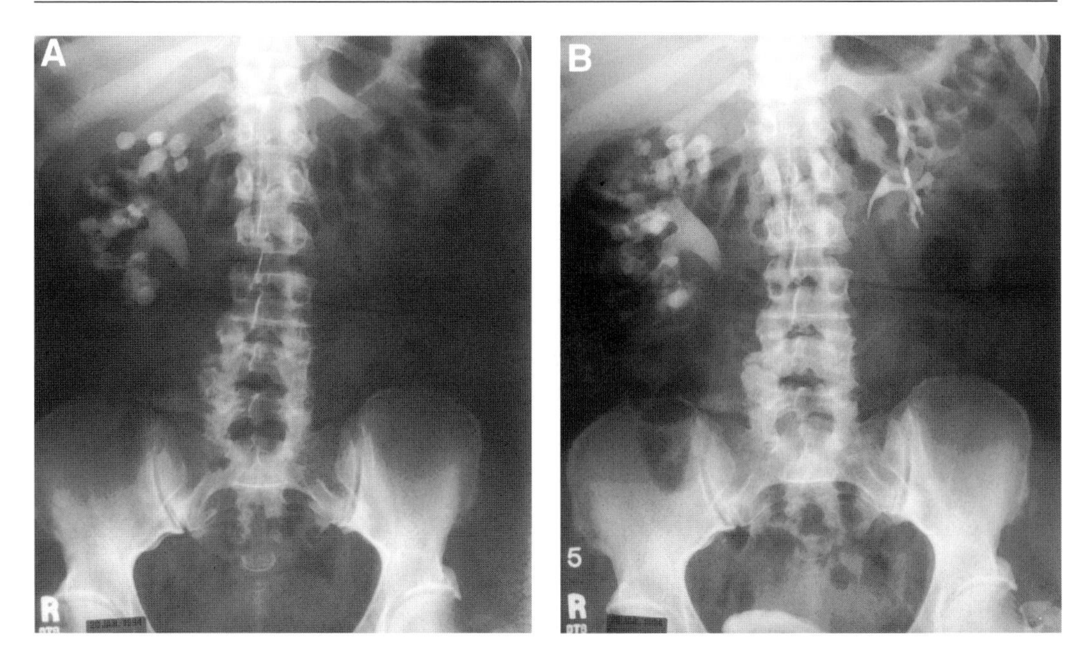

Fig. 5. This IVP demonstrates the importance of starting with a "scout" or plain abdominal x-ray before administering contrast. Note the right renal staghorn calculus in the first film **(A)**, performed without contrast. In the second film **(B)**, one can see that the left kidney is normal. Had a "scout" film not been obtained, one might have simply thought that the right kidney was hydronephrotic—the stone looks like contrast!

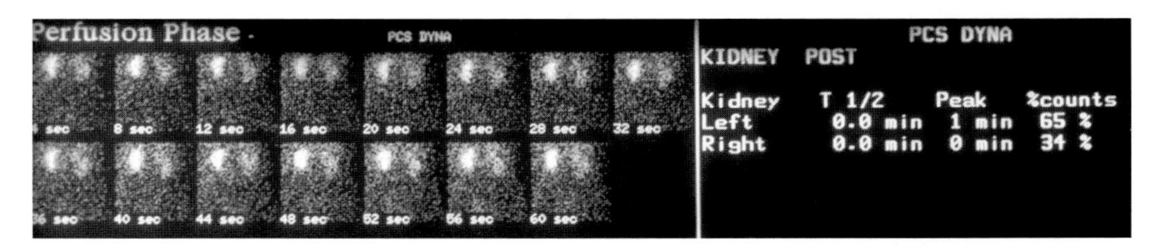

Fig. 6. A nuclear renal scan demonstrates, in sequence, the uptake by right and left kidneys in this patient with right renal staghorn calculus; note that the right kidney comprises 34% of total renal function.

Case 3

P.B. is a 72-yr-old male with a long history of hypertension. He experienced total, gross, painless hematuria but had a negative work-up, including IVP, cystoscopy, and urine cytology. Four years later he again experienced total, gross, painless hematuria and this time his urine showed positive cytology (squamous metaplasia). A renal flow scan (not shown) showed no renal function on the right, and a CT scan revealed a solitary left kidney (congenital absence of the right kidney) with hydronephrosis of the left upper pole collecting system and a mass in the central portion of the renal pelvis (Fig. 8A–D).

Fig. 7. *(Opposite page)* These pictures detail the surgery that was performed in order to remove the stones and reconstruct the kidney **(A–E)**. *Continued on page 110*

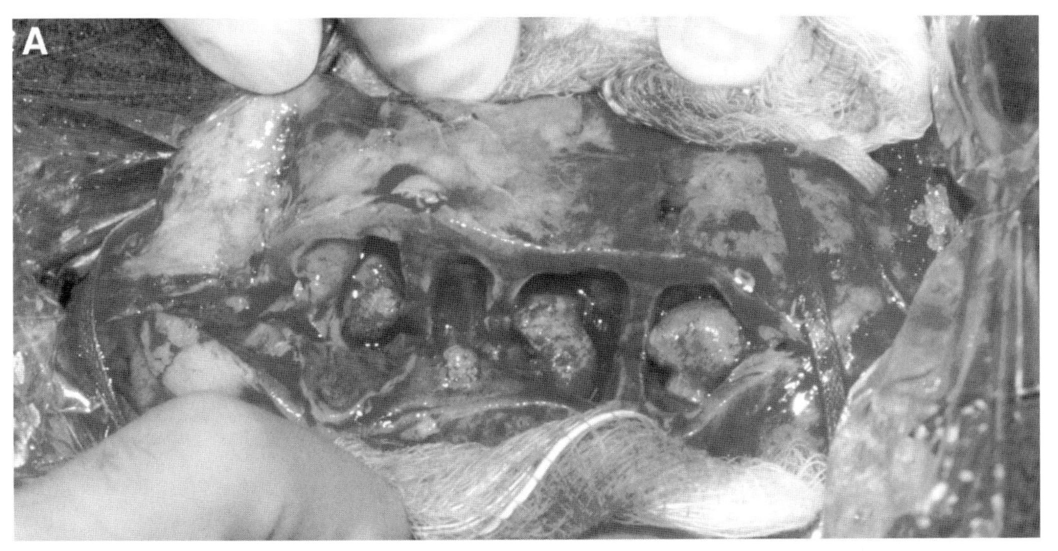
A

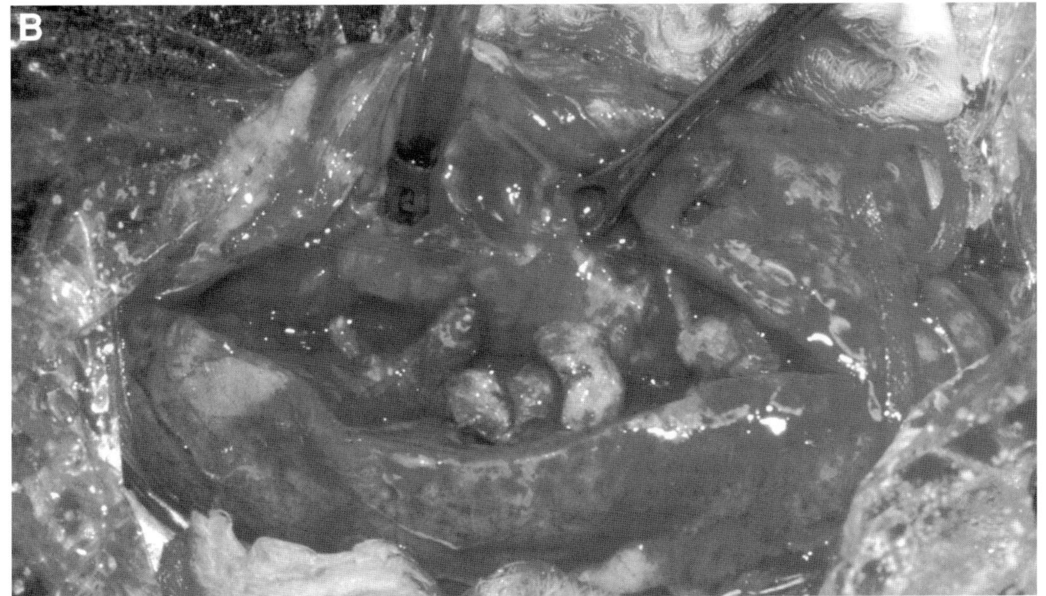
B

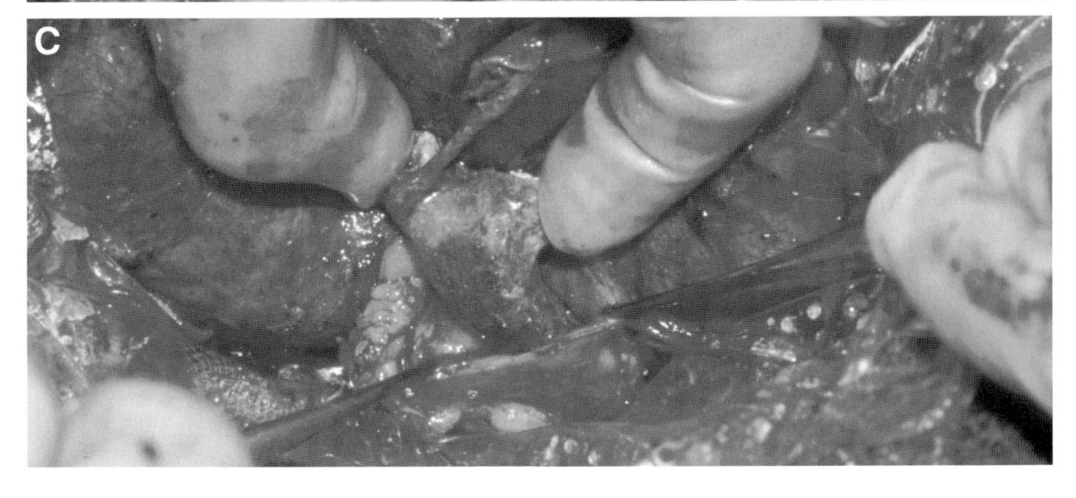
C

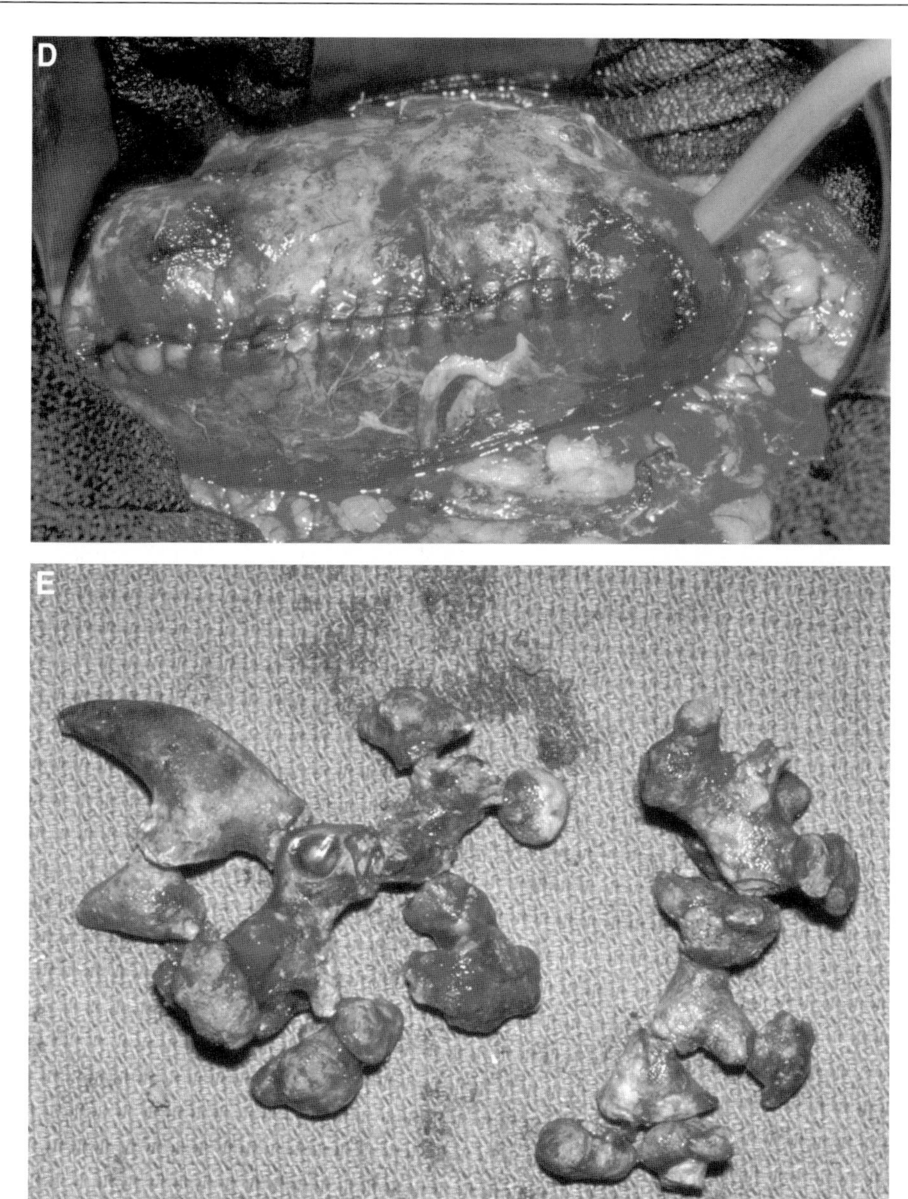

Fig. 7. *(Continued)* These pictures detail the surgery that was performed in order to remove the stones and reconstruct the kidney **(A–E)**.

A retrograde pyelogram showed effacement of the upper collecting system with only the lower portion filling with contrast (Fig. 9). An arteriogram demonstrated that the upper pole of the left kidney was hypovascular (Fig. 10A and B). An open surgical procedure was performed, including partial nephrectomy (50–60% removal) with reconstruction of the renal remnant. Frozen sections of the margins were negative, and pathology revealed a grade 3/3 papillary TCC without renal parenchymal involvement. The patient experienced an uneventful postoperative recovery and remains tumor-free with 4-yr follow-up.

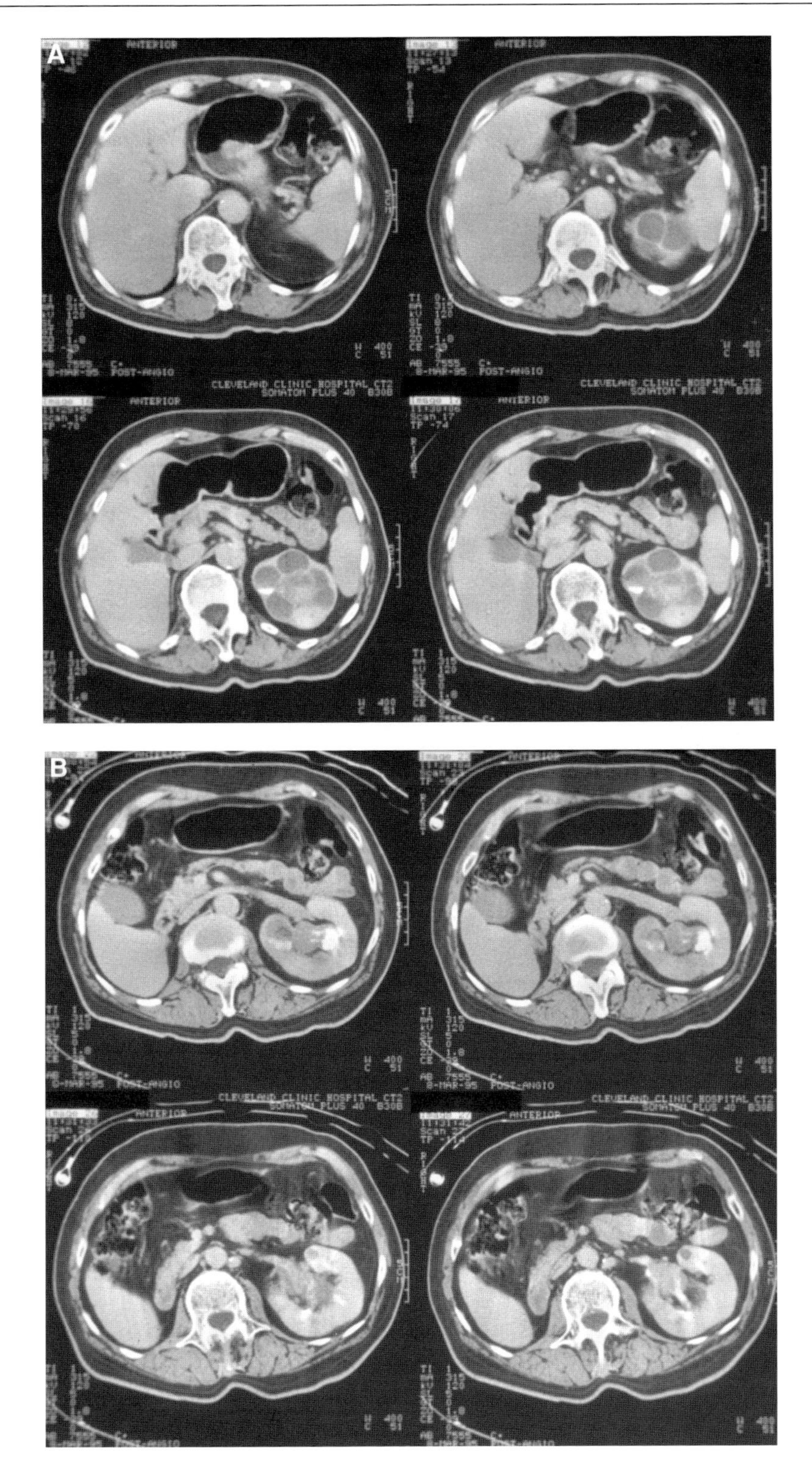

Fig. 8. This CT scan demonstrates the hydronephrosis of the left upper-pole collecting system and a mass in the central portion of the renal pelvis of this solitary left kidney. No kidney is demonstrable on the patient's right side **(A–D)**. *Continued on next page*

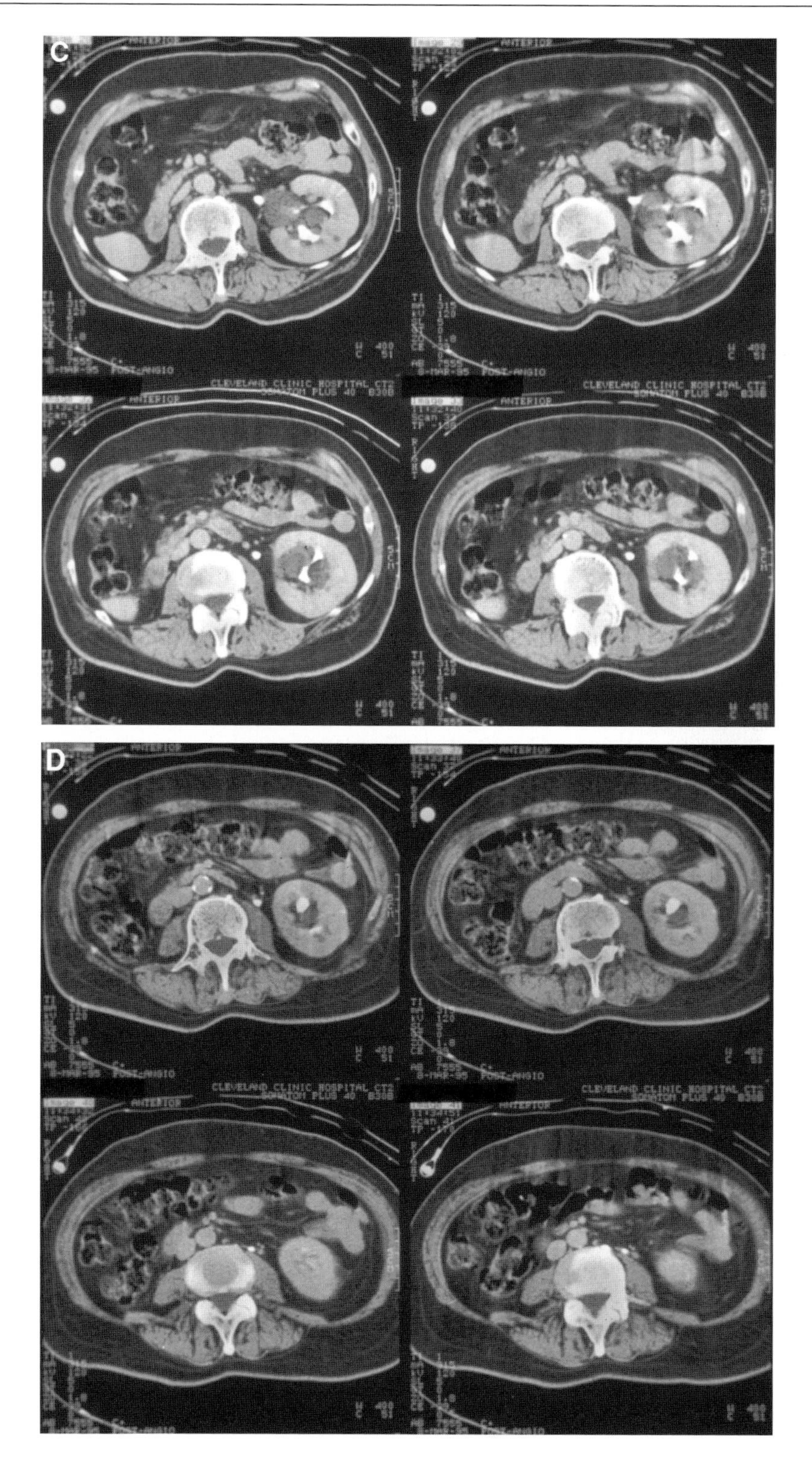

Fig. 8. *(Continued)* This CT scan demonstrates the hydronephrosis of the left upper-pole collecting system and a mass in the central portion of the renal pelvis of this solitary left kidney. No kidney is demonstrable on the patient's right side **(A–D)**.

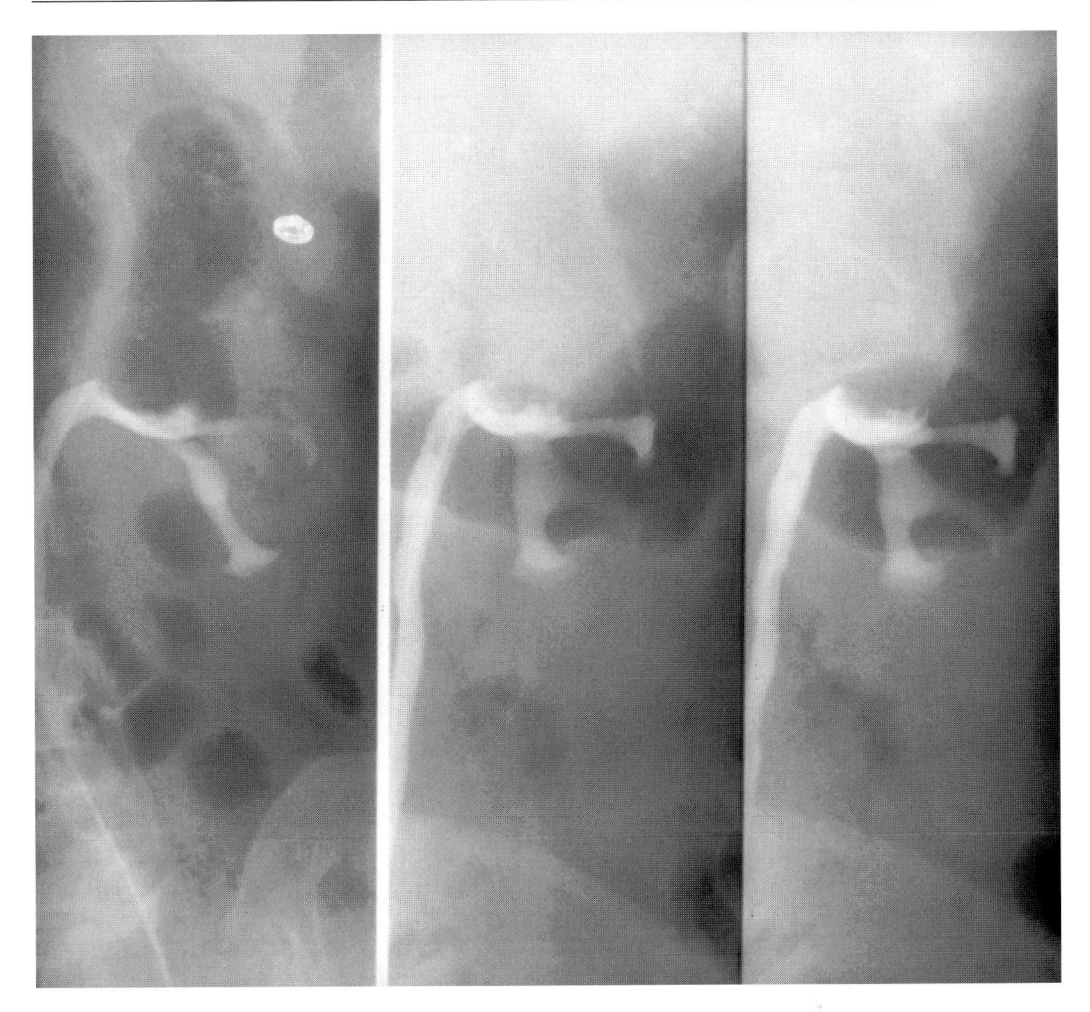

Fig. 9. Note the effacement of the upper collecting system with only the lower portion filling with contrast, as seen on this retrograde pyelogram.

Case 4

A 26-yr-old male who had previous EMT (paramedic) training was admitted to the hospital with a history of severe gross hematuria with clots occurring almost every day. He stated his hematuria was painless. He had a history of evaluation by three other urologists over the preceding 15 mo with no explanation for the hematuria despite thorough testing. Interestingly, the patient was not anemic. He underwent IVP, CT scan, renal arteriogram, and cystoscopy with retrograde pyelography. All tests were normal. Urine cytology demonstrated no evidence of cancer cells. The bleeding was so severe at times that the patient was placed on continuous bladder irrigation with a three-way Foley catheter. One morning, on rounds, the nurses noted the presence of a blood clot on the balloon injection port for the Foley catheter. Consultation with the hospital attorney ensued, and it was determined that:

1. The patient had given permission for evaluation and treatment of his hematuria, which included determination of the cause of the hematuria.

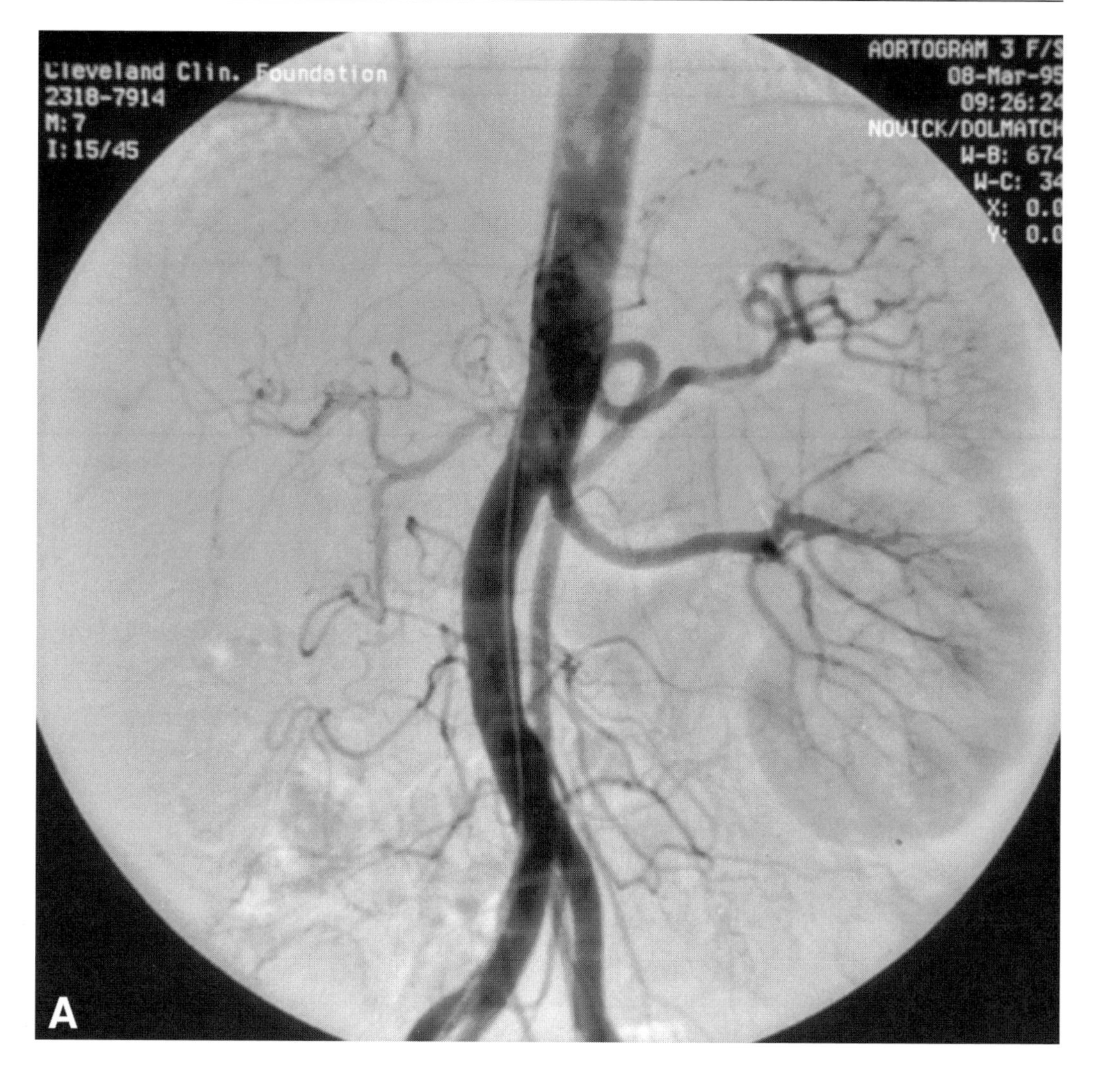

Fig. 10. Arteriography demonstrates the aorta with only an artery supplying the left kidney (absence of a right kidney; **A**) and selective contrast injection of the left renal artery (**B,** *see* facing page) reveals hypovascularity of the upper pole of the left kidney.

2. The only way to determine whether he was putting blood into his own urine was to search his belongings.
3. The hospital owned the patient's hospital room and closet and could certainly give permission to search these.

The patient's room and closet were therefore searched while he was in x-ray, and it was observed that paraphernalia were protruding from his jacket pocket (syringe with attached needle, plus a tourniquet). The patient was presented with this discovery and he at first denied, but then subsequently admitted, drawing his own blood and injecting it into urine containers and then into his Foley catheter to create convincing hematuria. It was his unfamiliarity with a three-way irrigation catheter that caused him

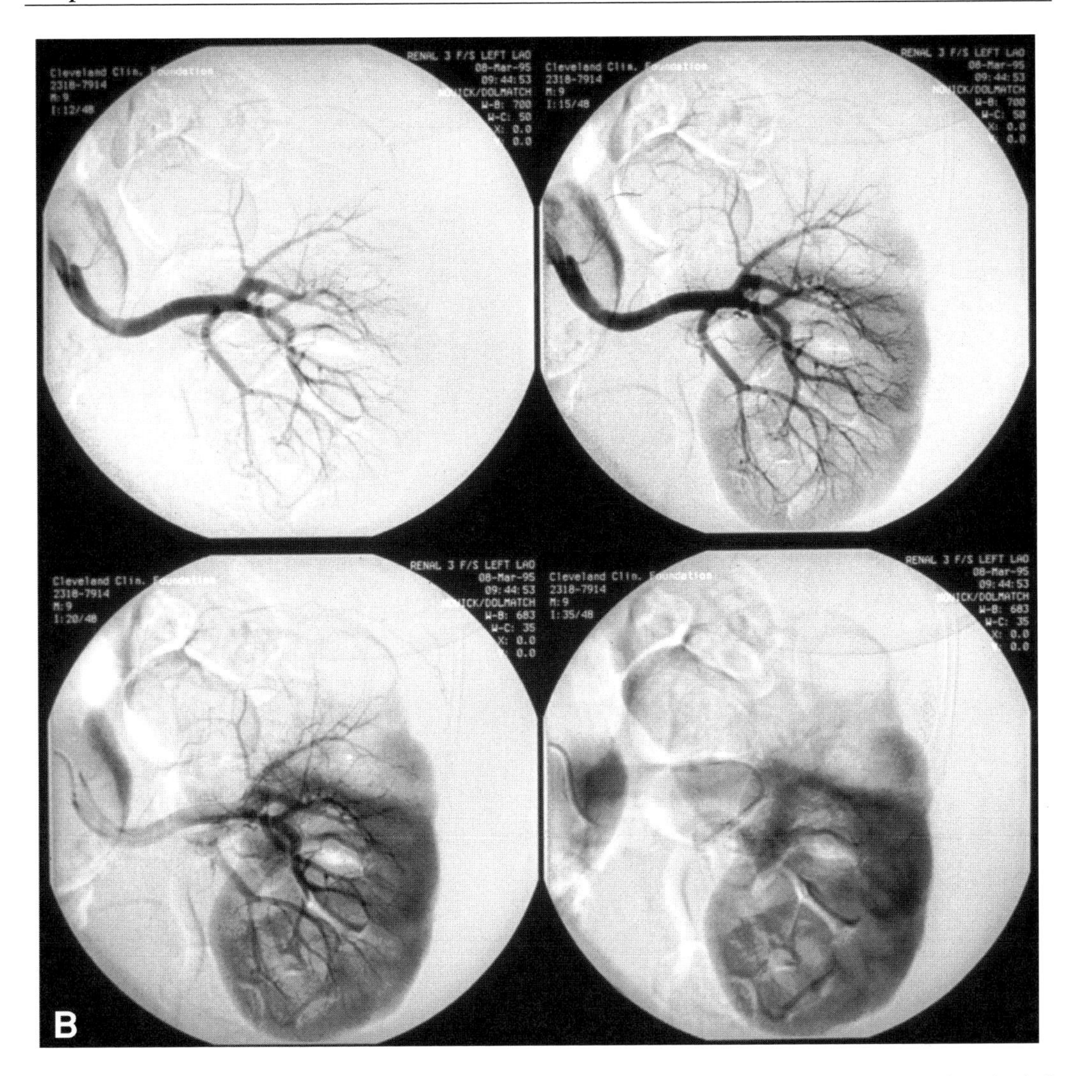

Fig. 10. *(Continued)* Arteriography demonstrates the aorta with only an artery supplying the left kidney (absence of a right kidney; **A**), and selective contrast injection of the left renal artery **(B)** reveals hypovascularity of the upper pole of the left kidney.

to err in his methodology. He was referred for psychiatric evaluation and treatment. No further gross hematuria occurred.

SUMMARY

This chapter presents an overview of the types of hematuria that may be encountered, the various methods to evaluate hematuria, some of the disorders that may commonly (and sometimes uncommonly) produce hematuria, and some of the major complications of hematuria. A summary of the current practice standard as set forth by the American Urological Association is included in a form designed to keep ideas as clear and as simple as possible. Although an entire textbook can be devoted to this subject, as it is a very broad one, one hopes that the reader at least has a better understanding of this subject that may enable improved care of patients presenting with hematuria. This, after all, is a major goal for any physician, whether he or she practices in family medicine or in some other specialty.

SUGGESTED READINGS

Abarbanel J, Benet AE, Lask D, Kimche D. Sports hematuria. J Urol 1990; 143: 887–890.

Ahmed Z, Lee J. Asymptomatic urinary abnormalities. Hematuria and proteinuria. Med Clin North Am 1997; 81: 641–652.

Banks RA, Stower M. Investigation of haematuria in adults. Br J Hosp Med 1989; 41: 476–480.

Bartlow BG. Microhematuria. Picking the fewest tests to make an accurate diagnosis. Postgrad Med 1990; 88: 51–55, 58, 61.

Benbassat J, Gergawi M, Offringa M, Drukker A. Symptomless microhaematuria in schoolchildren: causes for variable management strategies. Quar J Med 1996; 89: 845–854.

Bloom KJ. An algorithm for hematuria. Clin Lab Med 1988; 8: 577–584.

Bryden AA, Paul AB, Kyriakides C. Investigation of haematuria. Br J Hosp Med 1995; 54: 455–458.

Buntinx F, Wauters H. The diagnostic value of macroscopic haematuria in diagnosing urological cancers: a meta-analysis. Fam Pract 1997; 14: 63–68.

Copley JB. Isolated asymptomatic hematuria in the adult. Am J Med Sci 1986; 291: 101–111.

Corwin HL, Silverstein MD. Microscopic hematuria. Clin Lab Med 1988; 8: 601–610.

DeFelippo NP, Fortunato RP, Mellins HZ, Richie JP. Intravenous urography: important adjunct for diagnosis of bladder tumours. Br J Urol 1984; 56: 502–505.

Diven SC, Travis LB. A practical primary care approach to hematuria in children. Pediatr Nephrol 2000; 14: 65–72.

Feld LG, Waz WR, Perez LM, Joseph DB. Hematuria. An integrated medical and surgical approach. Pediatr Clin North Am 1997; 44: 1191–1210.

Foo KT. Surgical causes of haematuria—the diagnostic approach. Ann Acad Med Singapore 1987; 16: 235–237.

Gambrell RC, Blount BW. Exercised-induced hematuria. Am Family Phys 1996; 53: 905–911.

Grossfeld GD, Carroll PR. Evaluation of asymptomatic microscopic hematuria. Urol Clin North Am 1998; 25: 661–676.

Grossfeld GD, Wolf JS, Jr., Litwan MS, et al. Asymptomatic microscopic hematuria in adults: summary of the AUA best practice policy recommendations. Am Family Phys 2001; 63: 1145–1154.

Hall CL. The patient with haematuria. Practitioner 1999; 243: 564–566, 568, 570, 571.

Harper M, Arya M, Hamid R, Patel HR. Haematuria: a streamlined approach to management. Hosp Med 2001; 62: 696–698.

Hillman BJ. Digital imaging of the kidney. Radiol Clin North Am 1984; 22: 341–364.

Hillman BJ. Renal digital subtraction angiography. Urol Clin North Am 1985; 12: 699–713.

Kiel DP, Moskowitz MA. The urinalysis: a critical appraisal. Med Clin North Am 1987; 71: 607–624.

Lieu TA, Grasmeder HM III, Kaplan BS. An approach to the evaluation and treatment of microscopic hematuria. Pediatr Clin North Am 1991; 38: 579–592.

Mahan JD, Turman MA, Mentser MI. Evaluation of hematuria, proteinuria, and hypertension in adolescents. Pediatr Clin North Am 1997; 44: 1573–1589.

McCarthy JJ. Outpatient evaluation of hematuria: locating the source of bleeding. Postgrad Med 1997; 101: 125–128, 131.

Mokulis JA, Arndt WF, Downey JR, Caballero RL, Thompson IM. Should renal ultrasound be performed in the patient with microscopic hematuria and a normal excretory urogram? J Urol 1995; 154: 1300–1301.

Mota-Hernandez F, Munoz-Arizpe R, Lunar OR. Hematuria in children. Paediatrician 1979; 8: 270–286.

Mukherjee B. Haematuria. J Indian Med Assoc 1998; 96: 121–122.

Patel HP, Bissler JJ. Hematuria in children. Pediatr Clin North Am 2001; 48: 1519–1537.

Pollack HM. Some limitations and pitfalls of excretory urography. J Urol1976; 116: 537–543.

Restrepo NC, Carey PO. Evaluating hematuria in adults. Am Family Phys 1989; 40: 149–156.
Rockall AG, Newman-Sanders AP, al-Kutoubi MA, Vale JA. Haematuria. Postgrad Med J 1997; 73: 129–136.
Roth KS, Amaker B, Chan JC. Asymptomatic gross hematuria followed by persistent microhematuria. Acta Paediatr Taiwan 2000; 41: 2–5.
Roth KS, Amaker BH, Chan JC. Pediatric hematuria and thin basement membrane nephropathy: what is it and what does it mean? Clin Pediatr 2001; 40: 607–613.
Roy S III. Hematuria. Pediatr Ann 1996; 25: 284–287.
Roy C, Tuchmann C, Morel M, Saussine C, Jacqmin D, Tongio J. Is there still a place for angiography in the management of renal mass lesions? Eur Radiol 1999; 9: 329–335.
Sarosdy MF. The use of the BTA Test in the detection of persistent or recurrent transitional-cell cancer of the bladder. World J Urol 1997; 15: 103–106.
Schuster GA, Lewis GA. Clinical significance of hematuria in patients on anticoagulant therapy. J Urol 1987; 137: 923–925.
Segal AJ. Optimizing urography. World J Urol. 1998; 16: 3–8.
Shafer N, Shafer R. Factitious diseases including Munchausen's syndrome. N Y State J Med 1980; 80: 594–604.
Sizeland PC, Harris BH, Bailey RR. The patient with haematuria. N Z Med J1993; 106: 151–152.
Sokolosky MC. Hematuria. Emerg Med Clin North Am 2001; 19: 621–632.
Stapleton FB. Hematuria associated with hypercalciuria and hyperuricosuria: a practical approach. Pediatr Nephrol 1994; 8: 756–761.
Verstraete M. Psychogenic hemorrhages. Verh K Acad Geneeskd Belg 1991; 53 : 5–28.
Webb JA. Imaging in haematuria. Clin Radiol 1997; 52: 167–171.
Wood EG. Asymptomatic hematuria in childhood: a practical approach to evaluation. Indian J Pediatr 1999; 66: 207–214.
Woolhandler S, Pels RJ, Bor DH, Himmelstein DU, Lawrence RS. Dipstick urinalysis screening of asymptomatic adults for urinary tract disorders. I. Hematuria and proteinuria. JAMA 1989; 262: 1214–1219.

7 Evaluation and Medical Management of Kidney Stones

John C. Lieske, MD *and Joseph W. Segura*, MD

CONTENTS

INTRODUCTION

Urolithiasis is extremely common in Western societies, developing in up to 10% of men and 3% of women during their lifetimes *(1,2)*. The majority of stones (70–80%) are composed of calcium oxalate, either alone or admixed with calcium phosphate *(3)*. In many but not all individuals, the formation of calcium oxalate stones is associated with one or more urinary risk factors that include low urine volume, low pH, hypercalciuria, hyperuricosuria, or hyperoxaluria. Calcium phosphate is also a common constituent of stones, present to some extent in up to 80% *(4)*. However, less than 20% of stones are composed of more than half calcium phosphate, and pure calcium phosphate stones are rare, often seen in association with disorders of urinary acidification. Another 10% of stones are composed of uric acid, with or without a concurrent history of gout, or a mixture of uric acid and calcium oxalate. A similar percentage (10%) is composed of struvite, which develops in association with urinary tract infection caused by urease producing organisms, most often the *Proteus* species. Cystine stones comprise the remainder, probably no more than 1%, and arise only in patients with the autosomal-recessive disorder of cystinuria.

From: *Essential Urology: A Guide to Clinical Practice*
Edited by: J. M. Potts © Humana Press Inc., Totowa, NJ

Despite their common occurrence, the exact cellular mechanisms that mediate the formation of kidney stones remain poorly understood. Clearly, however, metabolic risk factors can be identified in many stone-forming individuals that increase stone-forming risk. In addition, treatment to correct those abnormalities that are identified can reduce the subsequent stone-forming rate. Therefore, in this chapter we will review metabolic risk factors and the corresponding treatment strategies for which there is strong evidence of clinical efficacy.

SUPERSATURATION PREDICTS STONE COMPOSITION

The importance of the urinary composition in the pathogenesis of stone disease is suggested by the observation that urinary supersaturation predicts stone composition. In a large study of patients with complete metabolic work-ups and known stone composition, those with calcium oxalate stones had supersaturated urine with respect to calcium oxalate, and those with calcium phosphate stones tended to be supersaturated with respect to that crystalline phase *(5)*. As a group, the urine of patients with brushite (BR) stones had a higher pH and low citrate concentration, whereas calcium oxalate stone-formers had more acidic urine. The urine of those with uric acid stones was most acidic of all. Individuals with mixed calcium oxalate and calcium phosphate stones had urine that was supersaturated with respect to both crystallization phases.

There were interesting differences between men and women in this study that, together with other studies, suggests that stone disease is a different process in the two sexes. The urine of normal men was supersaturated to almost the same extent as calcium oxalate stone-forming men, whereas the urine of calcium oxalate stone-forming women was also supersaturated to a similar extent *(5)*. In this respect, normal women formed a unique group with urine that was routinely undersaturated. The factors that produce supersaturation in stone-formers of both sexes also differed. The urine volume of stone-forming women was, on average, markedly lower than normal women, whereas the urinary volumes of calcium oxalate stone-forming men were not particularly low, and instead their supersaturation tended to be driven by overexcretion of stone-forming constituents, such as calcium. This study provides interesting clues as to why up to 80% of calcium oxalate stone-formers are men, since even "normal" men appear to have supersaturated "at-risk" urine, and also suggests that low urine volumes are an especially important risk factor for stone formation in women. Because supersaturation predicts stone composition, these data also provide good evidence that it is logical to use urinary supersaturation data to evaluate and treat patients with nephrolithiasis.

COST EFFECTIVENESS: WHY TREAT PROPHYLACTICALLY TO PREVENT STONES?

Medical prevention is widely accepted and recommended for patients with recurrent nephrolithiasis. However, an active treatment program requires laboratory evaluation, dietary changes, and medications and also entails a financial cost. Furthermore, although surgical intervention for symptomatic stones imposes definite risks, in the age of extracorporeal shock wave lithotripsy, ureteroscopic, and percutaneous procedures, the morbidity of surgical intervention is much reduced. In fact, it has been questioned whether medical evaluation and treatment to prevent stone formation can be justified on a financial basis alone. Such an evaluation does not take into consideration the pain and suffering that might be avoided by preventing acute stone events, factors that might, in and of themselves, justify preventative treatment, regardless of the financial analysis. Nevertheless, such a comprehensive analysis from the large stone clinic at the University of Chicago suggested that although medical evaluation and treatment of patients cost \$1068 per patient per year, \$3226 per patient per year was saved as a result of decreased stone events (and associated emergency room evaluations, hospitalizations, and procedures that were therefore not required; ref. *6*). The net savings were \$2158 per patient per year treated. The outcome of any such analysis will depend critically on the relative costs associated with evaluation, medications, and hospital procedures; however, several similar analyses also have suggested a net savings, albeit less quantitatively *(7)*. Nevertheless, medical evaluation and treatment to prevent kidney stones makes good economic sense, as well as medical sense.

DIETARY FACTORS

Nephrolithiasis has long been linked to affluence *(8)* and, hence, dietary factors have been implicated *(9)*. More recently, important epidemiological risk factors for stone formation have been identified in two large prospective studies of both men and women *(10,11)*. These were seminal studies because dietary data were prospectively obtained before the first stone event. Dietary factors that correlated with subsequent stone events included higher animal protein intake, lower potassium intake, lower fluid intake, and, somewhat surprisingly, lower calcium intake *(10)*. Although low dietary calcium appears to increase stone-forming potential, calcium supplements appear to increase stone risk *(12)*. Modest vitamin C supplementation did not increase stone-forming potential *(11,13)*, whereas pyridoxine (vitamin B_6) appeared to reduce stone forming potential, at least in women *(11)*. Somewhat surprisingly, and unexplained to date, use of grapefruit juice was associated with increased stone-forming potential in both groups *(14)*.

Physiological investigation suggests why some of these dietary habits may be associated with increased stone-forming potential. Dietary protein correlates with renal acid excretion, which in turn correlates with urinary calcium excretion *(15)*. Thus, a dietary protein load indirectly increases urinary calcium excretion. In a recent trial, dietary protein also increased urinary oxalate excretion in calcium oxalate stone formers, but not controls (Fig. 1). In addition, animal protein is the major dietary source of purines (Fig. 2), the precursors to uric acid; therefore, increased protein intake correlates with uric acid excretion *(16)*. Although the mechanism(s) are not clear, hyperuricosuria increases the risk of calcium oxalate stone formation. Uric acid solubility decreases dramatically at lower pH values *(17)* (Fig. 3). Metabolism of the sulfur-containing amino acids in a high protein diet reduces urinary pH; therefore, the excess uric acid generated from urine in a high protein diet will be excreted in an acid urine and be more likely to crystallize. Therefore, a high-protein diet appears to increase the stone-forming risk via several independent mechanisms.

Although there are good scientific reasons to predict that stone-formers should avoid a high-protein diet, patient outcome data to support this recommendation were lacking until recently. A randomized, long-term controlled trial of a low-animal protein, high-fiber diet was reported in which patients on the interventional diet actually formed significantly more stones than those advised to simply maintain a normal calcium intake and increase fluid ingestion *(18)*. The reasons for this unexpected outcome were not clear. More recently, however, a randomized, 5-yr trial compared

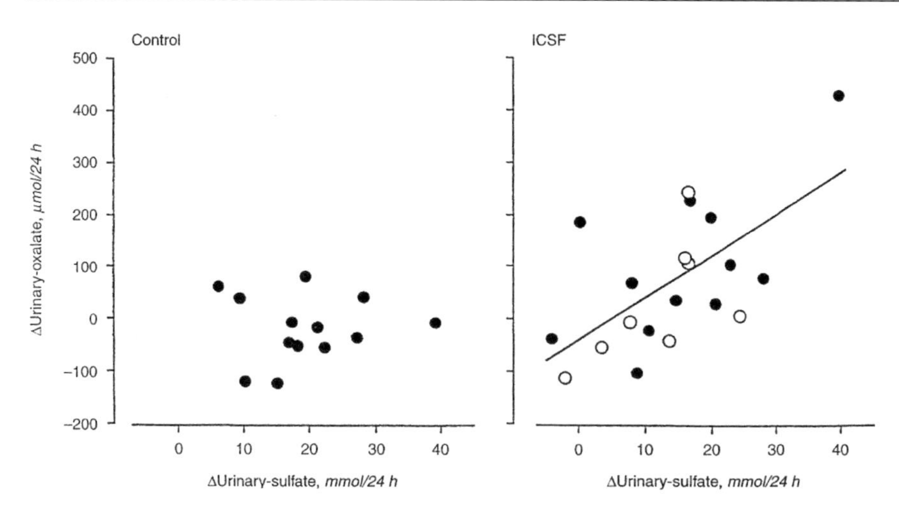

Fig. 1. Correlation between changes in urinary excretion of oxalate and sulfate in controls and idiopathic calcium stone-formers (ICSF). Increased urinary sulfate, an indicator of dietary protein intake, correlated with oxalate excretion in stone formers, but not controls. (From ref. *18a* with permission.)

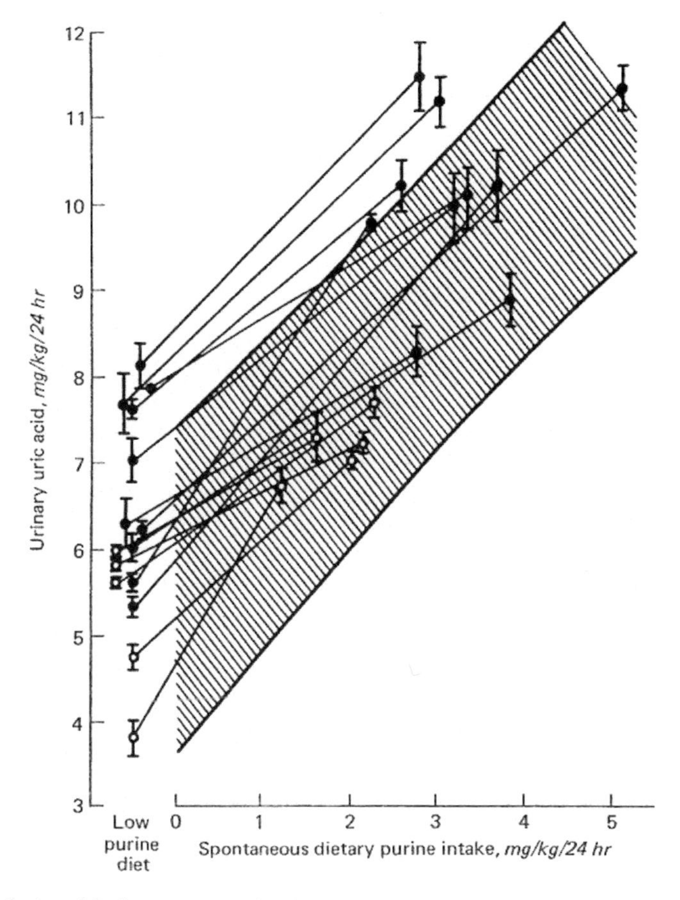

Fig. 2. Relationship between purine intake and uric acid excretion. There is a direct correlation between purine intake and uric acid excretion in both controls (○, open circles) and hyperuricosuric patients (●, closed circles). (From ref. *15* with permission.)

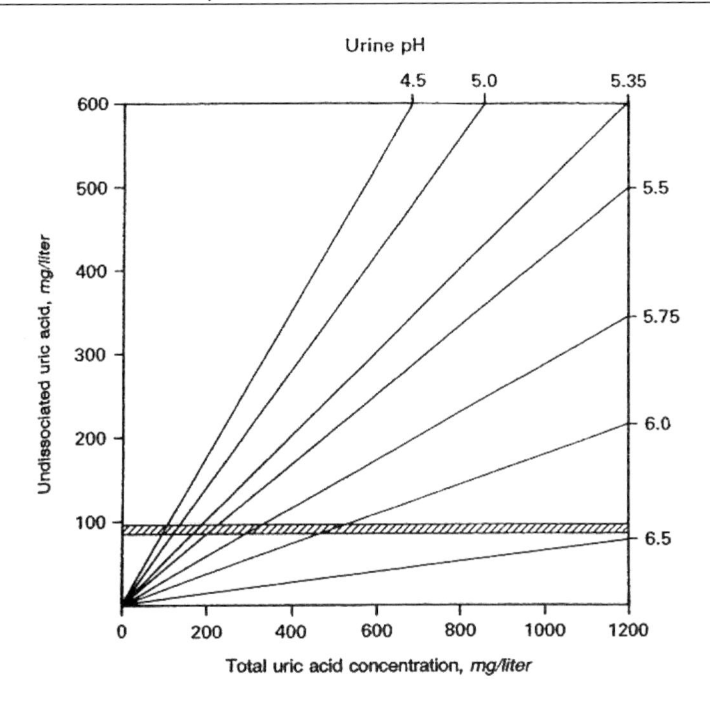

Fig. 3. Nomogram of undissociated uric acid concentration at values of urine pH and total uric acid concentration. The solubility limit for uric acid is indicated by the crosshatched bar. At a pH of 6.5, more than 1200 mg/L of total uric acid can remain in solution, whereas at a pH of 4.5 only 100 mg remains. (From ref. *17* with permission.)

stone recurrence in patients assigned to a low-calcium diet as compared with those on a normal calcium, low-protein, and low-sodium diet *(19)*. Both groups were advised to increase fluid intake. Those on the normal calcium, low-protein, and low-salt diet formed significantly less stones (Fig. 4). Urine chemistries disclosed lower urinary calcium and oxalate excretions in those on the normal calcium, low-protein diet, whereas those on the low-calcium diet had lower urinary calcium excretion but higher urinary oxalate levels. Therefore, not only are there good physiological reasons to recommend a diet low in protein and salt and normal in calcium to patients with idiopathic calcium urolithiasis, but this study now provides long-term outcome data to support its efficacy.

Sodium ingestion is another potential dietary risk factor for stone formation. Increased dietary sodium intake, and hence urinary sodium excretion, promotes calciuria both via renal mechanisms as well as increased calcium mobilization from bone *(20)*. Higher urinary sodium excretion also correlates with increased uric acid excretion and decreased citrate excretion, both of which promote crystallization. Therefore, although no controlled studies have demonstrated that sodium restriction alone can prevent stone formation, and sodium intake did not correlate with stone formation risk in a prospective study *(12)*, a recommendation that stone-formers modestly reduce dietary salt makes good sense *(19)*.

The importance of mild hyperoxaluria in stone pathogenesis remains controversial. In the absence of bowel disease, endogenous metabolism contributes a larger propor-

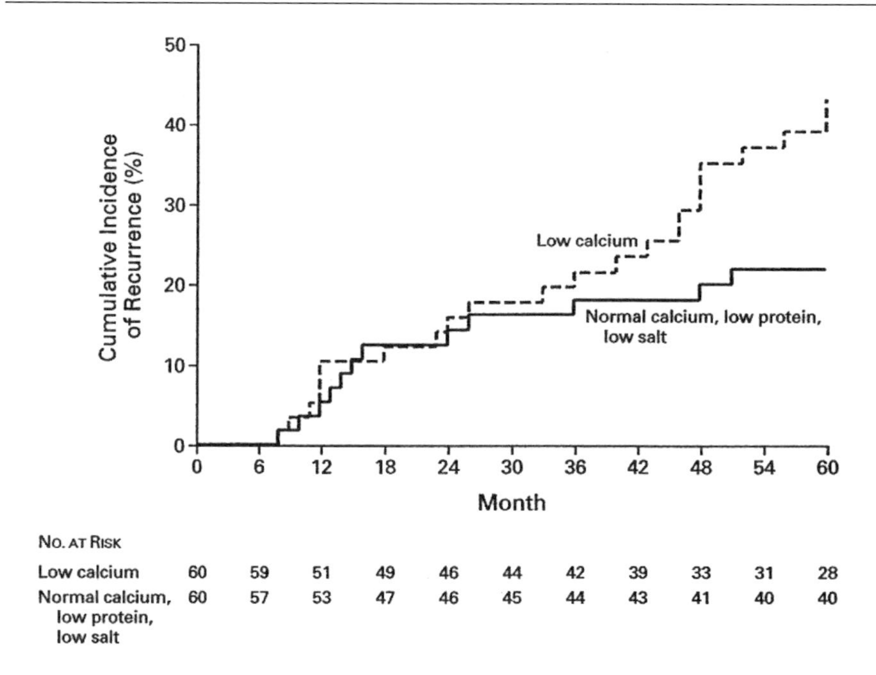

Fig. 4. Kaplan–Meier estimates of the cumulative incidence of recurrent stones, on controlled diets. After 60 mo, there were significantly less stone events in patients on the low protein, normal calcium, low salt diet compared to a low calcium diet ($p < 0.04$). (From ref. *19* with permission. Copyright © 2002, Massachusetts Medical Society. All rights reserved.)

tion of urinary oxalate than does dietary oxalate, and dietary calcium and/or other factors may influence absorption of oxalate to a greater extent that the amount of oxalate ingested *per se*. Furthermore, no epidemiological data link dietary oxalate to stone formation risk, and no studies suggest that dietary restriction reduces the stone formation rate. However, it is obviously prudent for all calcium oxalate stone forming patients to limit their intake of high oxalate foods. Finally, we must stress that it is essential for all patients with fat malabsorption (from any cause) to strictly adhere to a low-oxalate diet.

ENVIRONMENTAL FACTORS

Environmental or occupational factors, as well as the presence of any bowel disease associated with diarrhea and/or malabsorption, can each predispose to stone disease. For example, residents of the "stone belt" in the southeastern Untied States are at increased risk of stone disease *(21)*. In this case, two factors have been hypothesized: climate-induced perspiration resulting in a more concentrated urine, and sunlight-induced vitamin D conversion promoting calcium absorption from food.

THE STONE CLINIC EFFECT AND THE SINGLE STONE-FORMER

Many individuals will present after having passed a single kidney stone, with no other stones apparent on a radiologic study. What is the proper advice? The "stone clinic effect" is the well-described phenomenon that the severity of stone disease seems to decrease after evaluation in a stone clinic, even if medications are not prescribed *(22)*.

A large component of this effect appears to be a tendency to increase fluid intake, presumably based on advice received at the clinic visit. In a group of 108 calcium oxalate stone-formers treated conservatively with dietary recommendations, those 63 who remained metabolically inactive increased their urine volume on average 493 mL, whereas the urine volume did not change in the 45 patients who formed new stones *(22)*. These patients were also advised to limit meat intake to one meal daily and limit calcium to one serving of dairy products daily in addition to drinking fluids to maintain urine volumes 2.5 L (8–12 glasses daily, at least half being water), so these observations do not prove that increased fluid intake was responsible for the fall in stone activity. However, experimental evidence also suggests that increased urine dilution should be an effective measure to reduce stone-forming potential. When the mean urine volume of six stone-formers and two normal individuals was increased from 1.023 to 2.383 L/d (by ingesting excess distilled water), the supersaturation (urinary activity product ratio) for calcium phosphate, calcium oxalate, and uric acid all decreased, and the minimum supersaturation needed to elicit spontaneous calcium oxalate nucleation (formation product ratio) increased *(23)*. These data provide important in vivo evidence that drinking excess water increases urine dilution and diminishes urinary supersaturation.

Importantly, a controlled trial also supports the effectiveness of increased fluid intake to prevent stones. In a group of 220 first-time stone-formers, half were randomized to a program of increased water intake to maintain urine volumes greater than 2 L, whereas the remainder were told to continue with their ambient diet and habits (Fig. 5) *(24)*. Patients in the intervention group successfully maintained urine volumes greater than 2 L for the 5 yr of the study, up from a baseline of about 1000 mL in both groups. Urine supersaturation for calcium oxalate, calcium phosphate, and uric acid, as assessed by the computer program EQUIL2, fell on this regimen, and the 5-yr stone recurrence rate decreased from 27% in the control group to 12% in the intervention group. This important study clearly demonstrates that a program to increase urine volumes is achievable and effective.

After a single stone, approx 50% of patients will have a second stone within 10 yr and up to 80% within 20–30 yr *(25)*. The recurrence rate appears to accelerate after a second stone *(26)*. Therefore, there is a definite but perhaps modest risk of recurrence after a single stone attack, but the risk of recurrence increases after passage of a second. Because of these observations, metabolic evaluation and prescription of a medical regimen to prevent stone recurrence is often deferred in patients with single stones. It is important to remember, however, that the number of stone events before initiation of a treatment program worsens the outcome, that is, increases the likelihood of passing more stones. Therefore, how aggressively to evaluate and treat the single stone-former is to some extent a subjective consideration based on how complicated the first stone passage was and how motivated the patient is to prevent recurrence. One compromise approach to the single stone-former is a limited evaluation that includes a thorough history and physical, stone analysis (if possible), serum calcium (to screen for systemic conditions associated with hypercalcemia and stone disease), urinalysis (and culture if indicated, to screen for infection), and finally a good radiographic study (kidneys–ureters–bladder or computed tomography [CT]) to look for additional, asymptomatic stones *(27)*. If the patient indeed fits into that group of patients who have truly formed a single calcium stone, and this event was fairly uncomplicated, then a trial of conservative therapy consisting of dietary recommendations emphasizing increased fluid intake has a high likelihood of success *(22)*.

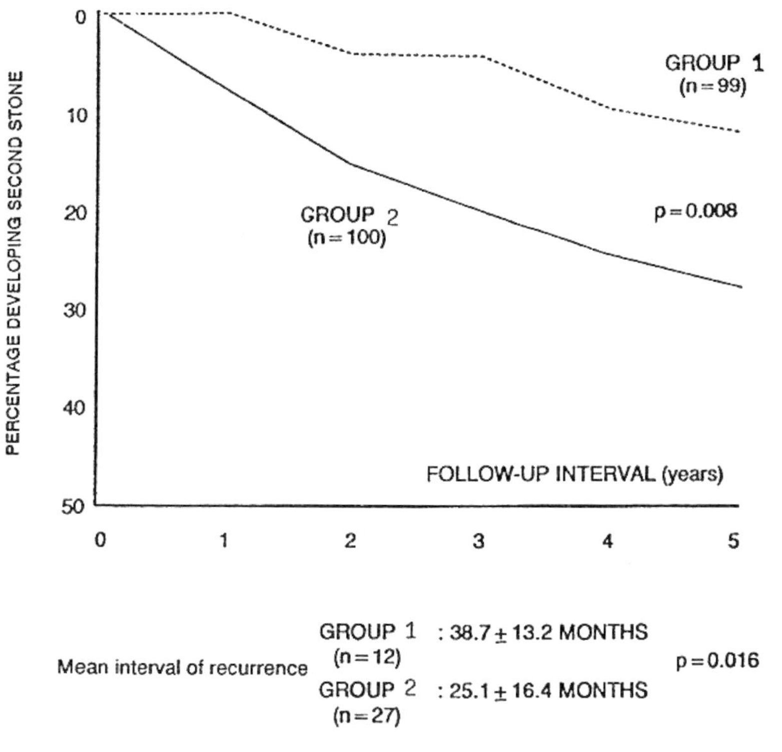

Fig. 5. Effect of increased water intake on stone recurrence rate over 5 yr. Increased water intake alone (group 2) can significantly reduce stone recurrence rate. (From ref. *24* with permission.)

EVALUATION OF THE RECURRENT STONE-FORMER

Serum Studies

As a baseline, renal function can be assessed via a serum blood urea nitrogen and creatinine level, and an electrolyte panel can be drawn to screen for acidosis or hypokalemia, both of which could contribute to hypocitraturia. A serum calcium and phosphorous can also be drawn to screen for hyperparathyroidism, because in the absence of hypercalcemia, hyperparathyroidism is extremely unlikely *(28)*. Finally, a serum uric acid level is useful to screen for a gouty diatheses, especially if allopurinol is considered a therapeutic option.

Urine Studies

A urinalysis should be performed to screen for pyuria, and hence, evidence of infection, and a 24-h urine obtained to identify metabolic risk factors for stone formation. Essential analytes include volume, pH, citrate, calcium, oxalate, uric acid, sodium (as a guide to salt ingestion, which can influence calcium excretion), and creatinine (as a guide to completeness of the collection). In known or suspected cystine stone-formers, cystine excretion should be quantitated, unless a stone analysis is available to exclude this possibility.

The supersaturation of urine can be assessed if one measures the concentration of all the ions that can interact, including calcium, chloride, citrate, magnesium, oxalate, pH, phosphate, potassium, sodium, sulfate, and uric acid *(29)*. Once the concentrations of all these relevant urinary ions are known, the iterative computer program EQUIL2 can calculate the theoretical supersaturation value with respect to the important crystalline phases *(29)*. EQUIL2 uses the measured concentrations of the ions and their known affinity constants for each other at the given pH, and calculates a supersaturation for each ion pair of interest (e.g., calcium oxalate, calcium phosphate, and uric acid). Knowledge of the relative supersaturations is useful in diagnosing and managing patients with kidney stones. Urine is often supersaturated with respect to crystalline stone constituents (e.g., calcium oxalate), even in the urine of nonstone-formers. However, on average the urine of those individuals who do form kidney stones is more saturated and the "normal" values are simply derived by comparing supersaturation values for the important stone-forming crystalline phases between a population of stone-formers and a population of nonstone-formers.

Because the supersaturation of urine correlated with stone type in a large series of patients (in the absence of an available stone analysis; ref. *5*), calculated supersaturation data can also be used to infer stone type. In addition, therapy is logically targeted towards decreasing those urinary supersaturations that are identified. During follow-up, changes in the urine supersaturation can be used to monitor the effectiveness of therapy in order to confirm that the crystallization potential has indeed decreased.

The number of 24-h urine collections that are necessary to identify important risk factors is not absolute. Clearly, metabolic abnormalities will be identified more frequently if three collections are considered (2.79 abnormalities per patient) than if only one (0.83 abnormalities per patient) or even two collections (approx 2.0 abnormalities per patient) are performed *(30)*, presumably because of dietary and other environmental factors. Individual analytes do, however, correlate quite significantly between 24-h samples *(31)*. Therefore, in many cases, a single 24-h urine sample may suffice to identify the most important metabolic abnormality, although in difficult or complicated cases two or even three samples might be necessary. If treatment is begun based on a single 24-h urine sample, or dietary and/or pharmacological changes are prescribed, a repeat 24-h urine study 4–6 weeks later is an important way not only to gauge the effect of therapy but also to screen for additional abnormalities that might have been missed.

Stone Analysis

Stone analysis is relatively inexpensive and should be performed for all first stones, and those that are passed by patients on a treatment regimen, especially if there is an associated infection. Typically analysis is accomplished on a pulverized sample of the stone by comparing an infrared spectrum profile to reference spectra of known stone components. Although most (>90%) are composed of calcium oxalate, calcium phosphate, uric acid, or an admixture of these components, stone analysis can confirm the presence of struvite stones (indicating infection), more unusual stone components such as cystine, or even drugs (e.g., Indinavir). An evaluation and treatment algorithm has been proposed based on stone composition alone *(32)* and, as a minimum, the stone composition is an important piece of data to be considered together with urinary studies to guide treatment strategies. For example, patients with calcium oxalate stones should be carefully screened for hypercalciuria, hyperoxaluria, and low urinary citrate, whereas those individuals with calcium phosphate stones should be evaluated for a urinary acidification defect (high urine pH and low urine citrate), in addition to hypercalciuria. The presence of uric acid, alone or combined with calcium oxalate, suggests that alkalinization with citrate might be an effective strategy to prevent future stones, given the marked increase in uric acid solubility at a higher pH (*see* below). Patients with cystine stones should have a 24-h urine to quantitate cystine excretion, as well as to assess urine volume and pH. The presence of struvite stones suggests that an aggressive surgical intervention will be required to remove all stone material, with close follow-up and a prolonged course of appropriate antibiotics.

Radiological Investigation

Helical CT scanning is the preferred method to screen for stones. Unlike calcium stones, uric acid stones are not visualized using routine radiography without contrast dye, although they will be seen on CT. In addition, helical CT scanning is faster and more sensitive than intravenous pyelography and may even be more cost effective *(33)*.

STONE-CAUSING SYNDROMES

Hypercalciuria

Hypercalciuria is a biological syndrome usually defined as a 24-h urinary calcium excretion greater than 0.1 mmol/kg or greater than 7.5 mmol in males and 6.25 mmol in females, in the absence of dietary manipulations *(34)*. Dietary imbalances and a number of endocrine, renal, and bone diseases can cause secondary hypercalciuria (Table 1; ref. *35*). If clinical and laboratory investigation fails to identify a cause, patients are classified as having idiopathic hypercalciuria. Overall, hypercalciuria is present in up to 50% of patients with calcium urolithiasis.

Primary Hyperparathyroidism

Primary hyperparathyroidism should be considered in all patients with calcium urolithiasis, especially if hypercalciuria is present. A serum calcium determination is a good screen because patients with primary hyperparathyroidism are unlikely to have normal serum calcium (Fig. 6). This distinction is not absolute, and if the serum calcium is high normal, and hyperparathyroidism remains a consideration, an intact PTH determination is the definitive test *(36)*. Other elements of the history and physical will suggest other more unusual causes of hypercalciuria, listed in Table 1.

Idiopathic Hypercalciuria

In general, the factors that can contribute to hypercalciuria are overabsorption of calcium from the intestine, mobilization of calcium from bone, and impaired reabsorption of calcium in the kidney. A classification scheme was developed to evaluate patients and determine which factor was prominent in each by measuring calcium excretion on high-, normal-, and low-calcium diets, as well as while fasting *(37)*. However, in general clinical practice the protocol is cumbersome to perform, and it is now recognized that there is considerable overlap among groups *(38)*. For example, many patients classified as "absorptive" hypercalciuria will assume a negative calcium balance when placed on a low calcium diet, suggesting that increased intestinal calcium absorption is not the only defect. Although this classification scheme is a valuable tool to characterize patients for research studies, it probably is not necessary or helpful during routine patient care *(39)*.

Urinary calcium is dependent on dietary calcium, and about 6% of intake is excreted in the urine *(40)*. This proportion increases two- to threefold in patients with idiopathic

Table 1
Causes of Hypercalciuria

Dietary causes • Excessive vitamin D and calcium supplements • Excessive salt intake (>6 g/d) • High animal protein intake	Increased intestinal calcium absorption • Sarcoidosis and other granulomatous diseases • Severe hypophosphatemia (Fanconi's syndrome)
Increased bone osteoclastic resorption • Immobilization • Bone metastases, myeloma • Paget's disease • Hyperthyroidism • Cushing's syndrome, glucocorticoid therapy • Renal tubular acidosis	Decreased renal tubular calcium reabsorption • Loop diuretics • Genetic renal tubular disorders: X-linked hypercalciuric nephrolithiasis (Dent's disease) *(177)*, mutations of calcium-sensing receptor *(178)* • Barter's syndrome
Primary hyperparathyroidism[a]	Idiopathic

[a] Acts via renal, intestinal, and bone mechanisms.

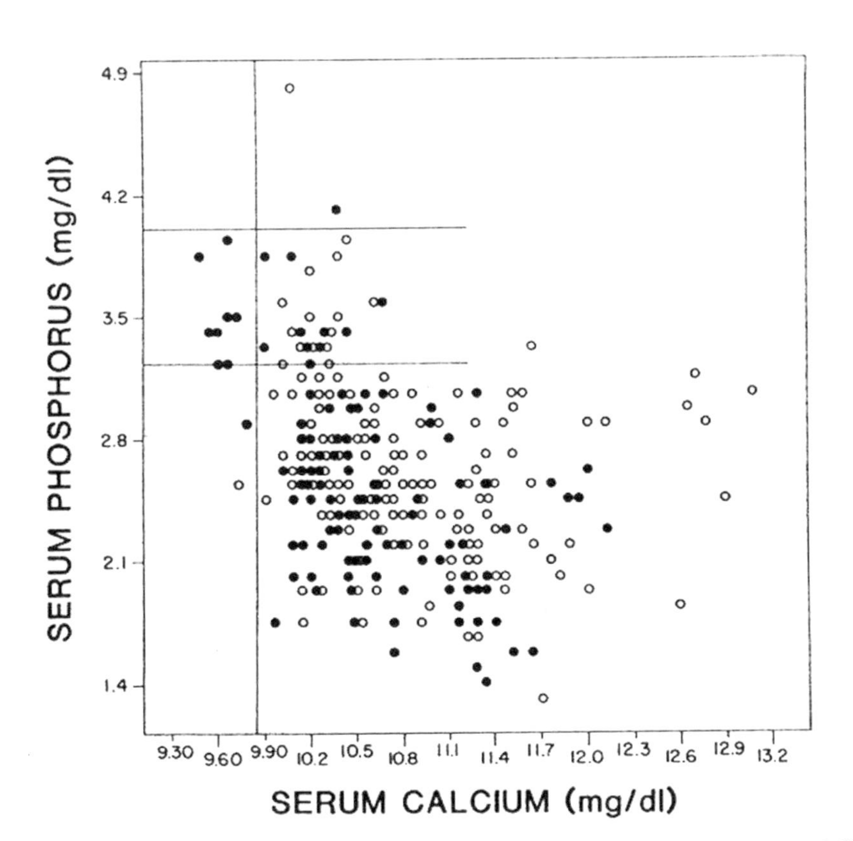

Fig. 6. Calcium and phosphorous values in surgically proven hyperparathyroidism. The vast majority exhibited hypercalcemia and hypophosphatemia. (From ref. *28* with permission.)

hypercalciuria because increased intestinal absorption of calcium is the distinguishing feature of idiopathic hypercalciuria *(41)*. Evidence supporting abnormalities of vitamin D action and/or the vitamin D receptor *(42)*, as well as renal tubular reabsorption of calcium *(43,44)*, have both been reported. However, the exact molecular defect that underlies the pathogenesis of hypercalciuria in the majority of these patients remains elusive.

There is evidence that bone mineral density is reduced in patients with idiopathic hypercalciuria, although in the majority of patients the loss is moderate *(45)*. In population-based studies of urolithiasis patients, the long-term risk of forearm fracture was not increased *(46)*, although the risk of vertebral fracture was *(47)*. These studies included stone patients with and without hypercalciuria, so that the effect of hypercalciuria on fracture risk may have been diluted. In a placebo-controlled trial, use of thiazide diuretics for 3 yr did help to preserve bone mass in a group of elderly men and women. By inference, use of thiazides may well help preserve bone mass in patients with hypercalciuria. Certainly, the presence of osteopenia, or other risk factors for osteoporosis, is an important consideration when electing whether or not to treat hypercalciuric stone patients with a thiazide diuretic.

Treatment of hypercalciuria starts with dietary recommendations. The calcium intake should be normal (approx 800–1000 mg per d) and not reduced. Lower calcium diets may cause bone mineral loss and even increase the stone forming risk *(12)*. Calcium pill supplements are, however, discouraged because they may increase stone-forming potential *(48)*. Moderation in dietary sodium (<200 mmol/d) and protein (<1mg/kg/day) are encouraged. In some individuals, these dietary measures may be sufficient, if long-term compliance is achieved.

If pharmacological intervention is required, a thiazide diuretic is the treatment of choice, especially since thiazides can improve calcium balance *(49)*. Two 3-yr placebo-controlled trials support the efficacy of thiazides to decrease stone-forming risk by about 50% *(50,51)*. Hydrochlorothiazide is effective but often must be dosed twice daily for a sufficiently sustained biologic effect. Chlorthalidone has a longer half-life and can be dosed once daily, but hypokalemia is also more likely. Adherence to a low-salt diet is essential to limit hypokalemia, as well as to maximize the hypocalciuric effects. Amiloride is a helpful adjunct if hypokalemia occurs. If a potassium supplement is needed, potassium citrate is preferred. It is essential to treat hypokalemia because hypokalemia can indirectly reduce urinary citrate excretion via effects on proximal tubular cells. In patients who cannot tolerate thiazides, Neutra-Phos (Ortho McNeil Pharmaceutical, San Bruno, CA; e.g., 500 mg QID) represents an alternative therapeutic option *(52)* because it decreases calcium excretion presumably via direct effects on renal tubular calcium reabsorption and/or on vitamin D production *(53)*. Thiazide may not suppress urinary calcium excretion indefinitely in certain patients with an absorptive form of hypercalciuria *(54)*, and Neutra-Phos represents a second option for these patients whose urinary calcium rises on thiazide. Although observational studies suggest benefit in stone formation risk *(55)*, no controlled trials have been performed to document the efficacy of Neutra-Phos. In addition, because of the gastrointestinal side effects and the requirement for multiple times per day dosing, it is not as well tolerated as thiazide diuretics. A newer preparation (UroPhos-K; Mission Pharmacol, San Antonio, TX) is under investigation, appears to be well tolerated and has short-term beneficial effects on urinary supersaturation in patients with idiopathic hypercalciuria *(56)*, but is not generally available yet. Calcium binders (e.g., sodium cellulose phosphate) have no proven utility and may result in diminished bone density.

Hyperoxaluria

Idiopathic Hyperoxaluria

The relative importance of hyperoxaluria as a cause of calcium oxalate stone disease remains controversial, especially in relationship to hypercalciuria. Many, but not all studies have identified mild hyperoxaluria in a large subset of these patients *(57)*. In addition, in normal urine the ratio of calcium to oxalate is usually equal to or greater than 5:1 (calcium to oxalate). Because the stoichiometric relationship between calcium and oxalate in calcium oxalate crystals is 1:1 and because the greatest crystalline mass is produced when they are closest to equimolar, increases in urinary oxalate should have a greater influence on crystalline mass than increase in oxalate *(3)*. Furthermore, in the normal urinary range, small changes in oxalate concentration influence supersaturation with respect to calcium oxalate far more than changes in calcium concentrations *(57)*. These predictions are supported by in vitro studies performed in urine because it is easy to initiate calcium oxalate crystallization by addition of oxalate, but difficult by adding excess calcium *(58)*.

Studies in the Arabian Peninsula strongly support an important role for hyperoxaluria in nephrolithiasis. Stone disease is fairly common in this population, affecting up to 20% *(57)*. Studies of patients there revealed relatively marked hyperoxaluria, and a lack of hypercalciuria. Compared with a typical Western diet, the typical Arabian diet is lower in calcium (approx 50%) and higher in oxalate (approx 250%; ref. *3*), allowing overabsorption of "free" oxalate from the intestine *(57)*. Because most common syndromes of idiopathic hypercalciuria are associated with overabsorption of calcium from the intestine, it has been proposed that, somewhat paradoxically, patients with idiopathic hypercalciuria may be predisposed to stone formation because of oxalate over absorption *(3)*. There is some in vivo evidence to support this hypothesis because in a study of 96 calcium oxalate stone-formers those with the greatest calcium absorption also had the highest oxalate excretion *(3)*. In addition, in a small group of normal controls, administration of spinach increased calcium oxalate supersaturation to greater extent than milk, and this effect was largely blunted when the milk and spinach were given together *(3)*. These limited studies support the importance of "free" intestinal calcium and oxalate in controlling oxalate absorption from the gut, and hence elimination in the urine.

Treatment of patients with idiopathic hyperoxaluria includes recommendations to avoid high oxalate foods, such as spinach, chocolate, and nuts. In metabolically active stone-formers without other identified abnormalities, potassium citrate can be used in addition to decrease the nucleation and growth of calcium oxalate crystals.

Enteric Hyperoxaluria

Patients with inflammatory bowel disease have a risk of nephrolithiasis that is 10–100 times the general population, ranging from 1 to 25% *(59)*. Enteric hyperoxaluria has been documented in other diverse malabsorptive states, including after jejunoileal bypass for obesity *(60–62)*, after gastric ulcer surgery *(61)*, and in the setting of chronic mesenteric ischemia *(61)*. Patients often have multiple stones and those with ileocolonic disease (9–17%) are more commonly affected compared with those with ileal (6–8%) or colonic disease (3–5%) alone. The kidney stones that form are primarily composed of calcium oxalate if the ileum is involved (e.g., ileocolonic Crohn's disease), or uric acid when patients have copious diarrhea or small bowel ostomies *(59)*.

Contributing factors include a low urinary pH, low urinary citrate concentration, and decreased urine volumes, all caused by the diarrhea and consequent loss of fluid and bicarbonate in the stool. In addition, increased intestinal oxalate absorption produces hyperoxaluria *(63)*. Two mechanisms of increased colonic oxalate uptake are commonly purported: (1) bile salt malabsorption caused by the ileal disease, resulting in fat malabsorption; increased colonic fats then bind to free calcium, increasing unbound oxalate that is able to cross the colonic mucosa; and (2) colonic permeability is increased by malabsorbed fatty acids and bile acids, perhaps induced by changes in epithelial tight junctions allowing oxalate to pass from the intestine into the blood stream. In malabsorptive states, the percentage of oxalate absorbed from the gut and excreted in urine can be markedly increased, and hyperoxaluria correlates with steatorrhea *(64)*. Unabsorbed bile acids may also exert damaging effects on intestinal oxalate-metabolizing bacteria, thereby increasing oxalate available for absorption *(65)*.

In the kidney, hyperoxaluria enhances calcium oxalate crystal formation and deposition. Possible contributing factors include low urinary volumes, low urinary citrate, and a low urinary pH. The low pH favors uric acid precipitation, which in turn can promote calcium oxalate crystal formation. In addition to calcium oxalate stones, chronic severe hyperoxaluria is associated with interstitial fibrosis and renal scarring *(66–68)*. Cellular responses to oxalate ion or calcium oxalate crystals may both contribute to this pathologic outcome *(66,69–71)*.

Treatment strategies for enteric hyperoxaluria depend largely on dietary modification. Important components include dietary restriction of oxalate (to limit its delivery to the colon); a low-fat diet (to limit fat malabsorption and the distal colonic effects of fatty acids and bile acids; refs. *72*, *73*); oral calcium (to bind oxalate; ref. *60*); and bile acid sequestrants, such as cholestyramine (to limit colonic irritation by bile acids; refs. *64*, *72*). Dietary recommendations are not always entirely effective because many patients cannot identify causative dietary constituents in their own diets *(74)*. In its entirety, this dietary regimen is quite rigorous for patients, and even if compliance is achieved, the therapy is not always effective. Therefore, newer treatment strategies are sorely needed.

Primary Hyperoxaluria

The primary hyperoxalurias, initially described in the 1920s, are now known to be caused by a deficiency of enzymes important in metabolic pathways of glyoxylate and other intermediates that lead to oxalate synthesis *(75)*. Increased understanding of the subcellular targeting of alanine glyoxylate transferase (AGT) has revealed heterogeneous causes of deficient AGT activity resulting in type I primary hyperoxaluria (PHI; ref. *76*), whereas the enzymology of type II primary hyperoxaluria (PHII) is just beginning to be understood *(77)* with identification of the causative gene (glyoxylate/hydroxypyruvate reductase) by two laboratories within the past few years (Fig. 7; refs. *78*, *79*). The molecular genetics of PHI is complex, and to date 25 separate mutations of the AGT complex have been implicated in type I primary hyperoxaluria *(80,81)*.

With increased understanding of the primary hyperoxalurias and availability of earlier and more reliable diagnostic techniques, the clinical heterogeneity of PHI and PHII is increasingly apparent. The initial clinical manifestations of the primary hyperoxalurias may occur in infancy, or not until mid- to late-adulthood *(82–85)*. A wide range of urine oxalate excretion rates is observed, from 0.8 mmol/1.73 m^2/d to as high as 3.8 mmol/1.73 m^2/d *(82,86)*. Long-term renal prognosis is widely variable, with some patients progress-

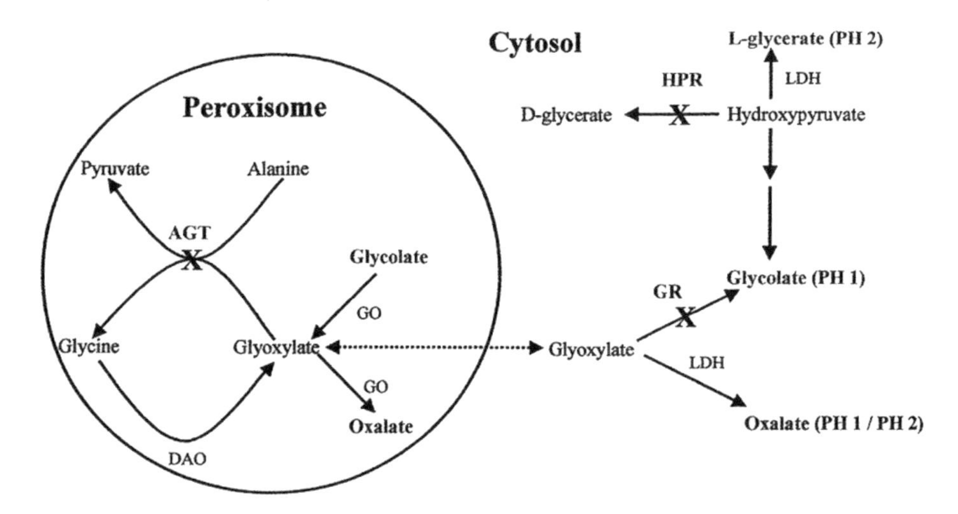

Fig. 7. Metabolic defects in primary hyperoxaluria. AGT activity is deficient in PHI, allowing excess conversion of glyoxylate to oxalate and glycolate. Pyridoxine is a cofactor for AGT. Glyoxalate/hydroxypyruvate reductase is defective in PHII, allowing excess conversion of hydroxypyruvate to L-glycerate and oxalate. (From ref. *85a* with permission.)

ing to end-stage renal disease in infancy or early childhood, whereas others retain satisfactory renal function even into the seventh decade of life *(82–84)*. Clinical experience suggests that patients with PHII have a more favorable long-term outcome than those with PHI *(86)*.

All PH patients should receive a trial of pyridoxine (5 mg/kg/d for 3 mo followed by 10 mg/kg/d for 3 mo), an important co-factor for AGT activity. Limited studies suggest that approximately one-third of patients with PHI will have improvement or normalization of urine oxalate excretion while receiving pharmacological doses of pyridoxine. Both neutral phosphate *(82)*, and potassium citrate *(87)* have been advocated for treatment of patients with primary hyperoxaluria to reduce urinary supersaturation with respect to calcium oxalate, and one or the other should be employed. Other important factors are strict adherence to a low oxalate diet and adequate fluid intake to maintain maximally dilute urine. Long-term clinical follow-up suggests that with careful clinical care, renal function can be preserved indefinitely in many patients *(82)*. If a patient progresses to end-stage renal failure, a combined kidney–liver transplant is curative *(88)*.

Low Urinary Citrate

Citrate retards crystallization of stone-forming salts in vitro because it inhibits spontaneous nucleation of calcium oxalate, retards agglomeration of calcium oxalate crystals, inhibits calcium phosphate crystal growth, and prevents heterogeneous nucleation of calcium oxalate by monosodium urate *(89)*. Hypocitraturia has been identified in a sizable number of patients with calcium urolithiasis, ranging from 19 to 63% in different series *(89)*.

Table 2
Causes of Low Urinary Citrate Excretion

Causes
Systemic acidosis
• Renal tubular acidosis
• Chronic diarrhea
Magnesium, potassium depletion
Excessive meat, protein intake
Idiopathic

Urinary citrate excretion is importantly influenced by the systemic acid-base status (Table 2). In renal tubular acidosis or chronic diarrheal states, filtered citrate is avidly reabsorbed in the proximal tubule, and returned to the circulation as bicarbonate *(90)*. Moderate hypocitraturia may result from intracellular acidosis in the proximal tubule during thiazide-induced hypokalemia *(91)*.

Dietary factors are probably the most important determinant of citrate excretion. In the absence of systemic acidosis, the single most important determinant of urinary citrate excretion is the net absorption of alkali from the diet *(92)*. In both normal and stone-forming individuals, there was a direct correlation between the gastrointestinal absorption of alkali and urinary citrate, with complete overlap between stone-formers and controls (Fig. 8). The net gastrointestinal absorption of alkali in turn reflects the combined effects of animal proteins, vegetables, and fruits. A diet rich in animal proteins tends to lower net alkali absorbed (relative excess of phosphate over cations), whereas a vegetable-rich diet tends to raise net alkali absorbed (relative excess of anions over cations) *(92)*. Ingestion of citrus fruits would tend to increase alkali absorption, and provide potassium but very little phosphate or chloride. The net effect is that ingestion of vegetables and fruits tends to increase citrate excretion, whereas animal proteins tend to lower citraturia. The critical determinant of citrate excretion may be the balance between the food groups rather than the absolute quantity of each. Other dietary factors may also influence citrate excretion, but probably to a lesser extent. An oral sodium load (250 mEq/d) reduces urinary citrate, commensurate with a slight fall in serum bicarbonate and a rise in urinary pH. These data suggest that the sodium loss is associated volume expansion, bicarbonaturia and consequent mild metabolic acidosis, resulting in the fall in urinary citrate. In addition, a small subset of patients may have a low urinary citrate on the basis of a renal abnormality in citrate reabsorption *(89)*. Finally, hormonal status also appears to influence urinary citrate excretion because citrate excretion is higher in women than men *(93)*, and is higher in those postmenopausal women that are administered replacement estrogens *(94)*.

Urinary citrate rises after oral administration of potassium citrate, presumably because of the alkali load. The urinary calcium excretion may also fall, especially if a systemic acidosis is corrected (e.g., renal tubular acidosis). These factors combine to reduce urinary supersaturations, and hence risk of crystallization. During long-term treatment of stone-forming women with potassium citrate, the mineral density of the radial shaft showed a small but significant increase *(89)*. Thus, long-term treatment with potassium citrate may also promote calcium retention and help to prevent bone mineral loss.

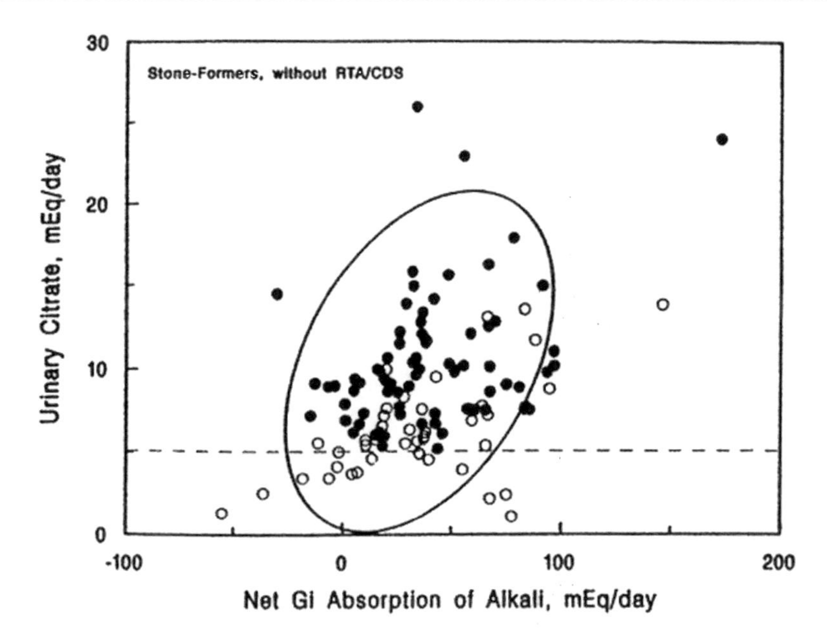

Fig. 8. Dependence of urinary citrate on net gastrointestinal (GI) absorption of alkali in stone forming patients without RTA or chronic diarrhea. GI alkali absorption determined urinary citrate excretion in a group of stone formers, whose response completely overlapped with the normal range (ellipse), suggesting that in this group without diarrhea or renal tubular acidosis, the low urinary citrate is caused by diet. (From ref. *92* with permission from the American Society for Bone and Mineral Research.)

In a 3-yr placebo-controlled trial, oral administration of potassium citrate (60 mEq per d) to hypocitraturic calcium stone-formers reduced the stone recurrence rate dramatically (0.1 vs 1.1 stones/patient/year) *(95)*. Sodium salts of alkali are to be avoided because, unlike potassium citrate, they do not reduce urinary calcium excretion and may instead increase it *(96)*. In addition, sodium alkali may also raise the urinary supersaturation for sodium urate, and sodium urate in turn promotes calcium oxalate crystallization. Patients with renal impairment, with type 4 renal tubular acidosis, or on potassium sparing diuretics must be monitored closely while receiving potassium citrate for hyperkalemia. Other side effects are primarily gastrointestinal and include bloating, nausea, indigestion, and diarrhea. These effects may be minimized by taking potassium citrate with food. Lemon juice is relatively replete with citrate, and consumption of lemonade (4 oz lemon juice in 2 L of water per day) was found to be an effective method to increase urinary citrate *(97)* and represents an alternative regimen for those patients who cannot tolerate potassium citrate.

More recently, a new formulation of potassium–magnesium citrate has been studied. This combination appears to more effectively raise the urinary pH and citrate concentration compared with potassium citrate alone and also raises urinary magnesium levels, which is of theoretical benefit to reduce calcium oxalate supersaturation. A placebo-controlled trial demonstrated the effectiveness of this preparation as the recurrence rate of calcium oxalate nephrolithiasis was reduced by 85% *(98)*. Potassium–magnesium citrate should be particularly useful in stone-forming states associated with hypomagnesemia, including magnesium loss because of thiazides or chronic diarrheal states.

Uric Acid Stones

Uric acid stones account for 5–10% of all those analyzed *(99)*, although this figure does not take into account passage of smaller fragments and gravel, which commonly occurs in patients with this stone type. The defining feature of uric acid crystallization is its strong pH dependence because the fully protonated form of the uric acid molecule that forms stones and the pK_a of this reaction is approx 5.35 in urine *(17)*. Therefore, uric acid stones form only when the urine is acidic (pH 5.5 or less), and they often dissolve in vivo when the urine pH is raised to levels that are easily achievable via administration of alkali (6.5–7; ref. *100*). For this reason, uric acid stones can often be medically managed, avoiding the need for surgical manipulations or other interventional procedures. In addition, uric acid stones are particularly amenable to medical preventative management.

Uric acid is the major end product of the degradation of the purines adenine and guanine. In humans, purines are derived from diet, *de novo* synthesis, and tissue catabolism. Uric acid is a weak acid with two dissociable protons, with pK_as of 10.3 and 5.57. In human plasma (pH 7.4), most uric acid is present as the monovalent form, and in gouty states it can deposit in tissues as monosodium urate. In human urine, the pK_a is approx 5.3, meaning that when the urine is maximally acidic (pH approx 5.0), the majority of uric acid is in the undissociated form (Fig. 3). For example, if a urine sample contains 800 mg of uric acid (a typical quantity), at the acidic pH of 5.0, approx 600 mg will be undissociated uric acid, whereas at a pH of 6.5 only about 100 mg will be in this form *(17)*. Because it is undissociated uric acid that is relatively insoluble and readily forms crystals and stones, the key role of urinary pH in uric acid stone formation becomes clear. Because a high sodium concentration can increase supersaturation with respect to monosodium urate, which is less soluble than monopotassium urate, and monosodium urate promotes calcium oxalate crystallization *(96)*, the use of potassium forms of alkali is the preferred treatment strategy.

From the above discussion, it is clear that when the urine is maximally acidic, uric acid stones are most likely to form. Chronic diarrhea (from any cause) or the presence of an ileostomy are potential causes because under these circumstances the kidney must excrete acid to compensate for stool bicarbonate losses. Patients without bowel disease who form uric acid stones appear to have urine that is acidic most of the time *(101)*. Many appear to excrete inappropriately low amounts of urinary ammonium *(102)*, and the daily acid load is therefore disproportionately titrated onto phosphate ions, in the process lowering the pH *(102)*. In this population of uric acid stone-formers, there also appears to be a tendency toward loss of the physiological "alkaline tide" after meals. In older patients in general, there is also a decrease in renal ammoniagenesis, resulting in a more acidic urine and consequent increased risk for uric acid stones *(103)*. Dietary factors are important in many patients as well because breakdown of ingested proteins contributes to uric acid stone formation in several ways. Animal proteins are high in purines, the precursor of uric acid *(104)*; glandular proteins such as liver are particularly rich in purines. Urinary uric acid excretion directly correlates with dietary protein ingestion (Fig. 2; ref. *16*). In addition, animal proteins are rich in sulfur containing amino acids, such as cystine and methionine, which are metabolized to sulfuric acids that must be excreted by the kidney, resulting in an acid urine *(105)*. Finally, amino acids increase urinary uric acid excretion by inhibiting its tubular reabsorption *(106)*. The net effect is that a high-protein diet increases the uric acid pool, increases uric acid excretion, and lowers the urine pH, all of which potentiate uric acid stone formation.

The incidence of uric acid stones is higher in patients with gout, perhaps approaching 20%. This combination of uric acid stones and gout has been termed a "gouty diathesis" *(107)*, and is characterized by a low urinary pH and low fractional excretion of uric acid and high serum uric acid. In this population group, the likelihood of passing a stone correlates with the absolute level of urinary uric acid excretion: those excreting less than 300 mg of uric acid per day had an 11% incidence of stones, whereas those excreting greater than 1000 mg per day had a 50% incidence *(108)*. Because urinary uric acid excretion correlated with serum uric acid levels, the tendency towards stones also correlated with serum uric acid levels. The gouty population as a group also tends to excrete an overly acid urine, perhaps because of defective renal ammoniagenesis *(108,109)*. Therefore, several mechanisms can promote stone formation in these patients. Uric acid stones are also associated with other secondary causes of uric acid overproduction, such as myeloproliferative disorders *(110)*, a rare genetic disorder of uric acid metabolism (Lesh–Nyhan syndrome; ref. *111*), and in association with glycogen storage disease type I in which a chronic acidosis is thought to inhibit reabsorption of uric acid.

Treatment of uric acid stones usually involves drinking water to maintain a dilute urine (ideally >2 L/d), a low-protein diet (<1 g/kg of ideal body weight per day), and oral potassium citrate to maintain a urine pH of 6.5–7.0. A higher urinary pH (>7.0) does not increase uric acid solubility further, and may increase the risk of apatite crystallization, which is an important consideration in certain clinical circumstances (e.g., tumor lysis syndrome). The amount of alkali necessary will depend on the diet, but is usually between 50 and 100 mEq/d. Potassium citrate is the preferred salt (*see* above). It is useful for patients to use pH strips to monitor their urinary pH on treatment, both to achieve the desired pH range and to aid with compliance. Every other day dosing with alkali to raise the urine pH to 7.0 or greater may be an alternative prophylaxis regimen *(112)*, although it is not recommended for dissolution of stones. This alternate day regimen has the advantage of improved potential for compliance, and patients with large gastrointestinal losses of base (e.g., those with an ileostomy) may be able to achieve an intermittent increase in urine pH better than a prolonged one.

Allopurinol, an inhibitor of xanthine oxidase, an enzyme in the pathway that converts purines to uric acid, is of limited utility for prevention of most pure uric acid stones. Allopurinol is, however, an appropriate therapy for prevention of gout, or in patients with large overproduction of uric acid (e.g., patients with myeloproliferative diseases on chemotherapy). If allopurinol is used, measures to alkalinize the urine are still necessary in most circumstances.

Hyperuricosuric Calcium Oxalate Kidney Stones

It is common for a patient to have mixed uric acid and calcium oxalate stones, or to pass uric acid stones at some times and calcium oxalate at others. Gout is often an associated feature *(101,113)*. Overall, approx 5% of all stones are mixed calcium oxalate and uric acid *(4)*. Excess excretion of uric acid in the urine is thought to be the pathologic link, and this syndrome has been named hyperuricosuric calcium oxalate nephrolithiasis *(114)*. In solution, crystals of uric acid and sodium hydrogen urate appear to promote calcium oxalate crystallization *(115,116)*. The exact mechanisms underlying this observation, and whether it occurs in human urine, remain controversial. Among proposed mechanisms uric acid and sodium hydrogen urate crystals appear to inactivate urinary calcium oxalate crystal growth inhibitors *(117)*, soluble uric acid appears to decrease spontaneous nucleation of calcium oxalate (by a "salting out" mechanism) *(118)*, and

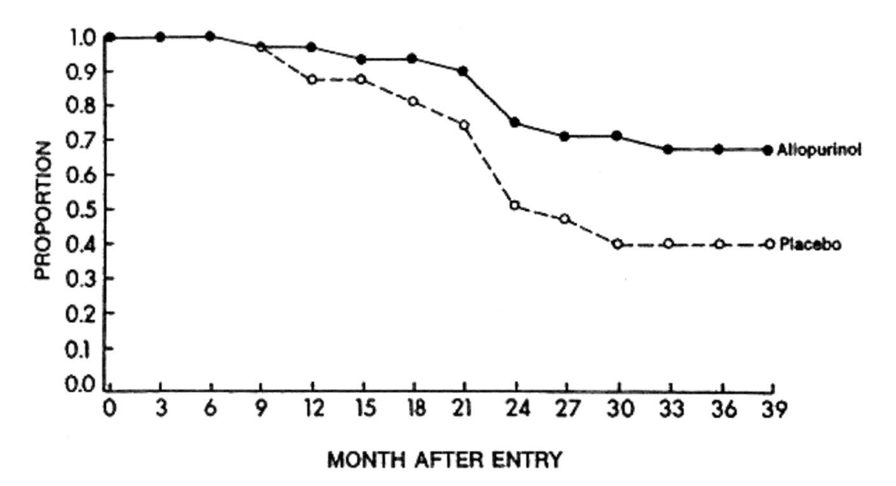

Fig. 9. Allopurinol treatment of hyperuricosuric calcium oxalate stone formers. After 39 mo, patients treated with allopurinol had significantly less recurrences. (From ref. *92* with permission. Copyright © Massachusetts Medical Society. All rights reserved.)

any uric acid crystals that form in the kidney could occlude tubules, promote stasis, and thereby promote retention of calcium oxalate crystals in the kidney *(119)*.

The urinary profile of patients who excrete mixed uric acid/calcium oxalate stones is intermediate between those who excrete pure calcium stones, and those who excrete uric acid stones. The average urinary pH is, on average, lower than that of pure calcium oxalate stone formers (pH 5.7 vs 6.0 *[117,120]*), favoring precipitation of uric acid, and perhaps indirectly promoting calcium oxalate crystallization (*see* above). Urinary citrate excretion is also reduced *(117)*. This more acidic urine, which is most pronounced in the early morning when urine is also maximally concentrated *(121)*, is likely to be at least as important as the absolute quantity of uric acid excreted.

Treatment includes high fluid intake and moderate ingestion of purines and animal protein. If hyperuricosuria cannot be controlled by diet alone, allopurinol is a useful treatment strategy. At a dose of 300 mg per d, a 30–40% reduction in uric acid excretion is typical. A 3-yr placebo-controlled trial clearly demonstrates that treatment of hyperuricosuric calcium oxalate stone-formers with allopurinol reduces the formation of new stones by 51% (Fig. 9; ref. *122*) . Because allopurinol does not alter other urinary constituents (e.g., oxalate or calcium) *(123)* and has no effect on calcium oxalate crystal growth *(124)*, it is overwhelmingly likely that the allopurinol is effective because it reduces urinary uric acid excretion. The major side effect of allopurinol is a hypersensitivity rash, which occurs in about 2% of patients. In a small number (0.01%) a severe, life-threatening reaction can develop. Typically, adverse effects occur in the first weeks, and all patients should be advised to stop the medication at the first sign of itching or rash. An alternative treatment strategy is oral citrate to raise the urinary pH, thereby preventing uric acid crystallization (Fig. 10). A preliminary study suggests that oral citrate may in fact be an effective strategy, although whether citrate would be an effective treatment in those hyperuricosuric calcium oxalate stone-formers with normal or high urinary citrate levels remains unknown. It may be possible to prescribe the citrate as a single nighttime dose (e.g., 30–60 mEq), to prevent an acidic urinary pH early in the morning

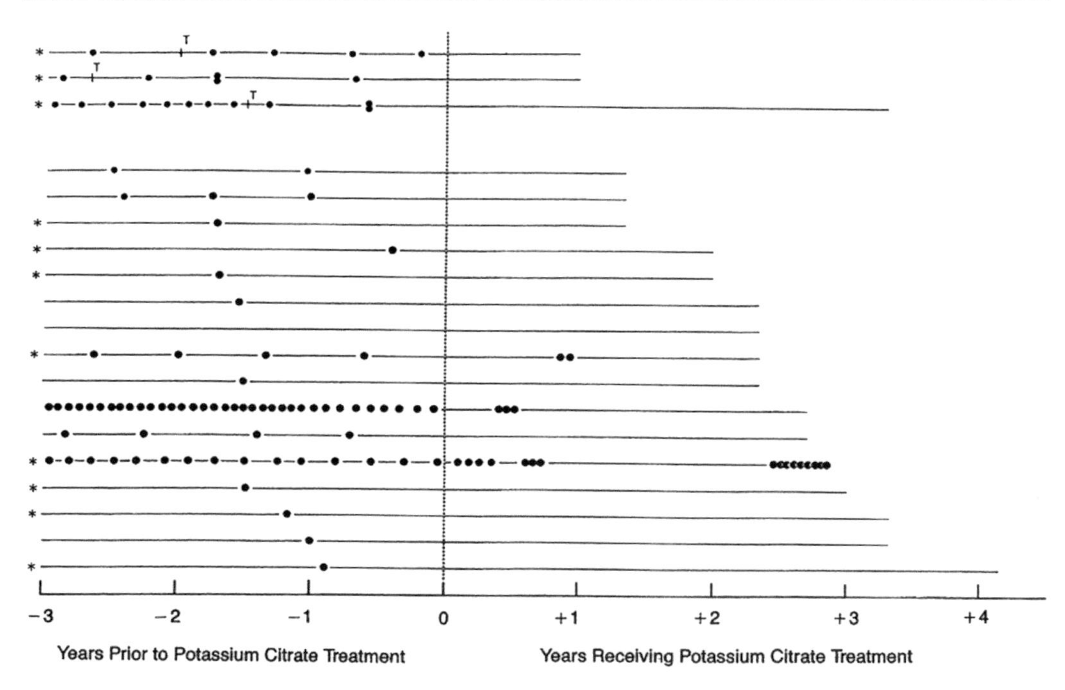

Fig. 10. Potassium citrate treatment of hyperuricosuric calcium oxalate stone-formers. Mildly hyperuricosuric calcium oxalate stone formers had less stone events (dots) once placed on oral potassium citrate, in this nonplacebo-controlled trial. (From ref. *124a* with permission. Copyright © 1986 from the American Medical Association.)

(112); however, this strategy has not been rigorously examined in hyperuricosuric calcium oxalate stone-formers, nor compared to other treatment strategies.

Calcium Phosphate Stones and Renal Tubular Acidosis

Viewed as a group, patients with calcium phosphate stones, or those with mixed calcium oxalate-calcium phosphate stones, tend to have a higher urinary pH than those with pure calcium oxalate stones *(125–128)*. In addition, those with calcium phosphate stones, pure or mixed with calcium oxalate, tend to have a lower urinary citrate, hypercalciuria, and experience more frequent stone events *(28,129,130)*. Some may have an "incomplete" form of distal renal tubular acidosis (dRTA), characterized by an abnormal urinary acidification response to an acid load but lacking systemic acidosis *(128)*.

The ambient pH has a profound effect on the supersaturation with calcium phosphate. The dissociation of $H_2PO_4^-$–HPO_4^{2-} has a pK_a of 6.8, whereas the pK_a of the further dissociation to PO_4^{3-} is 11.6. *(131)*. PO_4^{3-} is a constituent of amorphous calcium phosphate and hydroxyapatite (HA), whereas HPO_4^{2-} is a constituent of BR. Therefore, calcium phosphate crystallization is strongly favored by a pH of 6.5 or greater *(132)*, although mixed calcium oxalate/BR calcification can occur at lower pH values if the calcium concentration is high, and when the pH is 6.5 or greater even slight hypercalciuria strongly promotes BR crystallization (Fig. 11; *133*). Above a pH of 6.8, mixtures of BR and carbonated apatite form. HA is usually formed via conversion from amorphous

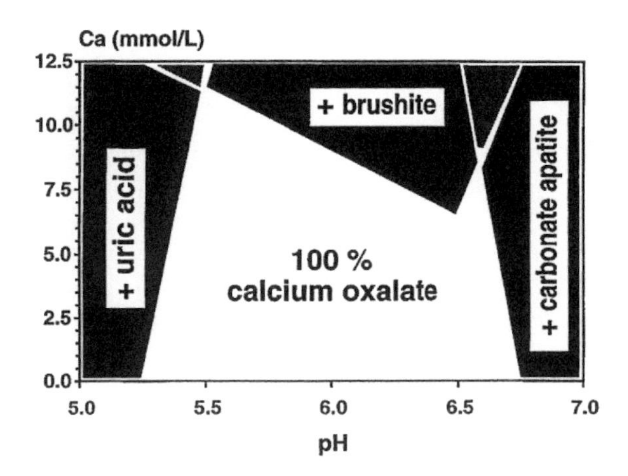

Fig. 11. Crystalline formation phase as a function of pH and calcium concentration. (From ref. *133* with permission. Copyright © 1999, Springer-Verlag.)

mixtures of BR and octacalcium phosphate, which are thermodynamically less stable precursors *(133)*; conversion to HA is strongly favored by a pH of 6.9 or greater. If carbonate ions are available, as is invariably the case in urine, carbonate is incorporated into the crystalline phase, resulting in carbonated hydroxyapatite *(133)*. The solubility of calcium phosphate crystals is also pH-dependent and greatly increased at pH of 6.2 or less. In general, BR is much more soluble than HA or octacalcium phosphate.

Given these considerations, it is not surprising that calcium phosphate stones are most commonly seen in patients with dRTA, a condition caused by specific defects in renal tubular hydrogen ion secretion *(130)*. However, because of the solubility characteristics discussed above (Fig. 11), stones that form in patients with dRTA often are not pure calcium phosphate but commonly contain calcium oxalate *(130,134)*. Causes of dRTA can be hereditary, idiopathic, or secondary to a variety of conditions. The most common secondary causes are autoimmune diseases, including Sjögren's syndrome or systemic lupus. Factors that favor calcium phosphate crystallization in dRTA include the abnormally alkaline urine, hypercalciuria, and low urinary citrate concentration *(130)*. The defect in urinary acidification can be incomplete, characterized by a high urinary pH and low urinary citrate but a lack of systemic acidosis. The low urinary citrate is thought to result from a combination of a decreased filtered load of citrate and increased proximal tubular reabsorption of citrate, presumably driven indirectly by the urinary loss of base *(130)*. Hypokalemia and hypomagnesemia, often associated with RTA, also stimulate proximal tubular reabsorption of citrate. Hypercalciuria can result from a systemic acidosis, if present, although idiopathic hypercalciuria is common and in many cases it may exist as a compounding independent trait (presumably in addition to the dRTA; ref. *130*). In fact, in certain individuals, it has been proposed that hypercalciuria is a cause of a secondary dRTA, perhaps because nephrocalcinosis damages distal tubules *(130,135,136)* . An incomplete form of proximal RTA has also been described in patients with hypercalciuria and stone disease, characterized by abnormal bicarbonaturia in response to a bicarbonate load *(137)*. In these patients, it is speculated that transient bicarbonaturia, especially if other risk factors such as hypercalciuria are present, promotes favorable conditions for the formation of a calcium phospate nidus.

Nephrolithiasis is common in patients with dRTA (up to 59% in on series *[138]*), and conversely patients with dRTA make up a sizable percentage of those seen in stone clinics (up to 8% in one large clinic *[28]*). In certain patients with dRTA, the stone formation rate can be accelerated *(138)*. Nephrocalcinosis is also common, affecting as many as 55% in certain familial cases *(135)*. The treatment is oral potassium citrate to indirectly increase urinary citrate excretion; a large clinical trial confirms the efficacy of this approach. *(134)*. In a group of dRTA patients treated with citrate, the relative supersaturation for BR increased because of a rise in urinary pH, whereas the supersaturation for calcium oxalate fell because of an increase in urinary citrate levels. Because stones associated with dRTA often contain some calcium oxalate, these data suggest that supersaturation with respect to calcium oxalate may be an important pathogenic factor in the stones that form. Urinary calcium excretion may fall with citrate administration; if not, this risk factor can be treated independently by addition of a thiazide diuretic. Urinary acidification via chronic ammonium chloride or L-methionine administration has been proposed for refractory patients with incomplete dRTA and without evidence for systemic acidosis (who typically present with pure brushite stones) *(133,139)* because a fall in urinary pH from 6.5 to 5.5 will markedly decrease BR supersaturations *(139)*. Because of concerns about long-term effects on bone, this strategy has not been widely used but is probably worthy of careful research protocols in those specific patients who do not respond well to citrate.

Infection Stones

Infection stones are most often composed of a mixture of magnesium ammonium phosphate (struvite) and carbonated apatite. Because of the presence of three cations (calcium, magnesium, and ammonium), they are often referred to as "triple phosphate" stones. Although struvite calculi represent a small percentage of stones, perhaps as few as 2–3% *(140)*, they cause disproportionate morbidity. Untreated, struvite stones are often progressive and grow quickly and tend to provoke repeated episodes of pyelonephritis and sepsis. The amorphous mixture of struvite and carbonated apatite can literally fill the renal calyces, forming a so-called "staghorn" calculus. Although cystine and uric acid stones can also form large staghorn stones, struvite is the most likely to do so *(140)*.

Struvite stones are more common in women than men, presumably because of more frequent urinary tract infections *(141)*. An underlying predisposition to stone formation or even a previous history of nonstruvite stones is common, especially in men *(142)*. In these circumstances, it is presumed that a preformed (nonstruvite) stone became colonized with a urease-producing organism, resulting in rapid overgrowth of struvite. Patients with abnormal urological drainage can, however, develop struvite stones without an underlying stone diathesis *(140)*. Examples include patients with ileal conduits or neurogenic bladders. Patients with spinal cord injury and bladder dysfunction are particularly predisposed to infection stones *(142)*; hypercalciuria because of immobilization and the need for bladder catheterization are important contributing factors.

For struvite to form, the urine must contain abundant ammonium ion and trivalent phosphate at the same time. Under physiological conditions, ammonium ion is excreted only when the urine is acidic, whereas trivalent phosphate (PO_4^{3-}) is virtually absent when the urine pH is <5.5 because of its pK_a. Conversely, when the urine is alkaline enough to contain PO_4^{3-}, tubular production of ammonium is minimal. Therefore, struvite crystals cannot form under physiological conditions. However, the action of bacterial

$$NH_2\text{–}CO\text{–}NH_2 \xrightarrow{\text{UREASE}} H_2CO_3 + 2\,NH_3$$

$$2\,NH_3 + H_2O \Rightarrow 2\,NH^{4+} = 2\,OH^-$$

$$H_2CO_3 \Rightarrow H^+ + HCO_3^- \Rightarrow 2\,H^+ + CO_3^{2-}$$

Fig. 12. Actions of bacterial urease. The net effect is the production of NH_4^+, HCO_3, and CO_3^{2-}, and an alkaline pH. Together with calcium, magnesium and phosphate, all abundant in urine, struvite stones are easily formed.

urease on urea creates the ideal combination of conditions for struvite crystallization *(143)*, resulting in an alkaline urine containing abundant ammonia (NH_4^+), carbonate, and bicarbonate ions (Fig. 12). Alkaline urine also contains abundant phosphorous in the form of PO_4^{3-}, as well as calcium, providing all the necessary ingredients for growth of struvite, as well as carbonated apatite.

Most struvite stones are caused by *Proteus* or *Providencia* species *(141)*, although many bacteria can at least occasionally synthesize urease, including *Haemophilus influenza*, *Staphylococcus aureus*, *Yersinia enterolitica*, and *Klebsiella pneumoniae (144)*. *Ureaplasma urealyticum* can also cause struvite stones, and because it is difficult to culture may be causative in many "culture negative" cases *(145)*. Biofilm produced by the offending organism can make it difficult to culture, as well as to eradicate infection *(146)*. Therefore, all organisms should be cultured from the urine, even if the total colony counts are low. It is also important to culture any stone material surgically removed because in many cases this may be the only way to identify the responsible bacteria *(147)*.

First and foremost, all stony fragments must be removed to cure infected stones. Although it is possible to sterilize small amounts of struvite with antibiotic therapy, exactly how much and under what circumstances remains indeterminate. Historically, at least, the outcome in patients with conservatively managed staghorn calculi was dismal, with 10-yr mortality rates as high as 28% (compared with 7% in those treated surgically) *(148)*. Those patients with struvite stones remaining in their kidney are at risk for recurrent urinary tract infection, abscess formation, and sepsis. Extracorporeal shock wave lithotripsy (ESWL) alone may be effective for small stones (<2.5 cm; ref. *149*), although larger stones must be treated with percutaneous lithotripsy (often in staged procedures), percutaneous lithotripsy followed by ESWL to dislodge any remaining fragments, or in some cases open surgery *(149)*. All appear equally effective at rendering a kidney stone free. Irrigation with the acidifying agent hemiacidrin was a mainstay of treatment in the past, and in select cases can still be useful for dissolution of residual fragments.

Close follow-up after hospital discharge, including frequent imaging studies, is a key to treatment success. Any new stones that develop should be treated promptly, lest a staghorn calculus regrow. Important adjunctive measures include intermittent catheterization in patients with bladder dysfunction, as opposed to the use of indwelling catheters. Suppressive antibiotics may be indicated to prevent recurrent urinary tract infections, and all patients should be routinely screened for asymptomatic infections.

Evaluation and treatment of any underlying metabolic risk factors for stone formation may prevent the formation of a nidus that could once again become secondarily infected.

Acetohydroxyaminic acid (AHA) is an effective urease inhibitor that can be given orally. AHA has demonstrated clinical efficacy to reduce the growth or struvite stones *(141)*, but it must be administered three times daily, is associated with a low-grade intravascular coagulation problem and the formation of deep vein thrombi in a significant number of patients, and may cause reversible neurological effects, such as headache. In addition, increased risk of toxicity precludes use of this drug in renal insufficiency (glomerular filtration rate <40). Given these considerations, AHA is probably useful only in very select circumstances where surgery is contraindicated. Use of a low-phosphorous, low-magnesium diet together with aluminum hydroxide gel (the Shorr regimen) may be able to reduce stone growth rates via substrate depletion *(150)*. However, this regimen is associated with significant side effects, including constipation, anorexia, bony pain, and hypercalciuria and is, therefore, not generally recommended. Urinary acidification with ascorbic acid, ammonium chloride, or L-methionine have all been proposed and on a pathophysiological basis make sense *(151)*. Although there is no strong evidence to support their efficacy of chronic urinary acidification, one series did demonstrate that L-methionine could maintain an acidic urine and favorable chemistries over a period of years *(152)*. Overall, however, in the group of patients where surgery is not an option, long-term suppressive antibiotics are probably the best choice.

Cystine Stones

Cystinuria is an autosomal recessive disorder in which cystine and the dibasic amino acids (lysine, arginine, and ornithine) are not properly absorbed in the proximal tubule and small intestine. The incidence is about 1:15,000 in the United States, but is higher in specific population groups (e.g., 1:2,500 in Libyan Jews) *(153)*. The only clinical consequence of this genetic defect is the formation of cystine stones because on average only approx 250 mg/L of cystine is soluble in urine (1 m*M*/L), *(154)*. Cystine stones are relatively hard, not easily amenable to fragmentation *(155)*, and can quickly grow into large, potentially organ-threatening staghorn calculi *(154)*. Therefore, medical therapy to prevent their formation is particularly important. About one-quarter of patient present in their first decade of life and another 30–40% as teenagers *(153)*.

Almost all (approx 99%) of cystine in the glomerular ultrafiltrate is normally reabsorbed by transporters located in the luminal brush border of proximal tubular cells. In patients with cystinuria, filtered cystine is not completely reabsorbed, and as tubular fluid is concentrated in the collecting duct it is concentrated, allowing crystals to form. Two gene mutations have been identified, *SLCA3A1*, the cystinuria type I gene, was identified in 1994. and *SLC7A9*, the gene causing nontype I cystinuria, was identified in 1999 *(156)*. Structural and functional evidence suggest that these genes encode heavy (*SLCA3A1*) and light (*SLC7A9*) subunits of the heteromultimeric amino acid transporter responsible for cystine reabsorption in the kidney and intestine *(156)*. A clinically distinguishing feature is that type I heterozygotes have normal urinary amino acid excretion, whereas nontype I heterozygotes have variably increased excretion of cystine and other dibasic amino acid in the urine. Recent studies have identified specific genetic mutations in affected individuals, and correlated the degree of transporter dysfunction in vitro and with the amount of cystinuria in vivo *(156) (157)*.

The average solubility of cystine in urine is approx 250 mg/L (1 m*M*/L) at pH 7.0 but can increase to as high as 500 mg/L (2 m*M*/L) at a pH 7.5 *(154)*, although maintaining a urinary pH this high (or higher) is not easy. These principles determine the mainstay of treatment for cystinuria: hyperdiuresis and maximal alkalinization of the urine *(158)*. Thiol derivatives, including D-penicillamine *(159)* and tiopronin *(160)*, cleave cystine into two cysteine moieties and combine with a single molecule of cysteine to form a highly soluble D-penicillamine–cysteine compound (or troponin–cysteine compound), reducing the total urinary cystine concentration in the process. Captopril acts in a similar fashion *(161)* and can be used in patients that cannot tolerate D-penicillamine or tiopronin *(162)*, although the molar quantities of captopril that can be achieved in the urine will be less because systemic effects (e.g., hypotension) limit the total dose of captopril that can be administered.

To treat cystinuric stone patients, the amount of urinary cystine excreted in a 24-h urine sample should first be quantitated. Based upon the predicted solubility of cystine, this value will give some guidance as to the total quantity of urine that is theoretically necessary to dilute the cystine and keep it in solution. In general, patients should be encouraged to drink water hourly while awake, and should need to arise at night at least once to urinate. Periodically collecting a 24-h urine and measuring the volume is a useful maneuver that can help provide feedback and encourage compliance. The importance of hyperdiuresis cannot be overemphasized because a patient's success in maintaining urine volumes greater than 3 L/d is the single factor that best predicts the success or failure of therapy *(154)*. Because the solubility of cystine in urine does not always follow a predictable pattern, the degree of supersaturation or undersaturation of urine with respect to cystine can be directly measured by adding cystine crystals to a sample and determining if they grow or dissolve *(163)*. Alkalinization of the urine is the next weapon in the treatment armamentarium. Potassium citrate can be administered but the urinary pH needs to be 7.5 or greater to have a significant benefit. Self-monitoring of urinary pH is useful to monitor the success of urinary alkalization, and to help in dosage adjustment. Finally, if these measures prove insufficient, addition of a sulfhydryl agent can be considered. In particular, if D-penicillamine or tiopronin are used, the total urinary cystine excretion should be monitored as the dose is titrated upward *(164)*, as the incidence of side effects is closely related to dose. The minimal dosage should be used that reduces urinary cystine to acceptable levels. A recent report documents the long-term efficacy of this program to recurrent stone formation rates *(154)*; however, success was linked to the ability of patients to maintain a dilute urine.

Drug Stones

Obtaining a drug history is important because some drugs are associated with stone formation (Table 3). Certain drugs are excreted in the urine and have low solubility, tending to form precipitates (e.g., triamterene and indinavir). Others increase urinary calcium excretion (e.g., calcium and vitamin D supplements). Loop diuretics clearly promote hypercalciuria and are associated with nephrocalcinosis in premature infants, although the pathogenesis of calcification in these circumstances is likely to be multifactorial *(165)*. Loop diuretics also promote calcium excretion in adults, but they are not known to be associated with stone disease in this population. Vitamin C can raise urinary oxalate excretion *(166)*, but only in high doses, and perhaps more so in certain individuals with abnormal metabolism of the vitamin *(167)*. Agents that raise the uri-

Table 3
Drugs Associated With Kidney Stone Formation

Raise urinary pH	Increase urinary oxalate excretion
• Acetazolamide	• High-dose vitamin C *(166,167)*
• Antacids	
• Zonisamide *(179)*	Precipitate "drug stones"
	• Allopurinol (Hypoxanthine)
Increase urinary calcium excretion	• Guaifenesin/ephedrine *(180)*
• Calcium and vitamin D supplements	• Sulfonamides
• Loop diuretics *(165)*	• Triamterene
• Antacids	• Indinavir *(181)*

nary pH, including carbonic anhydrase inhibitors, promote calcium phosphate precipitation (*see* discussion on calcium phosphate stones).

Medullary Sponge Kidney

Medullary sponge kidney (MSK) applies to pathologically dilated collecting ducts within one or more renal pyramids of one or both kidneys. MSK is almost always diagnosed radiographically, is of uncertain etiology, and presents a clinical spectrum varying from an asymptomatic, incidental finding on a radiologic exam a severely complicated stone forming condition *(168)*. The changes of MSK are most often bilateral (94%), and usually affect three or more pyramids (73%) *(169)*. It is estimated to occur in between 1:2000 and 1:20,000 persons in the general population *(170)*, and renal function remains normal in affected individuals throughout life. The pathogenesis is unclear, but studies suggest that it is a congenital syndrome, present in full form at birth, not progressing throughout life, and not passed on to children. MSK is associated with congenital hemihypertrophy in up to 25% of cases, and it has been speculated that the pathogenesis may be linked to a group of imprinted genes on chromosome 11 that have been implicated in associated congenital conditions such as the Beckwith–Wiedemann syndrome *(170)*. Kidney stone formation is the major clinical consequence of MSK, occurring in 50–60% of affected individuals *(171)*. Calcium oxalate or mixed calcium oxalate/calcium phosphate stones are most common. Stasis in the dilated distal collecting ducts is also thought to favor stone formation. A low urinary citrate, perhaps as part of an incomplete distal RTA, is also often present as an important contributory factor for stone formation. Nephrocalcinosis and urinary tract infection are more common in affected individuals than in the general population. Treatment of stones associated with MSK is the same as in the general population. Metabolic work-ups should be performed, and any risk factors that are identified treated accordingly.

Other Factors

Identification and treatment of known metabolic risk factors can reduce stone formation rate. The treatment recommendations for each stone type and risk factor are summarized in Table 4. However, many patients who form stones have no or only minimal metabolic risk factors, whereas others with marked abnormalities make few stones *(172)*.

Table 4
Summary of Treatment Strategies

Stone type	*Risk factor*	*Treatment or strategy*[a]	*Alternative/adjunctive strategies*	*Comment*
Calcium oxalate ± calcium phosphate	Hypercalciuria	Thiazide diuretic	Neutral phosphate Potassium citrate Low-protein diet Low-salt diet	Hypokalemia/hypomagnesemia should be treated if they result during thiazide treatment
Calcium oxalate ± calcium phosphate	Idiopathic hyperoxaluria	Low-oxalate/low-fat diet	Potassium citrate	
Calcium oxalate	Enteric hyperoxaluria	Low-oxalate/low fat-diet	Calcium with meals Bile acid resin Potassium citrate	
Calcium oxalate	Primary hyperoxaluria	Potassium citrate or neutral phosphate Pyridoxine	Low-oxalate diet Liver–kidney transplant (if end-stage renal disease)	Should be referred to a tertiary referral center
Calcium oxalate	Hypocitraturia	Potassium citrate	Low-protein diet	Any causes of chronic diarrhea should be investigated and treated if possible
Calcium oxalate ± calcium phosphate	None apparent	Potassium citrate		
Uric acid	Low urinary pH	Potassium citrate	Low-protein diet	
Calcium phosphate ± calcium oxalate	High urinary pH; hypocitraturia	Potassium citrate	Thiazide diuretic (if hypercalciuric)	Incomplete dRTA commonly present
Cystine	Cystinuria	Increased fluid intake to maintain urine volumes >3 L; potassium citrate	D-Penicillamine Tiopronin Captopril	Maintaining high urinary volumes is the most important component of therapy
Struvite	Infection with urease positive organism	Surgical removal of stone(s)	Appropriate antibiotics	Close follow-up for recurrence is essential

[a]Increased fluid intake to maintain urine volumes >2 L recommended for all.

Clearly, other factors remain to be identified. For example, it was recently reported that in patients with recurrent unilateral urolithiasis, sleep posture correlated with stone formation (i.e., stones commonly formed in the kidney that was dependent during sleep *(173)*). It was speculated that alterations in renal hemodynamics that are dependent on posture, presumably causing intermittent renal ischemia, might have played a role.

The urine of all individuals contains macromolecules that can inhibit the nucleation, growth, and aggregation of crystals, and studies suggest that these molecules could be abnormal in the urine of at least a subset of stone formers *(174)*. However, despite decades of work in countless labs, the most important of these urinary inhibitors remain to be identified, and abnormalities in the quantity or function of any individual protein have not been identified in the urine of a population of stone-formers to date. Recent investigation has also focussed on the processes that mediate crystal retention in the kidney, including adhesion and internalization of crystals by renal tubular cells *(175)*, as well as the role of novel and poorly understood calcifying microorganisms (nanobacteria) in stone pathogenesis *(176)*. Clearly, much work remains if we are to make any major advances in the potential therapies to reduce stone formation, which have changed little in the last 20 yr.

AKNOWLEDGMENTS

This work was supported by grants to J.C.L. from the National Institutes of Health (R01 DK 53399), the Oxalosis and Hyperoxaluria Foundation, and the Ralph Wilson Foundation. We thank Charlann Thompson for excellent secretarial assistance.

REFERENCES

1. Mandel NS, Mandel GS. Urinary tract stone disease in the United States veteran population. I. Geographical frequency of occurrence. J Urol 1989; 142: 1513–1515.
2. Sierakowski R, Finlayson B, Landes RR, Finlayson CD, Sierakowski N. The frequency of urolithiasis in hospital discharge diagnoses in the United States. Invest Urol. 1978; 15: 438–441.
3. Smith LH. Diet and hyperoxaluria in the syndrome of idiopathic calcium oxalate urolithiasis. Am J Kidney Dis 1994; 17: 370–375.
4. Herring LC. Observations on the analysis of ten thousand urinary calculus. J Urol 1962; 88: 545–555.
5. Parks JH, Coward M, Coe FL. Correspondence between stone composition and urine supersaturation in nephrolithiasis. Kidney Int 1997; 51: 894–900.
6. Parks JH, Coe FL. The financial effects of kidney stone prevention. Kidney Int 1996; 50: 1706–1712.
7. Colussi G, De Ferrari ME, Brunati C, Civati G. Medical prevention and treatment of urinary stones. J Nephrol 2000; 13 (suppl 3): S65–S70.
8. Andersen DA. Historical and geographical differences in the pattern of incidence of urinary renal stones considered in relation to possible aetiologicla factors. Proceedings of the Renal Stone Research Symposium, Churchill Livingstone, London, England, 1968.
9. Robertson WG, Peacock M, Heyburn PJ, Hanes FA. Epidemiological risk factors in calcium stone disease. Scand J Urol Nephrol 1980; (suppl. 53): 15–28.
10. Curhan GC, Willett WC, Rimm EB, Stampfer MJ. A prospective study of dietary calcium and other nutrients and the risk of symptomatic kidney stones (*see* comments). N Engl J Med. 1993; 328: 833–838.
11. Curhan GC, Willet WC, Speizer FE, Stampfer MJ. Intake of vitamins B6 and C and the risk of kidney stones in women. J Am Soc Nephrol 1999; 10: 840–845.
12. Curhan GC, Willett WC, Rimm EB, Stampfer MJ. A prospective study of dietary calcium and other nutrients and the risk of symptomatic kidney stones. N Engl J Med. 1993; 328: 833–838.
13. Curhan GC, Willet WC, Rimm EB, Stampfer MJ. A prospective study of the intake of vitamins C and B6, and the risk of kidney stones in men. J Urol 1996; 155: 1847–1851.

14. Curhan GC, Willett WC, Speizer FE, Stampfer MJ. Beverage use and risk of kidney stones in women. Ann Intern Med 1998; 128: 534–540.
15. Trinchieri A, Zanetti G, Curró A, Lizzano R. Effect of potential renal acid load of foods on calcium metabolism of renal calcium stone formers. Eur Urol 2001; 39 (suppl 1): 33–37.
16. Coe FL, Moran E, Kavalich AG. The contribution of dietary purine over-consumption to hyperuricosuria in calcium oxalate stone formers. J Chronic Dis 1976; 29: 793–800.
17. Coe FL. Uric acid and calcium oxalate nephrolithiasis. Kidney Int 1983; 24: 392–403.
18. Hiatt RA, Ettinger B, Caan B, Quesenberry CP, Duncan D, Citron JT. Randomized controlled trial of a low animal protein, high fiber diet in the prevention of recurrent calcium oxalate kidney stones. Am J Epidemiol 1996; 144: 25–33.
18a. Nguyen QV, Kalin A, Drouve U, Casez J-P, Jaeger P. Sensitivity to meat protein intake and hyperoxaluria in idiopathic calcium stone formers. Kidney Int 2001; 59: 2273–2281.
19. Borghi L, Schianchi T, Meschi T, et al. Comparison of two diets for the prevention of recurrent stones in idiopathic hypercalciuria. N Engl J Med 2002; 346: 77–84.
20. Paviar F, Low RK, Stoller ML. The influence of diet on urinary stone disease. J Urol 1996; 155: 432–440.
21. Curhan GC, Rimm EB, Willet WC, Stampfer MJ. Regional variation in nephrolithiasis incidence and prevalence among United States men. J Urol 1994; 151: 838–841.
22. Hosking DH, Erickson SB, Van Den Berg CJ, Wilson DM, Smith LH. The stone clinic effect in patients with idiopathic calcium urolithiasis. J Urol 1983; 130: 1115–1118.
23. Pak CYC, Sakahee K, Crowther C, Brinkley L. Evidence justifying a high fluid intake in treatment of nephrolithiasis. Ann Intern Med 1980; 93: 36–39.
24. Borghi L, Tiziana A, Amato F, Briganti A, Novarini A, Giannini A. Urinary volume, water, and recurrences in idiopathic calcium nephrolithiasis: a 5-year randomized prospective study. J Urol 1996; 155: 839–843.
25. Sutherland JW, Parks JH, Coe FL. Recurrence after a single renal stone in a community practice. Mineral Electrolyte Metabolism 1985; 11: 267–269.
26. Johnson CM, Wilson DM, O'Fallon WM, Malek RS, Kurland LT. Renal stone epidemiology: a 25-year study in Rochester, Minnesota. Kidney Int 1979; 16: 624–631.
27. Erickson SB. When should the stone patient be evaluated? Limited evaluation of single stone formers. Med Clin North Am 1984; 68: 461–468.
28. Coe FL, Parks JH. Nephrolithiasis: Pathogenesis and Treatment, 2nd Ed. Year Book Medical Publishers, Chicago, IL, 1988.
29. Werness PJ, Brown CM, Smith LH, Finlayson B. EQUIL2: a BASIC computer program for the calculation of urinary saturation. J Urol 1985; 134: 1242–1244.
30. Hess B, Hasler-Strub U, Ackerman D, Jaeger P. Metabolic evaluation of patients with recurrent idiopathic calcium nephrolithiasis. Nephrol Dial Transplant 1997; 12: 1362–1368.
31. Pak CYC, Peterson R, Poindexter JR. Adequacy of a single stone risk analysis in the medical evaluation of urolithiasis. J Urol 2001; 165: 378–381.
32. Kourambas J, Aslan P, Teh CL, Mathias BJ, Preminger G. Role of stone analysis in metabolic evaluation and medical treatment of nephrolithiasis. J Endourol 2001; 15: 181–186.
33. Spencer BA, Wood BJ, Dretler SP. Helical CT and ureteral colic. Urol Clin North Am 2000; 27:231–241.
34. Coe FL, Favus MJ, Crockett T, et al. Effects of low-calcium diet on urine calcium excretion, parathyroid function and serum 1,25(OH)2D3 levels in patients with idiopathic hypercalciuria and in normal subjects. Am J Med 1982; 72: 25–32.
35. Coe FL, Parks JH, Asplin JR. The pathogenesis and treatment of kidney stones— medical progress. N Engl J Med 1992; 327: 1141–1152.
36. Halabe A, Sutton RAL. Primary hyperparathyroidism as a cause of calcium nephrolithiasis. In: Coe FL, Favus MJ, eds. Disorders of Bone and Mineral Metabolism, 1st Ed. Raven Press, New York, NY, 1992, pp. 671–684.
37. Pak CYC, Kaplan R, Bone H, Townsend J, Waters O. A simple test for the diagnosis of absorptive, resorptive and renal hypercalciurias. N Engl J Med. 1975; 292: 497–500.
38. Breslau NA. Pathogenesis and management of hypercalciuric nephrolithiasis. Miner Electroly Metab. 1994; 20: 328–339.

39. Pak CY. Southwestern internal medicine conference: medical management of nephrolithiasis- a new simplified approach for clinical practice. J Med Sci 1997; 313: 215–219.
40. Lemann JJ, Adams ND, Gray RW. Urinary calcium excretion in human beings. N Engl J Med. 1979; 301: 535–541.
41. Lemann J Jr, Worcester EM, Gray RW. Hypercalciuria and stones. (review). Am J Kidney Dis 1991; 17: 386–391.
42. Xiao QL, Tembe V, Horwitz GM, Bushinsky DA, Favus MJ. Increased intestinal vitamin D receptor in genetic hypercalciuric rats: a cause of intestinal calcium absorption. J Clin Invest 1993; 91: 661–7.
43. Sutton RAL, Walker VR. Responses to hydrochlorothiazide and acetazolamide in patients with calcium stones. N Engl J Med 1980; 13: 709–713.
44. Hou SH, Bushinsky DA, Wish JB, Cohen JJ, Harrington JT. Hospital-acquired renal insufficiency: a prospective study. Am J Med 1983; 74: 243–248.
45. Jaeger P, Lippuner K, Casez JP, Hess B, Ackerman D, Hug C. Low bone mass in idiopathic renal stone formers: magnitude and significance. J Bone Miner Res 1994; 9: 1525–1532.
46. Mallmin H, Ljunghall S, Persson I, Bergstrom R. Risk factors for fractures of the distal forearm: a population-based case-controlled study. Osteoporos Int 1994; 4: 298–34.
47. Melton LJ, Crowson CS, Khosla S, Wilson DM, O'Fallon WM. Fracture risk among patients with urolithiasis: a population-based cohort study. Kidney Int 1998; 53: 459–464.
48. Curhan GC, Willett WC, Speizer FE, Spiegelman D, Stampfer MJ. Comparison of dietary calcium with supplemental calcium and other nutrients as factors affecting the risk for kidney stones in women. Ann Intern Med 1997; 266: 497–504.
49. Coe FL, Parks JH, Bushinsky DA, Langman CB, Favus MJ. Chlorthalidone promotes mineral retention in patients with idiopathic hypercalciuria. Kidney Int 1988; 33: 1140–1146.
50. Laerum E, Larsen S. Thiazide prophylaxis of urolithiasis: a double-blind study in general practice. Acta Med Scand 1984; 215: 383–389.
51. Ettinger B, Citron JT, Livermore B, Dolman LI. Chlorthalidone reduces calcium oxalate calculous recurrence but magnesium hydroxide does not. J Urol 1988; 139: 679–684.
52. van den Berg CJ, Kumar R, Wilson DM, Heath III H, Smith LH. Orthophosphate therapy decreases urinary calcium excretion and serum 1,25-dihydroxy vitamin D concentrations in idiopathic hypercalciuria. J Clin Endocrinol Metab 1980; 51: 998–1001.
53. Breslau NA, Brinkley L, Hill KD, Pak CY. Relationship of animal protein-rich diet to kidney stone formation and calcium metabolism. J Clin Endocrinol Metab. 1988; 66: 140–146.
54. Preminger GM, Pak CYC. Eventual attenuation of hypocalciuric response to hydrochlorothiazide in absorptive hypercalciuria. J Urol 1987; 137: 1104–1109.
55. Smith LH, Thomas WC Jr, Arnaud CD. Orthophosphate therapy in calcium renal lithiasis. In: Urinary Calculi. Int. Symp. Renal Stone Res., Madrid 1972. Karger, Basel, 1973, pp. 188–197.
56. Breslau NA, Padalino P, Kok DJ, Kim YG, Pak CY. Physicochemical effects of a new slow-release potassium phosphate preparation (UroPhos-K) in absorptive hypercalciuria. J Bone Miner Res 1995; 10: 394–400.
57. Robertson WG, Hughes H. Importance of mild hyperoxaluria in the pathogenesis of urolithiasis—new evidence from studies in the Arabian peninsula. Scanning Microsc 1993; 7:391–401.
58. Robertson WG, Peacock M, Nordin BEC. Activity products in stone-forming and non-stone-forming urine. Clin Sci 1968; 34: 579–594.
59. Pardi DS, Tremaine WJ, Sandborn WJ, McCarthy JT. Renal and urological complications of inflammatory bowel disease. Am J Gastroenterol 1998; 93: 500–514.
60. Hylander E, Jarnum S, Nielsen K. Calcium treatment of enteric hyperoxaluria after jejunoileal bypass for morbid obesity. Scand J Gastroent 1980; 15: 349–352.
61. Canos HJ, Hogg GA, Jeffery JR. Oxalate nephropathy due to gastrointestinal disorders. Can Med Assoc J. 1981; 124: 729–733.
62. Drenick EJ, Stanley TM, Border WA, et al. Renal damage with intestinal bypass. Ann Intern Med 1978; 89: 594–599.
63. Modigliani R, Labayle D, Aymes C, Denvil R. Evidence for excessive absorption of oxalate by the colon in enteric hyperoxaluria. Scand J Gastroent 1978; 13: 187–192.
64. McLeod RS, Churchill DN. Urolithiasis complicating inflammatory bowel disease. J Urol 1992; 148: 974–978.

65. Argenzio RA, Liacos JA, Allison MJ. Intestinal oxalate-degrading bacteria reduce oxalate absorption and toxicity in guinea pigs. J Nutr 1988; 118: 787–792.
66. Lieske JC, Spargo B, Toback FG. Endocytosis of calcium oxalate crystals and proliferation of renal tubular epithelial cells in a patient with type 1 primary hyperoxaluria. J Urol 1992; 148: 1517–1519.
67. Mandell I, Krauss E, Millan JC. Oxalate-induced acute renal failure in Crohn's disease. Am J Med 1980; 69: 628–632.
68. Gelbart DR, Brewer LL, Fajardo LF, Weinstein AB. Oxalosis and chronic renal failure after intestinal bypass. Arch Intern Med 1977; 137: 239–243.
69. Lieske JC, Walsh-Reitz MM, Toback FG. Calcium oxalate monohydrate crystals are endocytosed by renal epithelial cells and induce proliferation. Am J Physiol 1992; 262: F622–F630.
70. Hammes MS, Lieske JC, Pawar S, Spargo BH, Toback FG. Calcium oxalate monohydrate crystals stimulate gene expression in renal epithelial cells. Kidney Int. 1995; 48: 501–509.
71. Scheid C, Koul H, Hill WA, et al. Oxalate toxicity in LLC-PK1 cells, a line of renal epithelial cells. J Urol 1996; 155: 1112–1116.
72. Stauffer JQ. Hyperoxaluria and intestinal disease. The role of steatorrhea and dietary calcium in regulating intestinal oxalate absorption. Am J Dig Dis 1977; 22: 921–928.
73. Andersson H, Bosaeus I. Hyperoxaluria in malabsorptive states. Urol Int 1981; 36: 1–9.
74. Parivar F, Low RK, Stoller ML. The influence of diet on urinary stone disease. J Urol 1996; 155: 432–440.
75. Williams HE, Smith LH Jr. Primary hyperoxaluria. In: Stanbury JB, Wyngaarden JB, Fredrickson DS, eds. Metabolic Basis of Inherited Diseases, 4th Ed. McGraw-Hill, New York, NY, 1978.
76. Danpure CJ, Rumsby G. Enzymology and molecular genetics of primary hyperoxaluria type 1. Consequences for clinical management. In: Khan SR, ed. Calcium Oxalate in Biological Systems. CRC Press, Boca Raton, FL, 1995, pp. 189–205.
77. Giafi CF, Rumsby G. Primary hyperoxaluria type 2: enzymology. J Nephrol 1998; 11 (suppl 1): 29–31.
78. Cregeen DP, Rumsby G. Recent developments in our understanding of primary hyperoxaluria type 2. J Am Soc Nephrol 1999; 10(suppl 14): S348–S350.
79. Cramer SD, Ferree PM, Lin K, Milliner DS, Holmes RP. The gene encoding hydroxypyruvate reductase (GRHPR) is mutated in patients with primary hyperoxaluria type II [published erratum appears in Hum Mol Genet 1999; 8(13):2574]. Hum Mol Genet 1999; 8: 2063–2069.
80. Tarn AC, Vonschnakenburg C, Rumsby G. Primary hyperoxaluria type 1—diagnostic relevance of mutations and polymorphisms in the alanine-glyoxylate aminotransferase Gene (Agxt). J Inhert Metab Dis 1997; 20: 689–696.
81. Pirulli D, Puzzer D, Ferri L, et al. Molecular analysis of hyperoxaluria type 1 in Italian patients reveals eight new mutations in the alanine: glyoxylate aminotransferase gene. Hum Genet 1999; 104: 523–525.
82. Milliner DS, Eickholt JT, Bergstralh E, Wilson DM, Smith LH. Results of long-term treatment with orthophosphate and pyridoxine in patients with primary hyperoxaluria. N Engl J Med 1994; 331: 1553–1558.
83. Cochat P, Deloraine A, Rotily M, Olive F, Liponski I, Deries N. Epidemiology of primary hyperoxaluria type 1. Societe de Nephrologie and the Societe de Nephrologie Pediatrique. Nephro Dial Transpl 1995; 10 (suppl 8): 3–7.
84. Latta K, Brodehl J. Primary hyperoxaluria type I. Eur J Pediatr 1990; 149: 518–522.
85. Milliner DS, Wilson DM, Smith LH. Clinical expression and long-term outcomes of primary hyperoxaluria types 1 and 2. J Nephrol 1998; 11 (Special Issue 1):56–59.
85a. Leumann E, Hoppe B. The primary hyperoxalurias. J Am Soc Nephrol 2001; 12(9): 1986–1993.
86. Milliner DS, Wilson DM, Smith LH. Phenotypic expression of primary hyperoxaluria types I and II. Comparative features. Kidney Int 2001; 59: 31–36.
87. Leumann E, Hoppe B, Neuhaus T. Management of primary hyperoxaluria: efficacy of oral citrate administration. Pediatr Nephrol 1993; 7: 207–211.
88. Saborio P, Scheinman JI. Transplantation for primary hyperoxaluria in the United States. Kidney Int 1999; 56: 1094–1100.
89. Pak CYC. Citrate and renal calculi: an update. Miner Electrolyte Metab. 1994; 20: 371–377.

90. Pak CY, Fuller C, Sakhaee K, Preminger GM, Britton F. Long-term treatment of calcium nephrolithiasis with potassium citrate. J Urol. 1985; 134: 11–19.
91. Pak CYC, Peterson R, Sakhaee K, Fuller C, Preminger GM, Reisch J. Correction of hypocitraturia and prevention of stone formation by combined thiazide and potassium citrate therapy in thiazide-unresponsive hypercalciuric nephrolithiasis. Am J Med 1985; 79: 284–288.
92. Sakhaee K, Williams RH, Oh MS, et al. Alkali absorption and citrate excretion in calcium nephrolithiasis. J Bone Miner Res 1993; 8: 789–794.
93. Parks JH, Coe FL. Urine citrate and calcium in calcium nephrolithiasis. Adv Exp Med Biol 1986; 208: 445–449.
94. Dey J, Creighton A, Lindberg JS, et al. Estrogen replacement increased the citrate and calcium excretion rates in postmenopausal women with recurrent urolithiasis. J Urol 2002; 167: 169–171.
95. Barcelo P, Wuhl O, Servitge E, Rousaud A, Pak CYC. Randomized double-blind study of potassium citrate in idiopathic hypocitraturic calcium nephrolithiasis. J Urol 1993150: 1761–1764.
96. Sakhaee K, Nicar M, Hill K, Pak CY. Contrasting effects of potassium citrate and sodium citrate therapies on urinary chemistries and crystallization of stone-forming salts. Kidney Int 1983; 24: 348–352.
97. Seltzer MA, Low RK, McDonald M, Shami GS, Stoller ML. Dietary manipulation with lemonade to treat hypocitraturic calcium nephrolithiasis. J Urol 1996; 156: 907–909.
98. Ettinger B, Pak CY, Citron JT, Thomas C, Adams-Huet B, Vangessel A. Potassium-magnesium citrate is an effective prophylaxis against recurrent calcium oxalate nephrolithiasis. J Urol 1997; 158: 2069–2073.
99. Mandel NS, Mandel GS. Urinary tract stone disease in the United States veteran population. II. Geographical analysis of variations in composition. J Urol 1989; 142: 1516–1521.
100. Rodman JS, Williams JJ, Peterson CM. Dissolution of uric acid calculi. J Urol 1984; 131: 1039.
101. Gutman AB, Yu TF. Uric acid nephrolithiasis. Am J Med 1968; 45: 756.
102. Yu T. Urolithiasis in hyperuricemia and gout. J Urol 1981; 126: 424–430.
103. Rodman JS. Management of uric acid calculi in the elderly patient. Geriatr Nephrol Urol 1991; 1: 129.
104. Loffler W, Grobner W, Zollner N. Influence of dietary protein on serum and urinary uric acid. Adv Exp Biol Med 1980; 122A:209.
105. Gibson T, Hannan SF, Hatfield PJ, et al. The effect of acid loading on renal excretion of uric acid and ammonium in gout. Adv Exp Biol Med. 1977; 76B:46.
106. Matzkies F, Berg G. The uricosuric action of amino acids in men. Adv Exp Biol Med. 1977; 76B: 36.
107. Pak CYC, Sakahee K, Peterson RD, Poindexter JR, Frawley WH. Biochemical profile of idiopathic uric acid nephrolithiasis. Kidney Int 2001; 60: 757–761.
108. Yu TF, Gutman AB. Uric acid nephrolithiasis in gout: predisposing factors. Ann Intern Med 1967; 67: 1133.
109. Gutman AB, Yu TF. A three-component system for regulation of renal excretion of uric acid in man. Trans Assoc Am Phys 1961; 74: 353.
110. Yu TF, Weinreb N, Wittman R, Wasserman LR. Secondary gout associated with chronic myeloproliferative disorders. Semin Arthritis Rheum 1976; 5: 247.
111. Kelley WN, Beardmore TD. Allopurinol: alteration in pyrimidine metabolism in man. Science 1970; 169: 388–390.
112. Rodman JS. Prophylaxis of uric acid stones with alternate day doses of alkaline potassium salts. J Urol 1991; 145: 97–99.
113. Prien EL, Prien ELJ. Composition and structure of urinary stone. Am J Med 1968; 45: 654.
114. Coe FL. Hyperuricosuric calcium oxalate nephrolithiasis. Kidney Int. 1978; 13: 418–426.
115. Pak CYC, Waters O, Arnold L, Holt K, Cox C, Barilla DE. Mechanism for calcium urolithiasis among patients with hyperuricosuria. J Clin Invest 1977; 59: 426–431.
116. Coe FL, Lawton RL, Goldstein RB, Tembe V. Sodium urate accelerates precipitation of calcium oxalate in vitro. Proc Soc Exp Biol Med 1975; 149: 926–929.
117. Robertson WG, Knowles F, Peacock M. Urinary acid mucopolysaccharide inhibitors of calcium oxalate crystallization. In: Fleisch H, Robertson WG, Smith LH, et al., eds. Urolithiasis Research, 1st Ed. Plenum, London, England, 1976, pp. 331–340.
118. Grover PK, Ryall RL, Marshall VR. Dissolved urate promotes calcium oxalate crystallization: epitaxy is not the cause. Clin Sci (Colch) 1993; 85: 303–307.

119. Finlayson B, Newman RC, Hunter PC. The role of urate and allopurinol in stone disease: a review. In: Schwille PO, Smith LH, Robertson WG, et al., eds. Urolithiasis and Related Research. Plenum, New York, NY, 1985, pp. 499–503.
120. Millman S, Strauss AL, Parks JH, Coe FL. Pathogenesis and clinical course of mixed calcium oxalate and uric acid nephrolithiasis. Kidney Int 1982; 22: 366–370.
121. Tiselius HG, Larsson L. Urinary excretion of urate in patients with calcium oxalate stone disease. Urol Res 1983; 11: 279–283.
122. Ettinger B, Tang A, Citron JT, Livermore B, Williams T. Randomized trial of allopurinol in the prevention of calcium oxalate calculi. N Engl J Med 1986; 315: 1386–1389.
123. Tiselius HG, Larsson L, Hellgren E. Clinical results of allopurinol treatment in prevention of calcium oxalate stone formation. J Urol 1986; 136: 50–53.
124. Finlayson B, Burns J, Smith A, Du Bois L. Effect of oxipurinol and allopurinol riboside on whewellite crystallization: in vitro and in vivo observations. Invest Urol 1979; 17: 227–229.
124a. Pak CY, Sakhaee K, Fuller C. Successful management of uric acid nephrolithiasis with potassium citrate. Kidney Int 1986; 30(3): 422–428.
125. Robertson WG. Epidemiology of urinary stone disease. Urol Res 1990; 18:S3–S8.
126. Berg C, Tiselius HG. The effect of pH on the risk of calcium oxalate crystallization in urine. Eur Urol 1986; 12: 59–61.
127. Peacock M, Robertson WG, Marshall RW. Disorders associated with renal calcium-stone disease. Endocrinology 1979; 2:823–827.
128. Gault MH, Chafe LL, Morgan JM, et al. Comparison of patients with idiopathic calcium phosphate and calcium oxalate stones. Medicine 1991; 70: 345–358.
129. Tiselius H-G, Larsson L. Calcium phosphate: an important crystal phase in patients with recurrent calcium stone formation. Urol Res 1993; 21: 175–180.
130. Buckalew VM. Nephrolithiasis in renal tubular acidosis. J Urol 1989; 141: 731–737.
131. Robertson WG. Factors affecting the precipitation of calcium phosphate in vitro. Calcified Tissue Res 1973; 11: 311–322.
132. Tiselius HG. A simplified estimate of the ion-activity product of calcium phosphate in urine. Eur Urol 1984; 10: 191–195.
133. Hesse A, Heimbach D. Causes of phosphate stone formation and the importance of metaphylaxis by urinary acidification: a review. Q World J Urol 1999; 17: 308–315.
134. Preminger GM, Sakhaee K, Skurla C, Pak CY. Prevention of recurrent calcium stone formation with potassium citrate therapy in patients with distal renal tubular acidosis. J Urol 1985; 134: 20–23.
135. Buckalew VM, Purvis LM, Shulman MG, Herndon CN, Rudman D. Hereditary renal tubular acidosis: a report of a 64 member kindred with variable clinical expression including idiopathic hypercalciuria. Medicine 1974; 53: 229–254.
136. Hamed IA, Czerwinski AW, Coats B, Kaufman C, Altmiller DH. Familial absorptive hypercalciuria and renal tubular acidosis. Am J Med 1979; 67: 385–391.
137. Tessitore N, Ortalda V, Fabris A, et al. Renal acidification defects in patients with recurrent calcium nephrolithiasis. Nephron 1985; 41: 325–332.
138. Caruana RJ, Buckalew VMJ. The syndrome of distal (type 1) renal tubular acidosis. Clinical and laboratory findings in 58 cases. Medicine (Baltimore) 1988; 67: 84–99.
139. Dick WH, Wilson DM, Bucki JJ. Ammonium chloride treatment for brushite calculi. Urolihtiasis, Dallas, TX, 1996.
140. Rodman J. Struvite stones. Nephron 1999; 81 (suppl): 50–59.
141. Williams JJ, Rodman JS, Peterson CM. A randomized double blind study of acetohydroxamic acid in struvite nephrolithiasis. N Engl J Med 1984; 311: 760–764.
142. Stewart AF, Adler M, Byers CM, Segre GV, Broadus AE. Calcium homostatis in immobilization: an example of resorptive hypercalciuria. N Engl J Med 1982; 306: 1136–1140.
143. Williams HE. Nephrolithiasis. N Engl J Med 1974; 290: 33–38.
144. Cohen TD, Preminger GM. Struvite calculi. Semin Nephrol 1996; 16: 425–434.
145. Petterson S, Brorson JE, Grenabo I, Hedelin H. *Ureaplasma urealyticum* in infection urinary tract stones. Lancet 1983;i:526–527.
146. Nickel JC, Emtage J, Costerton JW. Ultrastructural microbial ecology of infection induced urinary stones. J Urol 1985; 133: 622–627.

147. Lewi H, Hales DSM, Dunsumir R. Netilmicin sulfate prophyllaxis in the surgical treatment of renal stones. Surg Gynecol Obstet 1984; 159: 357–362.
148. Blandly J, Singh M. The case for a more aggressive approach to staghorn stones. J Urol 1976; 115: 505–506.
149. Segura JW. Staghorn calculi. Urol Clin North Am 1997; 24: 71–80.
150. Lavengood RW, Marshall VF. The prevention of renal phosphatidic calculi in the presence of infection by the Shorr regimen. J Urol 1972; 108: 368.
151. Schwartz BF, Stoller ML. Nonsurgical management of infection-related renal calculi. Urol Clin North Am 1999; 26: 765–778.
152. Jarrar K, Boedeker RH, Weidner W. Struvite stones: long term follow up under metaphylaxis. Ann Urol 1996; 30: 112–117.
153. Goodyer P, Boutros M, Rozen R. The molecular basis of cystinuria: an update. Exp Nephrol 2000; 8: 123–127.
154. Barbey F, Joly D, Rieu P, Mejean A, Daudon M, Jungers P. Medical treatment of cystinuria: critical reappraisal of long-term results. J Urol 2000; 163: 1419–1423.
155. Hernandez-Graulau JM, Castenada-Zuniga W, Hunter D. Management of cystine nephrolithiasis by endourologic methods and shock-wave lithotripsy. Urology 1989; 34: 139.
156. Font M, Feliubadalo L, Estivil X, et al. Functional analysis of mutations in SCL7A9, and genotype-phenotype correlation in non-Type I cystinuria. Hum Mol Genet 2001; 10: 305–316.
157. Bisceglia L, Purroy J, Jimenez-Vidal M, et al. Cystinuria type I. Identification of eight new mutations in *SLC3A1*. Kidney Int 2001; 59: 1250–1256.
158. Dent CE, Senior B. Studies on the treatment of cystinuria. Br J Urol 1955; 27: 317.
159. Crawhall JC, Scowen EF, Watts RW. Effects of penicillamine on cystinuria. Br J Med 1963; 5330: 588.
160. Lindell A, Denneberg T, Jeppsson JO. Urinary excretion of free cystine and the tiopronin-cysteine-mixed disulfide during long term tiopronin treatment of cystinuria. Nephron 1995; 71: 328.
161. Streem SB, Hall P. Effect of captopril on urinary cystine excretion in homozygous cystinuria. J Urol 1989; 142: 1522–1524.
162. Perazella MA, Buller GK. Successful treatment of cystinuria with captopril. Am J Kidney Dis 1993; 21: 504–507.
163. Nakagawa Y, Asplin JR, Goldfarb DS, Parks JH, Coe FL. Clinical use of cystine supersaturations. J Urol 2000; 164: 1481–1485.
164. Coe FL, Clark C, Parks JH, Asplin JR. Solid phase assay of urine cystine supersaturation in the presence of cystine binding drugs. J Urol 2001; 166: 688–693.
165. Pope JC, Trusler LA, Klein A, M., Walsh WF, Yared A, Brock JW. The natural history of nephrocalcinosis in premature infants treated with loop diuretics. J Urol 1996; 156: 709–712.
166. Wandzilak TR, D'Andre SD, Davis PA, Williams HE. Effect of high dose vitamin C on urinary oxalate levels. J Urol 1994; 151: 834–837.
167. Auer BL, Auer D, Rodgers AL. Relative hyperoxaluria, crystalluria and hematuria after megadose ingestion of vitamin C. Eur J Clin Invest. 1998; 28: 695–700.
168. Kuiper JJ. Medullary sponge kidney. In: Gardner KD, ed. Cystic Diseases of the Kidney. John Wiley & Sons, New York, NY, 1976, pp. 151–171.
169. Sage MR, Lawson AD, Marshall VR, Ryall RL. Medullary sponge kidney and urolithiasis. Clin Radiol 1982; 33: 435–438.
170. Rommel D, Pirson Y. Medullary sponge kidney—part of a congenital kidney. Nephrol Dial Transplant 2001; 16: 634–636.
171. Indridason OS, Thomas L, Berkoben M. Medullary sponge kidney associated with congenitla hemihypertrophy. J Am Soc Nephrol 1996; 8: 1123–1130.
172. Porile JL, Asplin JR, Parks JH, Nakagawa Y, Coe FL. Normal calcium oxalate crystal growth inhibition in severe calcium oxalate nephrolithiasis. J Am Soc Nephrol 1996; 7: 602–607.
173. Shekarriz B, Lu H-F, Stoller ML. Correlation of unilateral urolithiasis with sleep posture. J Urol 2001; 165: 1085–1087.
174. Asplin JR, Parks JH, Chen MS, et al. Reduced crystallization inhibition by urine from men with nephrolithiasis. Kidney Int 1999; 56: 1505–1516.
175. Lieske JC, Deganello S, Toback FG. Cell-crystal interactions and kidney stone formation. Nephron 1999; 81: S8–S17.

176. Ciftcioglu N, Bjorklund M, Kuorikoski K, Bergstrom K, Kajander EO. Nanobacteria: an infectious cause for kidney stone formation. Kidney Int 1999; 56: 1893–1898.
177. Scheinman SJ. X-linked hypercalciuric nephrolithiasis: clinical syndromes and chloride channel mutations. Kidney Int 1998; 53: 3–17.
178. Pearce SHS, Williamson C, Kifor O, et al. A familial syndrome of hypocalcemia with hypercalciuria due to mutations in the calcium-sensing receptor. N Engl J Med 1996; 335: 1115–1122.
179. Kubota M, Nishi-Nagase M, Sakakihara Y, et al. Zonisamide-induced urinary lithiasis in patients with intractable epilepsy. Brain Dev. 2000; 22: 230–233.
180. Assimos DG, Langenstroer P, Leinbach RF, Mandel NS, Stern JM, Holmes RP. Guaifenesin- and ephedrine-induced stones. J Endourol 1999; 13: 665–667.
181. Rich JD, Ramratnam B, Chiang M, Tashima KT. Management of indinavir associated nephrolithiasis. J Urol 1997; 158: 2228.

8 Management of Female Urinary Incontinence

Raymond R. Rackley, MD
and Joseph B. Abdelmalak, MD

Contents

INTRODUCTION

Urinary incontinence (UI) is generally defined as the involuntary loss of urine from the bladder through the urethral meatus. More than 13 million people in the United States—male and female, young and old—experience incontinence. UI is the second-leading cause of institutionalization of the elderly in the United States *(1)*, and the cost of managing this condition was approx $16 billion in 1994 *(2)*. UI is often temporary and always results from an underlying medical condition. Women experience incontinence two times more often than men do, most likely as a result of pregnancy, childbirth, menopause, and the structure of the female urinary tract. Additionally, older women experience incontinence more frequently than younger women. Despite one's age, incontinence is treatable and often curable.

Incontinence in women usually occurs because of problems with the muscles that help to hold and release urine. Normally during urination, muscles in the wall of the bladder contract, forcing urine out of the bladder and into the urethra. At the same time,

From: *Essential Urology: A Guide to Clinical Practice*
Edited by: J. M. Potts © Humana Press Inc., Totowa, NJ

sphincter muscles surrounding the urethra relax, letting urine pass out of the body. Incontinence occurs if the bladder muscles suddenly contract or if the muscles surrounding the urethra suddenly relax. UI should not be considered a disease, but rather a sign of an underlying problem with the muscles. Traditionally, UI has been classified into six categories, based on specific underlying etiologies, evaluation, and management *(3)*.

Transient (reversible) incontinence is common in elderly and hospitalized patients. It may be the result of medications, urinary tract infections, mental impairment (delirium or confusional state), restricted mobility, stool impaction (severe constipation), or excessive urine output (congestive heart failure, hyperglycemia).

Overflow incontinence is rare in women and reflects an overdistension of the bladder resulting from bladder-outlet obstruction (caused by stricture or overcorrective surgery for incontinence or vaginal prolapse), an acontractile detrusor (caused by diabetes, multiple sclerosis), or psychogenic retention. Patients usually present with frequent and constant dribbling of urine and a non-normal voiding pattern.

Total incontinence reflects continuous urine leakage without the sensation of bladder fullness or the urge to void. It may be caused by urinary tract fistulas, congenital anomalies, overflow incontinence, or severe intrinsic sphincteric deficiency.

Stress urinary incontinence (SUI) is defined as urinary leakage secondary to an increase in abdominal pressure (coughing, laughing, and sneezing). It is classified by bladder neck/urethral hypermobility and intrinsic sphincteric deficiency (ISD). Urethral hypermobility accounts for 85% of SUI and develops with aging, hormonal changes, traumatic or prolonged delivery, and pelvic surgery. ISD represents 15% of SUI in females. It may be caused by damage to the bladder neck after previous pelvic or anti-incontinence procedures, pelvic radiation, trauma, or neurogenic disorders that result in bladder neck denervation.

Urge incontinence is defined as urinary leakage associated with an abrupt (urge) desire to void that cannot be suppressed or inhibited. It is usually idiopathic and affects the elderly. However, other causes of unstable bladder, such as bacterial cystitis, bladder tumors, bladder stones, outlet obstruction, or neurological diseases, must be excluded before making this diagnosis.

Mixed incontinence is common in 50 to 60% of patients who present for evaluation of SUI. It is refers to the association of SUI and urge incontinence. Proper management requires recognition and evaluation of each anatomical and neurologic component that contributes to UI.

EVALUATION

The goals of the basic evaluation are to confirm UI and to identify factors that may be contributing to or resulting from UI. The general evaluation of UI should include a history, fluid intake/voiding diary, physical examination, urinalysis, urine culture, and a measurement of postvoiding residual urine. For selected patients, a blood test (urea and creatinine), urodynamic evaluation, cystoscopy, and imaging studies of the urinary tract and/or the central nervous system may be recommended.

HISTORY

A patient's history should include the problem's onset, duration, progression, evolution, and precipitating factors (Valsalva maneuvers, change of position). Important associated urinary symptoms, such as pain, burning, frequency, urgency, hesitancy, postvoid dribbling, nocturia, nocturnal enuresis, hematuria, constipation, fecal incontinence, sexual dysfunction, dyspareunia, and prolapse symptoms should also be recorded.

A thorough review of the patient's medical history is recommended to find any conditions that might interfere with urinary output, such as renal insufficiency, diabetes mellitus, congestive heart failure, pelvic radiation therapy for treatment of cancer, and/or neurological diseases, such as multiple sclerosis, Parkinson's disease, or stroke. All medications taken by the patient, including antihypertensive drugs, diuretics, sedatives, hypnotics, analgesics, and antidepressants, must be documented. A review of the patient's obstetric history is also important. This includes parity, types of delivery, perineal repairs, and difficult deliveries. Finally, the surgical history should include all genitourinary surgical interventions for treatment of incontinence and/or pelvic prolapse.

FLUID INTAKE/VOIDING DIARY

A fluid intake/voiding diary should be distributed to document the amount and type of fluid consumed by the patient, the volume and time of voiding and leakage, and the number and type of pads used per day and per night.

PHYSICAL EXAMINATION

A complete physical examination is essential, and special emphasis should be given to the abdominal, pelvic, genital, and neurological examinations.

Abdomen

The abdomen should be inspected for surgical scars and obesity and palpated for any abdominal or retroperitoneal masses or bladder distension.

Genitals

The external genitalia should be inspected for any abnormalities (Bartholin's cyst, condyloma, adhesion, and scar formation) and for atrophy of the vaginal epithelium (shiny cell wall or loss of rugae). In addition, inspect for periurethral and urethral lesions (mucosal prolapse, carbuncle, condyloma, Skein's abscess, or stenosis) and palpate for scaring, fibrosis, or tenderness that suggests urethritis or urethral diverticulum. Measure the urethral hypermobility by placing a Q-tip in the urethra to the level of the bladder neck while the patient is placed in the lithotomy position. Ask the patient to cough and strain. A deflection of the Q-tip greater than 30° suggests significant urethral hypermobility. The absence of a hypermobile urethra based on the Q-tip test in the presence of incontinence with coughing or straining suggests intrinsic sphincteric deficiency. Determine the postvoid residual urine by bladder ultrasound or by straight catheterization. Inspect the anterior, posterior, and apical aspects of the vaginal vault with the posterior blade of a Grave's speculum. Palpate the pelvic floor muscles while the patient is at rest and after she strains. Determine the various components of prolapse (cystocele, rectocele, enterocele, or uterine prolapse).

Provocation Test

Fill the patient's bladder with 200–300 cc of sterile water using a sterile catheter. Withdraw the catheter and ask the patient to strain or cough in various positions (supine, sitting, or standing). A leakage event indicates stress urinary incontinence.

Neurologic Examination

Examine the general neurologic status, perineum, and lower extremities for the presence of tremor, loss of cognitive function, weakness, or gait abnormality. Examine the back for asymmetry bone contours, skin dimples, or scar. Evaluate the S2–S4 nerve roots by the bulbocavernosus reflex (contraction of the external anal sphincter when sensation is applied to the clitoris). Evaluate lower extremities by testing typical sensory patterns and evaluating deep-tendon and primitive reflexes that may suggest anatomic and etiologic significance. A stocking pattern of sensory loss may be indicative of metabolic neuropathies such as diabetes or alcoholism. The Babinski sign (primitive reflex) and ankle clonus suggest suprasacral cord lesions. Deep tendon reflexes of the quadriceps (L4) and Achilles tendon (S1) can demonstrate segmental spinal cord function as well as suprasegmental function.

LABORATORY TESTS

The following are the laboratory tests that may be performed.

1. Urinalysis: Urinalysis is performed to exclude hematuria, pyuria, bacteriuria, glycosuria, and proteinuria.
2. Urine culture: A urine culture is obtained for evidence of bacteriuria or pyuria.
3. Urine cytology: Urine cytology is indicated to screen for bladder cancer if there is evidence of hematuria with frequency or urgency.
4. Blood urea nitrogen (BUN) and serum creatinine level: BUN and serum creatinine level determinations are indicated in patients with a history or findings of severe voiding dysfunction. Furthermore, the consumption of excess fluid intake may be reflected in an abnormally low level of BUN.
5. Vaginal swabs: Vaginal swabs are used for culturing ureaplasma and chlamydia.

Other Procedures

The following procedures are for selected patients with a history or physical findings suggestive of underlying urological disease, prolapse, hematuria, recurrent infection, or recent history of an abdominal or pelvic procedure.

Urodynamics

Urodynamics (evaluating the dynamic interaction of the bladder muscle and sphincter) may be performed at different levels of sophistication and complexity to identify bladder compliance, unstable bladder contractions, and voiding bladder pressures that influence the overall management of the patients voiding dysfunction. The levels of urodynamics testing used are as follows:

1. Simple cystometrography (CMG) is performed by filling the patient's bladder with 200–300 cc of sterile water using a sterile catheter. Withdrawing the catheter and asking the patient to strain or cough in various positions (supine, sitting, or standing) may lead to leakage, which indicates stress urinary incontinence.
2. Single-channel CMG uses a single catheter in the bladder to measure pressure during filling, which reflects bladder compliance.
3. Multichannel CMG typically measures the urine flow rate and bladder pressure through a catheter in the bladder, and intraabdominal pressure via a catheter in the rectum. This type of test is necessary in the management of mixed incontinence or for failures after

anti-incontinence procedures. It documents bladder compliance and instability as well as dynamic intrinsic sphincteric competency by determining the Valsalva pressure needed to cause urinary leakage. It also measures bladder pressure during voiding.

4. Videourodynamics use a combination of fluoroscopy and multichannel urodynamics to provide simultaneous anatomic and functional assessments of the bladder.
5. Ambulatory urodynamic monitoring provides continuous documentation of bladder pressure and voiding. It is generally restricted for research purposes and difficult cases of refractory bladder overactivity.
6. Electromyography testing measures the electrical activity of either the external urethral sphincter or anal sphincter to document denervation of the pelvic floor muscles or urinary sphincter, or abnormal coordination of the bladder and external urinary sphincter. It is mainly used in patients with an abnormal neurologic finding (multiple sclerosis and spinal cord disease, injury, or surgery).
7. Urethral pressure profile is the static measurement of pressure along the length of the urethra. It has a very little value in determining the dynamic cause and type of female urinary incontinence.
8. Abdominal leak point pressure is determined by having the patient perform a slow Valsalva maneuver while in the upright position to determine the level of abdominal pressure that allows urine to escape. This is an important dynamic test in the evaluation of women with stress incontinence.

Cystoscopy

Cystoscopy has a limited role in the evaluation of patients with a straightforward, isolated SUI. However, it is needed to evaluate other causes of UI or concurrent urologic diseases identified in the history and physical examination, especially in patients with urge incontinence. Examination of the urethra may reveal a diverticulum, fistula, stricture, or urethritis. The bladder is inspected for mucosal or trigonal abnormalities, trabeculation, foreign bodies, and stones. Bladder-neck hypermobility and intrinsic sphincteric deficiency may also be reassessed by having the patient cough or strain with the scope in the midurethra.

Urinary Tract Imaging

Urinary tract imaging has a very limited role in the evaluation of the uncomplicated case of female incontinence. Intravenous pyelography (IVP), voiding cystourethrography (VCUG), and ultrasound studies are commonly used for evaluation of the upper and lower urinary tract but are never first-line studies in the assessment of UI.

IVP

IVP is indicated if the patient's history suggests the presence of an ectopic ureter, hematuria, or recurrent urinary tract infections and if hydroureteronephrosis is found during ultrasound or computed tomography studies.

Ultrasonography

Ultrasonography is useful for the evaluation of the upper urinary tract, particularly to detect hydronephrosis due to elevated bladder pressure in patients with neurogenic bladder-sphincteric dysfunction. In addition to the study of pelvic pathology, ultrasound has been used for determining a postvoid residual volume and for detecting urethral diverticulum.

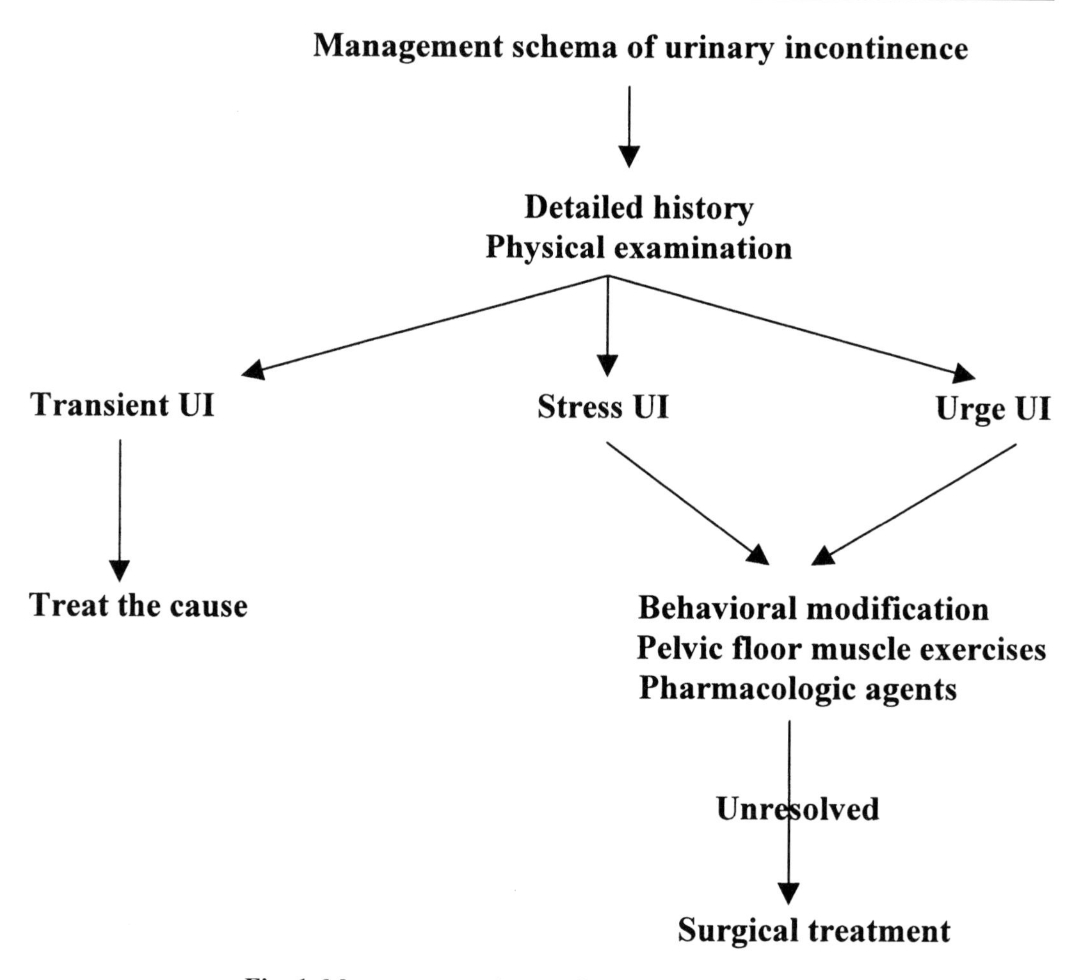

Fig. 1. Management schema of urinary incontinence.

VCUG

VCUG is a simple, safe, and reliable study to evaluate the integrity of the female lower urinary tract when one suspects bladder or urethral pathology, such as vesicovaginal or urethrovaginal fistulas, urethral diverticulum, or bladder prolapse. Although urethral hypermobility may be detected on rest and strain views, there is a limited role for the VCUG in determining conclusive evidence of ISD because the bladder pressure is not recorded during the examination.

MANAGEMENT

There are three major categories of therapy for female UI (*see* Fig. 1): behavioral, pharmacological, and surgical. Patients should be informed of all the treatment options and should receive information on the expected outcomes and risks, benefits of each, given their particular case *(3)*.

Treatments are usually staged with the least invasive forms (behavioral modification and pelvic floor retraining) being offered first, followed by the introduction of pharmacologic agents when indicated. Finally, after optimization of the pelvic floor and bladder physiology, reconstructive surgery may be recommended to obtain continence and normal voiding function.

Behavioral Interventions

Behavioral Interventions may be easily initiated. They include a range of behavioral modifications that are dependent on the type of voiding dysfunction diagnosed. For patients with incontinence, the awareness of the quantity of fluid intake, timing of fluid intake, and avoidance of bladder stimulants, such as caffeine, can achieve modest improvement in urinary symptoms. Avoidance of diuretics before recumbency and emptying the bladder before reaching maximum functional capacity (timed voiding) are also taught. Patients with congestive heart failure and/or fluid retention in the lower extremity benefit from promoting a diuretic phase before periods of recumbency by elevating the lower extremities while sitting, initiating light walking programs for muscle pumping of congested veins in the leg, using pressure-gradient stockings, and by the judicious use of diuretics and an avoidance of high-salt diets. The use of a bedside commode, adjustment of garments for easier undressing, and provision of mobility aids will prevent many episodes of urge incontinence in patients with cognitive dysfunction, mobility problems, and physical handicaps.

Bladder Retraining

Bladder retraining teaches patients methods of inhibiting the urge sensation to void to gradually expand the voiding interval. These methods rely on the sympathetic mediated negative feedback inhibition augmented by the somatic mediated contraction of the external urinary sphincter on bladder contractions. This means, by voluntary contraction of the external urinary sphincter, most patients are able to extinguish low-level bladder contractions (urgency). Retraining or improving a patient's ability to increase her external urinary sphincter tone with a voluntary effort may aid in the treatment of urge and urge incontinence, lead to less urinary frequency, and improve functional bladder capacity. Other methods to inhibit the urge sensation include distraction techniques and biofeedback using deep breathing and relaxation exercises. All of these techniques of bladder retraining appear to work best in patients who have forms of urge or mixed incontinence and who are cognitively intact, properly motivated, and who have the capacity to understand and follow instructions.

Pelvic Floor Muscle Rehabilitation

Pelvic floor muscle rehabilitation exercises the pelvic floor muscles (the levator ani muscles), resulting in decreased urethral hypermobility and increased urethral resistance, which prevent stress incontinence. Although many patients can be instructed to identify the proper muscle groups for pelvic floor muscle exercises in the office, the best results are achieved by repetitive training, use of biofeedback, and consultation or initiation of therapy by a physical therapist or a nurse with specialized training.

Current devices for pelvic floor muscle rehabilitation include intravaginal weighted cones *(4)* and the use of electrical stimulation (rectal or vaginal electrode; ref. *5*). Although the side effects of these devices are minimal, the results appear to last only as long as the device is used, and may not demonstrate any added advantage over properly performed exercises. We strongly emphasized the rehabilitation of the obturator interns muscle as well, which shares a common fascial insertion with the levator ani muscles called the arcus tendinous muscularis. Although pelvic floor rehabilitation may appear useful for all patients, stress UI that results from traumatic peripheral neuropathy can lead to muscle atrophy and dysfunction. Standard rehabilitation techniques require at least partial innervation to the muscle groups of interest unless the nerves are bypassed by an electrical stimulator. Thus, behavioral therapy does not work for all cases.

Currently, there is no reproducible neurological test to determine which patients are likely to benefit from a standard approach, yet the low risk of this noninvasive therapy makes pelvic floor exercises an acceptable first-line therapy for all patients except those with ISD.

Pharmacological Agents

Pharmacological agents have been used with variable success to treat UI. They work best when used as an adjuvant to behavioral interventions. Drug therapy for UI is generally used to inhibit the bladder smooth muscle contractions in urge incontinence, increase bladder outlet resistance in stress incontinence, or decrease outlet resistance and increase bladder smooth muscle contractions in overflow incontinence.

Bladder contractions are mediated primarily by the parasympathetic nervous system; therefore, pharmacologic therapies that inhibit contractions are used. These include drugs with anticholinergic activity. However, anticholinergics are contraindicated in patients with documented narrow-angle glaucoma.

Oxybutynin (Ditropan)

Oxybutynin (Ditropan XL) has anticholinergic as well as direct relaxation effects on the smooth muscle of the bladder. For patients with urge incontinence caused by bladder instability, these agents may provide at least partial relief of symptoms. Relaxation of the bladder muscle increases the volume that stimulates a bladder contraction, increases total bladder capacity, and decreases the strength of a normal bladder contraction. In general, patients with smaller bladder capacities respond well to oxybutynin. The recommended dose of oxybutynin (Ditropan) is 2.5 to 5.0 mg taken orally two to four times a day while Ditropan XL is given in doses of 5, 10, or 15 mg/once daily. Side effects and toxicity of these drugs may include dry mouth, blurred vision, constipation, elevated intraocular pressure, cardiac disturbances, and delirium *(6)*. A transdermal delivery formulation of oxybutynin is also available.

Dicyclomine

Dicyclomine is an anticholinergic drug indicated in patients with large capacity bladders. The recommended dose is 10 to 20 mg one to four times a day, and the side effects are the same as oxybutynin.

Tolterodine (Detrol)

Tolterodine is a potent muscarinic receptor antagonist that has been specifically developed for the treatment of overactive bladder with symptoms of urgency, frequency, and/or urge incontinence. It has two forms: Tolterodine immediate release tablets given in a bid dosage regimen of 2 mg/d, and Tolterodine extended release with a dose of 4 mg/d. Side effects are dry mouth, blurred vision, and constipation *(7)*.

Imipramine

Imipramine, a tricyclic antidepressant, has dual actions. It decreases bladder contractions through its anticholinergic effects while increasing bladder-neck resistance through its α-agonist properties. Although only approved by the Food and Drug Administration for enuresis in children, the usual adult dosage is 10 to 25 mg one to three times daily. Side effects may include postural hypotension and cardiac conduction disturbances in the elderly.

Hyoscyamine and Hyoscyamine Sulfate

Hyoscyamine and hyoscyamine sulfate are similar to other anticholinergic agents but generally appear to have less potent effects and fewer side effects. The adult doses of hyoscyamine range from 0.15 to 0.3 mg one to four times a day; the hyoscyamine sulfate dosage is 0.375 mg one to two times a day.

Propantheline

Propantheline, an antimuscarinic and ganglionic-blocking agent, is less popular for treating urge incontinence. The recommended adult dose is 15 to 30 mg every 4 to 6 h; the side effects are similar to those of oxybutynin.

α-Adrenergic Blocking Agents

Pseudoephedrine and Phenylpropanolamine

Pseudoephedrine and phenylpropanolamine are the most commonly used agents for stress incontinence because of the sympathetic control of the intrinsic sphincter and bladder-neck region. The usual adult dosage of phenylpropanolamine is 25 to 100 mg in sustained-release form, given orally twice a day; that of pseudoephedrine is 15 to 30 mg three times a day. Side effects include high blood pressure, stomach cramping, and central nervous system symptoms of excitation and drowsiness. These drugs must be used with caution in patients with hypertension, angina, hyperthyroidism, and diabetes.

Terazosin and Doxazosin

Terazosin and doxazosin are used for the treatment of overflow incontinence. They have been shown to reduce outlet resistance to urine flow and have synergistic effects with the use of estrogen therapy. Side effects may include dizziness, vertigo, fatigue, and rarely, hypotension. The dosage of doxazosin is 1 to 4 mg at bedtime.

Cholinergic Drugs

Cholinergic drugs (bethanechol) are used to treat patients with associated bladder hypocontractility, which may or may not be associated with moderate to large postvoid residuals. They are contraindicated in patients with asthma, bradycardia, and Parkinson's disease and have side effects of sweating and excessive salivation.

Estrogen Therapy

Estrogen therapy (ET) has recently been shown to have beneficial effects for the treatment of all types of incontinence. Through the restoration of the integrity of the urethra, bladder neck, and vaginal epithelium, the use of ET has been recommended as an adjuvant to pharmacological and surgical treatment of incontinence. Clinical studies have revealed its usefulness in conjunction with behavioral interventions and pharmacological agents. ET may augment the effects of anticholinergics and α-adrenergic receptor agents by promoting upregulation of neurotransmitter receptor function. Therefore, ET is recommended as baseline therapy for all forms of incontinence. Even in the case of overflow incontinence caused by urethral obstruction by scarring, fibrosis, or stenosis, estrogens play an adjunctive role in decreasing the impedance of urine flow by restoring mucosal, vascular, and muscle integrity to the urethra. Estrogens are used either orally, transdermally, or topically. Topical estrogen application should be considered first because of its low systemic absorption and preferential local uptake; in some cases, topical therapy is recommend in additional to oral or transdermal estrogen. This occurs when mild atrophic changes of the vaginal epithelium are noted on pelvic examination. Side effects of estrogens include endometrial cancer, fluid retention, depression, nausea, vomiting, elevated blood pressure, gallstones, and cardiovascular effects, such as stroke and myocardial infarction. The dosage of conjugated estrogens is 1.25 to 2.5 mg a day applied topically at bedtime. Estradiol is given at 0.3 mg/d to 0.625 mg/d orally. Yearly pap smears and breast examinations should be performed when placing or following patients on ET. Estrogens are restricted in patients with a history of deep venous thrombosis, embolization, and gynecologic malignancies *(8–10)*.

Botulinum Toxin

Botulinum Toxin is a potent muscarinic receptor antagonist that is approved for the treatment of muscle spasticity. Botulinum toxin injections into the external urethral sphincter have been described in the treatment of detrusor sphincter dyssynergia in spinal cord injury patients as a means to paralyze the sphincter muscle's activity and to relieve urethral obstruction *(11)*. This procedure is repeated three times at 4-wk intervals. In 2000, Schurch et al. *(12)* reported the injection of Botulinum toxin into the detrusor muscle in spinal cord injured patients in order to treat detrusor hyperreflexia. The side effects are sensitivity to the drug, mild hematuria, and local pain.

Intravesical Instillation of Capsaicin and Resiniferatoxin (Under Trial)

Capsaicin, the main pungent ingredient in hot peppers, is a specific neurotoxin that desensitizes C fiber afferent neurons. A dose of 50 to 100 mL of 2 m*M* capsaicin dissolved in 30% ethanol in saline is instilled in the bladder and left for about 30 min. It is very painful. Resiniferatoxin is 1000 times more potent than capsaicin and does not cause the initial pain sensation. The recommended form is 1 n*M* to 10 μ*M (13)*.

Sacral Nerve Stimulation (InterStim System, Medtronic, Minneapolis, MN)

The detrusor, levator ani, and external sphincter muscles share the sacral nerves as a common innervation. Sacral nerves contain a mixture of autonomic and somatic fibers (afferent and efferent). Afferent nerve fibers are sensory, and efferent fibers are motor. Stimulation of these nerves by InterStim system activates or inhibits muscle action, influences pelvic floor behavior, and modulates neural reflexes. This technique is safe and effective in treating refractory urge UI *(14)*.

SURGICAL MANAGEMENT

Surgical management is mainly for treatment of SUI, which may be the result of anatomic hypermobility or intrinsic sphincteric deficiency of the urethral closure mechanism. Clinical experience with objective urodynamic evaluations supports this classification. The aims of surgical treatments are (1) restoration of the urethra to its proper resting position and stabilization of this position during increases in intra-abdominal pressure; (2) augmentation of intraurethral pressures for restoration of intrinsic urethral closure, or (3) a combination of both restoration of support and augmentation of urethral closure.

Implants

Periurethral and transurethral injections of bulking agents at the level of the proximal urethra have been used extensively for years to increase the outflow resistance of the urethra for the treatment of SUI caused by ISD. Injectables are able to increase urethral closure function without significantly resulting in increases of urethral closure pressure, which would lead to a rise in voiding pressure. The overall effect is to correct the incompetent urethral closure mechanism without clinically disturbing voiding function *(15)*.

Many choices for injectable substances exist; they include sclerosing solutions, polytetrafluoroethylene paste, glutaraldehyde cross-linked bovine collagen (GAX collagen), carbon particles (Durasphere), autologous fat, silicone particles, and many more. Currently, the only injectable materials acceptable for use in the United States are autologous materials such as fat, xenogenic collagen, Contigen TM (C. R. Bard Inc., Covington, GA) and carbon particles known as Durasphere (Carbon Medical Technologies, Inc., St. Paul, MN). The ideal material is still being sought and should combine ease of administration with minimal tissue reaction, no material migration, and persistence over time. Placing the bulking agents between the 5 and 7 o'clock position is warranted to preserve a coapted urethral closure mechanism despite anatomic movement or location. All patients may receive this therapy in the office or in an outpatient surgical setting under a local block. There are no postprocedure restrictions.

Autologous Fat

Autologous fat *(16)* provides the advantages of easy accessibility, availability, affordability, and biocompatibility; however, the efficacy is abysmal because of poor graft neovascularity and long-term viability. Fat is usually harvested from the patient's lower abdomen with a liposuction-type technique. The cellular matrix is washed to remove debris and blood. Injections can be performed transurethrally or periurethrally.

GAX Collagen

GAX collagen is a purified bovine collagen that is cross-linked with glutaraldehyde in phosphate-buffered saline. The product is a sterile, nonpyogenic, low-viscosity formulation. Injections can be performed either transurethrally or periurethrally. Most patients require subsequent injections to achieve persistent continence. Skin testing is performed 4 to 6 wk before the procedure to rule out allergic reactions. Results with GAX collagen vary, with a cure rate averaging from 40 to 60%. If the improvement rates are also considered in the overall outcome, then the therapy is considered successful in 68–90% of cases using a mean of two injections sessions with an average follow-up of 22 mo *(15)*.

Carbon Particles

Carbon particles (Durasphere) are pyrolytic carbon-coated zirconium oxide beads suspended in a water-based carrier gel containing betaglucan. The Food and Drug

Administration recently approved this product for use as an injectable therapy. Unlike GAX collagen, no skin testing is required and the particles do not migrate distally because of their large size (>100 μm). Injections can be performed either transurethrally under direct observation into the submucosal area of the urethra or periurethrally. In a randomized study of 355 women, the use of the carbon particle injectables achieved a cure rate of 66% at 12 mo follow-up *(17)*.

Bladder-Neck Suspension Procedures

Retropubic approaches for bladder-neck suspensions are indicated in patients who have not undergone previous surgeries and in whom stress incontinence is predominantly caused by hypermobility of the bladder neck and urethra with high abdominal leakpoint or urethral pressure profiles.

Marshall-Marchetti–Krantz Procedure

The sutures for this suspension are placed close to or into the anterior urethra with subsequent high retropubic fixation to the symphysis pubis.

Burch Bladder-Neck Suspensions

Burch bladder-neck suspensions are modifications of retropubic bladder-neck suspensions that include stable suture fixation into Cooper's ligament and lateral placement of the suspending sutures into the periurethral tissue at the level of the bladder neck. The open abdominal Burch procedure has satisfactory long-term outcomes (83–85% long-term objective success rate), and is considered one of the gold standards in the surgical treatment of anatomic stress incontinence.

Transvaginal Needle Suspensions

Transvaginal needle suspensions were first introduced by Pereyra in 1959 *(18)*, who described a transvaginal approach to bladder-neck suspensions. This technique was later modified by Raz and is now referred to as the Pereyra–Raz procedure. The disadvantage of this procedure is the breakdown of the native supporting endopelvic fascia entering the retropubic space. By 1973, Stamey *(19)* introduced the concept of preserving the native endopelvic fascia support by using a ligature carrier, which is negotiated through the retropubic space under endoscopic control.

Percutaneous Bladder-Neck Suspensions

Percutaneous bladder-neck suspensions were introduced by Benderev *(20)* to duplicate a retropubic procedure from a transvaginal approach using a stable suture fixation provided by bone anchors into the pubic symphysis.

Laparoscopic Approaches for Bladder-Neck Suspensions

Laparoscopic approaches for bladder-neck suspensions were developed to treat stress UI and have increased in prevalence because of reduced patient morbidity and improved convalescence as compared to traditional open, retropubic bladder-neck suspensions *(21)*.

Sling Procedures

Sling procedures are specifically designed to address both anatomic hypermobility and intrinsic sphincteric deficiency components of stress UI.. The long-term success rate of 83% combined with the report of general medical and surgical complication rates equal those of transvaginal or retropubic bladder-neck suspension techniques. They are technically easier to perform than bladder-neck suspensions. Sling procedures have traditionally been performed from an abdominal–perineal approach and more recently through laparoscopic methods. The use of bone anchors into the undersurface of the inferior pubic rami or areas of the pubic symphysis in order to fix the supporting sling sutures can be placed from a transvaginal approach.

Rectus fascia pubovaginal slings were introduced by McGuire and Lyton in 1978. Autologous fascia has the advantages of durability and decreased removal rate secondary to infection and erosion *(22)*.

Allograft and synthetic materials are often considered as a substitute sling choice based on ease of acquisition and surgeons preference for performing quicker operative procedures *(23)*.

In situ vaginal wall slings were introduced by Raz et al. *(24)* and have been accepted for use in patients with acceptable tissue quality and vaginal capacity, especially those with concomitant poor detrusor function.

Tension-free vaginal tape (TVT; Gynecare, Johnson & Johnson, Somerville, NJ) was introduced by Ulmsten et al. *(25)*, who used a synthetic sling placed via a transvaginal, retrograde, retropubic passage of the supporting sling to the level of the rectus fascia. Because of the coefficient of friction between the sling material and all the intervening tissue, no effort is made to tie down the sling material to the rectus fascia in an attempt to reduce urethral obstruction from hypersuspension of the sling. The complications include retropubic hematoma, bladder perforation, and urinary retention.

Percutaneous vaginal tape is a polypropylene mesh (a non-absorbable synthetic material) that is placed at the level of the midurethra via an antegrade using a percutaneous ligature carrier (suprapubic approach). It has the advantages of short operative time, ease of technical performance, minimal patient discomfort, and a high rate of early return of normal voiding function. The complications include obstructive voiding, *de novo* instability, and urinary retention *(26)*.

Other Surgical Procedures for Urinary Incontinence

Artificial urinary sphincters permit intermittent urethral compression for maintenance of continence with voluntary reduction of urethral resistance during voiding. Indications for use include adequate manual dexterity, mental capacity, motivation to manipulate the device each time for voiding, normal detrusor function, and normal bladder compliance. It is technically difficult to insert both transvaginally and abdominally, and is usually reserved for patients with complex etiologies of stress urinary incontinence *(27)*.

Augmentation cystoplasty has proved its efficacy for the treatment of refractory overactive bladder conditions, as well as for improving quality of life and protecting the upper urinary tract from high intravesical pressure. However, the morbidity and postoperative discomfort associated with the open laparotomy incision is a major deterrent. For people with pre-existing debilitating neurologic and other co-morbid conditions, the open procedure significantly prolongs hospital stays, increases the metabolic needs for wound healing, and delays postoperative recovery.

Laparoscopic augmentation cystoplasty has distinct advantages when compared with open surgical procedures. These include decreased postoperative pain and morbidity, improved cosmesis, a shorter hospital stay and decreased convalescence *(28)*.

SUMMARY

Successful management of female UI begins with a thorough evaluation and is followed by the selection of individualized behavior modifications as well as pharmacologic supplementation. Reconstructive surgery should be considered only for patients who have failed to achieve an acceptable continence status with nonsurgical management and who have maximized their potential for overall pelvic floor rehabilitation and voiding function. A report in 1994 of a 10-yr expected cost per elderly patient with chronic stress incontinence revealed that untreated incontinence is the most expensive health care choice ($86,726) in America.

Comparative costs are lowest for surgical therapies and the highest for behavioral therapy (bladder-neck suspensions $25,388; pharmacologic therapy $62,021; and behavioral therapy $68,924; ref. *29*). Through continued advances in prevention, patient evaluation, and optimization of the pelvic floor and bladder function, the current and future potential for increased long-term effectiveness of all management options for patients who seek an acceptable continence status to improve their quality of life will continue to have a favorable impact on the overall cost.

REFERENCES

1. Resnick N, Yalla S, Laurino E. The pathophysiology of urinary incontinence among institutionalized elderly persons. N Engl J Med 1989; 320: 1–7.
2. Hu T, Gabelko K, Weis K, et al. Clinical guideline and cost implications-the case of stress urinary incontinence. Geriatr Nephrol Urol 1994; 4: 85–91.
3. Rackley RR, Appell RA. Evaluation and medical management of female urinary incontinence. Cleveland Clin J Med 1997; 64:83–92.
4. Wilson DP, Borland M. Vaginal cones for the treatment of genuine stress incontinence. Aust N Z J Obstet Gynaecol 1990; 157–160.
5. Jonasson A, Larsson, Pschera H, Nylund L. Short-term maximal electrical stimulation: a conservative treatment of urinary incontinence. Gynecol Obstet Invest 1990; 30: 120–123.
6. Anderson RU, Mobley D, Blank B, Saltzstein D, Susset J, Brown JS. Once daily controlled versus immediate release Oxybutynin chloride for urge urinary incontinence. J Urol 1999; 161: 1809–1812.
7. Van Kerrebebroeck P, Kreder K, Jonas U, Zinner N, Wein A, Tolterodine Study Group. Tolterodine once-daily: superior efficacy and tolerability in the treatment of the overactive bladder. Urology 2001; 57: 414–421.
8. Fantl JA, Cardozo L, McClish DK. Estrogen therapy in the management of urinary incontinence in postmenopausal women: a meta-analysis. First report of the hormones and urogenital therapy committee. Obstet Gynecol 1994; 83: 12–18.
9. Walter S, Kjaergaard B, Lose G, et al. Stress urinary incontinence in postmenopausal women treated with oral estrogen (estriol) and an alpha adrenoceptor-stimulating agent (phenylpropanolamine): a randomized double blind placebo controlled study. Int Urogynecol J 1990; 1: 74.
10. Goldstein F, Stampfer MJ, Colditz GA, et al. Postmenopausal hormone therapy and mortality. N Engl J Med 1997; 336: 1769–1775.
11. Dyskstra DD, Sidi AA. Treatment of detrusor-sphincter dyssynergia with botulinum A toxin: a double blind study. Arch Phys Med Rehabil 1990; 71: 24–26.
12. Schurch B, Hauri D, Rodic B, Curt A, Meyer M, Rossier B. Botulinum A Toxin as a treatment of detrusor-sphincter dyssynergia: a prospective study in 24 spinal cord injury patients. J Urol 1996; 155: 1023–1029.
13. Chancellor MB, de Groat WC. Intravesical capsaicin and resinferatoxin therapy: spicing up the ways to treat the overactive bladder. J Urol 1999; 162: 3–11.
14. Schmid RA, Jonas U, Oleson KA, et al. Sacral nerve stimulation for treatment of refractory urinary urge incontinence. J Urol 1999; 162: 352–357.

15. Dmochowski RR, Appell RA. Delivery of injectable agents for treatment of stress urinary incontinence in women evolving techniques. Tech Urol 2001; 7: 110–117.
16. Gonzales GS, Jimeno C, York M, Gomez P, Borruell S. Endoscopic autotransplantation of fat tissue in the treatment of urinary incontinence in the female. J Urol 1989; 95: 363–366.
17. Lightner D, Denko A, Synder J, et al. Study of Durasphere in the treatment of stress urinary incontinence: a multi-center, double blind randomized, comparative study. J Urol 2000; 163: 166.
18. Pererya AJ. A simplified surgical procedure for the correction of stress incontinence in women. J Urol. 2002; 167(2 Pt 2):1116–1118; discussion 1119.
19. Stamey TA. Endoscopic suspension of the vesical neck for urinary incontinence in females. Report on 203 consecutive patients. Ann Surg 1980; 192: 465–471.
20. Benderev TV. Anchor fixation and other modifications of endoscopic bladder neck suspension. Urology 1992; 40: 409–418.
21. Polascik TJ, Moore RG, Rosenberg MT, Kavoussi LR. Comparison of laparoscopic and open retropubic urethropexy for treatment of stress urinary incontinence. Urology 1995; 45: 647–652.
22. McGuire EJ, Lytton B. Pubovaginal sling procedures for stress incontinence. J Urol 1978; 119: 82–84.
23. Wright JE, Iselin CE, Carr LK, Webster GD. Pubovaginal sling using cadaveric allograft fascia for the treatment of intrinsic sphincter deficiency. J Urol 1998; 160: 759–762.
24. Raz S, Siegel AL, Short JL, Snyder JA. Vaginal wall sling. J Urol 1989; 141: 43–46.
25. Ulmesten U, Henriksson P, Johnson P, Varhos G. An ambulatory surgical procedure under local anesthesia for treatment of female urinary incontinence. Int Urogynecol J Pelvic Floor Dysfunct 1996; 7: 81–85; discussion 85–86.
26. Rackley RR, Abdelmalak JB, Tchetgen, MB, Madjar S, Jones S, Noble M. Tension-free vaginal tape and percutaneous vaginal tape sling procedures. Tech Urol 2001; 7: 90–100.
27. Elliot DS, Barrett DM. The artificial urinary sphincter in the female: Indications for use, surgical approach, and results. Int Urogynecol J Pelvic Floor Dysfunct 1998; 9: 409–415.
28. Rackley RR, Abdelmalak JB. Laparoscopic augmentation cystoplasty: surgical technique. Urol Clin North Am 2001; 28: 663–670.
29. Ramsey SD, Wagner TH, Bavendam TG. Estimated costs of treating stress urinary incontinence in elderly women according to the AHCPR clinical practice guidelines. Am J Manage Care 1996; 2: 147.

9 Interstitial Cystitis

Kenneth M. Peters, MD

CONTENTS

INTRODUCTION

Interstitial cystitis (IC) was first described more than 80 yr ago *(1)* and is one of the most common missed diagnoses in urology. The presentation may be variable; however, the key symptoms are urinary frequency, urgency, and pelvic pain *(2)*. Sixty percent of IC sufferers complain of pain with sexual intercourse, many so severe they abstain altogether *(3–5)*. Most IC patients have been treated with antibiotics for recurrent infections, although a review of medical records usually fail to document infections. Patients with IC often have other associated disorders, such as fibromyalgia, irritable bowel symptoms, and migraine headaches. Many IC patients have seasonal allergies and sensitivities to medications and foods *(6)*. The symptoms may have been present for many years or developed acutely. Undiagnosed IC patients are often managed for years without directed therapy and will seek evaluation from many different physicians to help determine the cause and an effective treatment for their symptoms. Patients with IC have been told that their symptoms are in their head and that there is nothing wrong with them. IC patients have been counseled to seek psychiatric help for their disease, and many patients suffer unduly until a diagnosis is made. When a patient is found to have IC, justifying the symptoms by determining a diagnosis is often therapeutic. Once the diagnosis is made, specific therapy can be initiated for this disease.

The impact of IC on a patient cannot be underestimated. IC patients scored worse on quality of life questionnaires than patients on dialysis. Fifty percent of patients with IC are unable to work full time. On average, $170 million per year is spent for medical care of IC. Combining lost wages and medical expenses, the economic impact of IC has been estimated to be $1.7 billion per year *(3)*. Until recently, IC has been thought to be a

From: *Essential Urology: A Guide to Clinical Practice*
Edited by: J. M. Potts © Humana Press Inc., Totowa, NJ

disease predominantly of women; however, more men are now being diagnosed with this disease. Men presenting with symptoms of genital pain, perineal pain, frequency, or dysuria are often labeled as having chronic, abacterial prostatitis. In fact, the majority of these men have characteristic findings of IC upon cystoscopy and hydrodistension and will respond to standard IC therapies *(7–10)*. IC is more prevalent in men than previously thought and it is imperative that the health care worker has a high index of suspicion for IC in the man with chronic prostatitis symptoms.

The difficulty with IC is that it is a diagnosis of exclusion, and there are no specific objective tests to determine whether a subject has IC or to monitor disease progression. For one to diagnose a patient with IC, the disease must be in the health care worker's differential diagnosis. The cause of IC is unknown despite a century of study.

INITIAL PRESENTATION OF IC AND DIFFERENTIAL DIAGNOSIS

The typical IC patient presents with complaints of urinary frequency, nocturia, pelvic pain, low back pain, dyspareunia, and small voided volumes. These symptoms may wax and wane, but rarely will resolve completely. It is striking in the IC population that many patients can recall the exact time their symptoms began. IC should be considered a syndrome, and not all patients with IC will have all the symptoms associated with this disease. It is appropriate to characterize the type and degree of symptoms, the duration of the symptoms, and to determine whether a specific event led to their onset. There may be an association of IC with documented urinary tract infections or previous pelvic or bladder surgery. In premenopausal women, endometriosis needs to be in the differential diagnosis and, if suspected, an appropriate evaluation, which may include hormonal manipulation or laparoscopy, should be considered. It is imperative if blood is found in the urine of a patient with irritative voiding symptoms that bladder cancer is ruled out by an evaluation of the upper urinary tract, bladder (cystoscopy), and urine cytology. Dietary factors, such as the amount of caffeine, alcohol, and acidic food consumption, should be characterized, along with their affect on bladder symptoms. A history of back pain or previous bladder or pelvic surgery may lead one to suspect a neurological cause for the symptoms. Obtaining a complete list of medical problems, including diabetes, neurological diseases, and malignancies, is important. Assessing whether the patient has received therapies that may affect the bladder, such as therapeutic radiation or chemotherapies (i.e., Cytoxan), will aid the clinician in determining the cause of their bladder symptoms.

Recognizing IC

The primary care physician is often the first to see patients with complaints of urinary frequency, urgency, and pain and has an important role in identifying patients who may suffer from IC. In addition, the primary care physician can begin education regarding this disease, initiate behavioral therapy, and secure the appropriate urological referral. Bladder-specific antibiotics and anticholinergics are the usual initial course of therapy. If the symptoms persist after a course of antibiotics or a urine culture fails to document an infection, IC should be considered.

Even before the diagnosis of IC is made, the primary care physician can initiate behavioral therapy that can often improve the symptoms of an irritative bladder. Many IC patients are sensitive to various food items *(11)*. Caffeine and alcohol should be removed from the diet, along with any other foods, such as tomatoes or citrus, which may

Table 1
Foods to Avoid in IC

Aged cheeses	Chocolate	Nitrates/nitrites	Salad dressing
Alcohol	Citrus	Nuts	Sour cream
Anchovies	Coffee	Onions	Sourdough bread
Apples	Corned beef	Peaches	Soy sauce
Apricots	Cranberries	Pineapples	Spicy foods
Aspartame	Cranberry juice	Plums	Tea
Avocados	Fava beans	Pomegranates	Tobacco
Bananas	Grapes	Processed meats and fish	Tofu
Caffeinated beverages	Junk food		Tomatoes
Cantaloupes	Lima beans	Rhubarb	Vinegar
Carbonated beverages	Mayonnaise	Rye bread	Yogurt
Caviar	Nectarines	Saccharine	

worsen their bladder symptoms (Table 1). Calcium glycerophosphate (Prelief®) is an over-the-counter food supplement that neutralizes the acid in foods, and many patients feel this helps their IC symptoms, although no supporting clinical trials have been published *(12)*. Most subjects with irritative voiding symptoms dehydrate themselves in the hope that they will void less. In IC, the protective barrier of the bladder is likely compromised, and this may allow the irritative solutes in the urine, such as potassium, to infiltrate the detrusor muscle, causing bladder irritation and nerve upregulation. Thus, patients who may have IC should be encouraged to increase their water intake, which will dilute the urine and cause less bladder irritation. Stress has been shown to worsen the symptoms of IC, and stress reduction may help alleviate pain, urgency, and frequency associated with IC *(13)*. Finally, the primary care physician can initiate pain relief with appropriate analgesics tailored to the severity of the pain.

Diagnosing IC

One can often suspect IC on history alone after ruling out other causes that can mimic the disease, such as documented bacterial cystitis, overactive bladder, endometriosis, bladder cancer, and urethral diverticulum. Unfortunately, there are no available urine or serum markers for this disease, although several promising markers are under investigation *(14–18)*. In 1987 and 1988, the National Institutes of Arthritis, Diabetes, Digestive and Kidney Diseases (NIDDK) held workshops on IC and developed a research definition for IC *(19)* (Table 2). The NIDDK criteria were found to be far too restrictive to be used as a clinical diagnosis for IC *(20)*. IC is a disease that may present as mild irritative symptoms to severe symptoms refractory to all standard therapies. Treating the disease early often leads to rapid improvement in symptoms; thus, it is important to recognize IC early so that therapy can be initiated.

A referral to a urologist interested in IC is the first step in securing a diagnosis. A physical exam, including a good pelvic and neurological exam, should be performed. A postvoid residual should be obtained to rule out urinary retention. When performing a vaginal exam, the anterior vaginal wall, including the urethra and bladder floor, should be carefully palpated. Urethral fullness, tenderness, or expression of pus may suggest a urethral diverticulum requiring further work-up. Often in IC, tenderness to palpation of

Table 2
NIDDK Research Criteria for IC

Inclusion criteria
1. Glomerulations or Hunner's ulcer on cystoscopic examination after hydrodistension under anesthesia
2. Pain associated with the bladder or urinary urgency
Exclusion criteria
1. Awake cystometric bladder capacity greater than 350 cc
2. Absence of intense urge to void with bladder filled to 100 cc of gas or 150 cc of water during cystometry, at fill rate of 30–100 cc/min
3. Demonstration of involuntary bladder contractions on cystometry
4. Duration of symptoms less than 9 mo
5. Absence of nocturia
6. Symptoms relieved by antimicrobials, urinary antiseptics, anticholinergics, or antispasmodics
7. Frequency of urination, while awake of less than eight times per day
8. Diagnosis of bacterial cystitis or prostatitis within 3 mo
9. Bladder or lower ureteral calculi
10. Active genital herpes
11. Uterine, cervical, vaginal, or urethral cancer
12. Urethral diverticulum
13. Cyclophosphamide or any type of chemical cystitis
14. Tuberculous cystitis
15. Radiation cystitis
16. Benign or malignant bladder tumors
17. Vaginitis
18. Age less than 18 yr of age

the anterior vaginal wall is noted at the level of the bladder trigone. Palpating the levator muscles may elicit tenderness, suggesting pelvic floor spasm. The patient's ability to contract and relax the pelvic floor muscles may suggest pelvic floor dysfunction. The degree of pelvic relaxation and prolapse should be determined. A rectal examination can rule out any rectal abnormalities or masses and in men, the prostate should be palpated to assess for any palpable prostate disease.

A urinalysis, urine culture, and cytology should be performed to exclude active infection or evidence of carcinoma *in situ*. Sterile pyuria should prompt urine tuberculosis cultures. If microscopic hematuria is present, a work-up, including upper-tract imaging, cystoscopy, and cytology, should be performed to rule out bladder cancer or stone disease. A voiding diary with both fluid intake (amount and kind) and urine output, including voided volumes, daytime frequency, and nocturia, should be completed. The voiding diary allows one to determine the average voided volume and to document the amount of daytime frequency and nocturia. Validated IC questionnaires are available to monitor other IC symptoms, including pain *(21–23)*. Sequential voiding diaries and symptom questionnaires allow one to determine the impact of various treatments for IC.

A cystometrogram may be performed to rule out uninhibited contractions and to determine the functional bladder capacity. The usual cytometric finding in IC is a small capacity bladder of the sensory/urgency type without uninhibited bladder contractions. Once all medical reasons for the bladder symptoms are ruled out and anticholinergics have failed to relieve the symptoms, other diagnostic tests should be undertaken. The gold standard for the diagnosis of IC has been bladder hydrodistension under a general or regional anesthetic *(24,25)*. A hydrodistension may not only aid in the diagnosis of IC but also may improve symptoms. This procedure is performed in an operating room setting, where a complete cystoscopy is used to assess the urethra and bladder. This will help rule out bladder cancer or urethral diverticulum. After inspection of the bladder, the bladder is filled by gravity drainage at 80–100 cm/H_20 pressure to its capacity. Upward pressure along each side of the urethra is often needed to maximally distend the bladder to prevent leakage around the cystoscope. The bladder is distended until no further water will run into the bladder, and this water is allowed to dwell for 2 min. The bladder is drained into a pitcher and the volume measured. Typically with IC, there is terminal hematuria seen when the bladder is drained. The average normal bladder capacity under an anesthetic is 1115 cc, and the average IC bladder capacity is 575 cc; however, in nonulcerative or early IC the bladder capacity can be normal *(26)*. Upon reinspecting the bladder, the vast majority of patients will have glomerulations seen in all sectors of the bladder suggestive of IC. Approximately 15% of IC patients will have deep cracks or ulcers in their bladder called Hunner's ulcers, which are associated with more severe symptoms *(27)*. If ulcerative lesions are present, these should be biopsied and the entire involved area should be gently cauterized, which often leads to improvement in symptoms. The vast majority of patients with the symptoms of IC will have the classic cystoscopic findings; unfortunately, these are not pathognomonic for IC and glomerulations can be seen in the asymptomatic patient *(28)*. Thus, one must make a clinical decision based on symptoms and the cystoscopic findings when diagnosing IC. A bladder biopsy can be performed for pathological evaluation and to rule out bladder cancer. Unfortunately, there are no classic pathological findings associated with IC. Mast cells have been implicated in the pathogenesis of IC by releasing multiple substances that can lead to inflammation in the bladder, such as histamine, kinins, vasoactive peptides, and prostaglandins. Studies have not consistently shown an elevation in bladder mast cells in IC. The role that mast cells play in IC is currently under intense investigation *(29–33)*.

Patients with IC should be informed that their symptoms may worsen for 2–3 wk after a hydrodistension, after which they usually return to their baseline, or a marked improvement in symptoms may occur, which can last for many months. If an IC patient responds well to a hydrodistension, this can be repeated in the future as a part of their multimodality treatment.

A second test that is becoming popular for the diagnosis of IC is the potassium (KCL) sensitivity test. This test is based on the hypothesis that there is increased epithelial permeability in the bladder of IC patients and that instilling a potassium solution in the bladder will provoke symptoms of urgency, frequency, and pain *(34–36)*. To perform this test, two solutions are placed in the bladder for 3–5 min. The first solution is 45 cc of sterile water and the second solution contains 400 mEq/L of KCL. After instilling the solution, the patient is asked whether it provokes symptoms on a scale of 0 to 5. If the patient does not react to water but states the KCL caused symptoms to increase two points or more on this scale, this is considered a positive test. Studies have shown that 70% of IC subjects have a positive test, whereas 4% of control subjects responded to potassium instillation. The pain caused by this test can be alleviated by rinsing the bladder with water and instilling heparin and bupivacaine hydrochloride into the bladder. The benefit of the potassium sensitivity test is that it can be performed in an office setting, does not require cystoscopy, and may lead to a more rapid initiation of treatment for the IC. The downside is that it does not allow one to inspect the bladder for other causes of symptoms, it evokes acute pain in the nonanesthetized patient, and it does not provide the patient the opportunity to have a clinical improvement in symptoms from a hydrodistension.

TREATMENT OF IC

Justifying a patient's symptoms by making a diagnosis of IC is usually therapeutic. Success in treating IC is based on the patient's understanding that this is a chronic condition that may flare and remit and empowering the patient with knowledge about the disease. The patient must understand all treatment options and be proactive in which treatment pathway to pursue. A multimodality approach is the most effective means of treating IC. Behavioral therapies must be stressed such as fluid management, pelvic floor exercises, dietary restrictions, and relaxation therapy *(37)*. Many IC patients suffer from pelvic floor spasm, which causes pelvic pain, dyspareunia, and urinary hesitancy. Treatment by a therapist knowledgeable in myofascial release techniques may be of benefit. Once behavioral therapy is optimized, oral medication is a reasonable first-line treatment for IC.

Oral Therapy

The only Food and Drug Administration (FDA)-approved oral therapy for IC is pentosan polysulfate sodium (Elmiron®). Pentosan polysulfate (PPS) is a glycosaminoglycan that binds tightly to the bladder mucosa. One theory of IC is that the bladder mucosa is "leaky," allowing the toxic substances in the urine to enter the bladder muscle, leading to inflammation and upregulation of nerve fibers. PPS may help rebuild the natural bladder barrier, leading to improvement in symptoms. PPS has been studied in several double-blind, placebo-controlled trials in the United States, and in subjects meeting the NIDDK criteria for IC, 38% of those receiving PPS at a dose of 100 mg three times per day for 3 mo reported a 50% reduction in bladder pain compared with 18% of placebo treated subjects *(38)*. An open-label physician usage study that enrolled 2809 patients from 1986 to 1996 demonstrated that 61% of patients on PPS for a minimum of 3 mo developed improvement in pain or discomfort and this improvement was sustained while subjects were taking PPS *(39)*. An IC patient must commit to taking PPS for 3–6 mo before determining that it is ineffective and, in addition, if symptom improvement is achieved, PPS may need to be continued indefinitely to maintain the improvement. PPS is a well-tolerated drug with 1–4% of patients complaining of alopecia (reversible upon discontinuation), gastrointestinal upset, headache, liver function abnormalities, or abdominal pain. PPS should not be given in conjunction with routine use of therapeutic doses of aspirin or nonsteroidal anti-inflammatories. PPS appears to help a subset of IC patients and has a good side-effect profile. PPS should be considered a first-line therapy for IC; however, because it may require several months before any clinical improvement is seen, it should not be used as a single agent for the treatment of IC.

Hydroxyzine is an antihistamine used primarily in the treatment of atopic dermatitis, urticaria, and allergic rhinitis. There is some evidence that mast cells may be involved in the pathogenesis of IC *(40)*. Hydroxyzine can reduce bladder mast cell degranulation, and anecdotal evidence suggests it may be effective in the treatment of IC *(33,41–44)*. This can be used in conjunction with PPS as part of a multmodality treatment regimen. Hydroxyzine may be more effective in IC patients who are found to have increased mast cells on bladder biopsy or those with seasonal allergies. Hydroxyzine is also sedative and in the short-term often improves quality of sleep and decreases nocturia. With prolonged use, both daytime and nighttime IC symptoms may improve. Hydroxyzine should be started at a dose of 25 mg at night and titrated based on side effects to 75 mg per night. The dose may need to be increased during allergy season. No controlled clinical studies on the efficacy of hydroxyzine for IC have been published.

Antidepressants can aid in the treatment of IC *(45–47)* and can be combined with Elmiron® as an initial treatment regimen. Patients with chronic pain and sleep deprivation often develop clinical depression *(48)*. In addition, tricyclic antidepressants have been used for chronic pain disorders by increasing the pain threshold. Low-dose Amitriptyline (10–75 mg) taken at night can be very effective in improving sleep and diminishing urinary frequency and bladder pain. Patients should be cautioned that tricyclic antidepressants could cause weight gain and daytime sedation. The sedative side effects will usually diminish with continued usage. The dose should be slowly titrated to minimize symptoms. Some IC patients will benefit from serotonin uptake inhibitors, such as fluoxetine hydrochloride or sertraline hydrochloride. These are nonsedative and should be given once per morning. No good controlled clinical trials on the use of antidepressants for IC have been performed; however, they clearly can provide some symptomatic relief for the treatment of IC.

Patients with IC often develop pelvic floor dysfunction, leading to tenderness of the pelvic floor muscles, urinary hesitancy, pelvic pain, and dyspareunia. Muscle relaxants, such a Valium or low-dose baclofen, may aid a subset of IC patients.

Finally, patients should have "rescue" medications available to them to be used as needed for symptom flares. These may include urinary analgesics, such as Pyridium or Urised, anticholinergics, and pain medications. These medications can be used as needed by the patient to control symptom flares.

Pain Management

Chronic pain is recognized as a legitimate complaint and should be treated aggressively *(49)*. Pain control is a serious problem for the IC patient and should be an integral component of the treatment regimen *(48,50)*. Once the pain is under control, treatments directed at IC are usually more effective. Narcotics are sometimes required to treat the pain associated with IC. Physicians treating IC must be comfortable prescribing narcotics and if they are not, then a referral to a pain specialist is in order. Medications combining both a narcotic and nonnarcotic analgesic such as codeine plus acetaminophen (Tylenol® 3), hydrocodone plus acetaminophen (Vicodin®, Lorcet®, Norco®), or propoxyphene napsylate plus acetaminophen (Darvocet®), can be the initial pain medication used. It is recommended that a total daily dose of acetaminophen should not exceed 4 g/d to prevent liver toxicity. Thus, one must be aware of the amount of acetaminophen in each tablet prescribed and be certain that the number of pills taken per day does not exceed the recommended dose (Table 3). In addition, the patients need to be educated on the proper dosage of these medications and cautioned about the sedative and constipating side effects. If patients require higher doses of narcotics to control the pain, oxycodone or morphine can be prescribed and carefully titrated until adequate pain relief

Table 3
Acetaminophen Levels in Commonly Prescribed Narcotic Compounds

Trade Name	*Narcotic*		*Acetaminophen*	*Max pills/d*
Tylenol #3	Codeine	30 mg	300 mg	12
Darvocet N-100	Propoxyphene	100 mg	650 mg	6
Vicodin	Hydrocodone	5 mg	500 mg	8
Vicodin-ES	Hydrocodone	7.5 mg	750 mg	5
Lorcet 10/650	Hydrocodone	10 mg	650 mg	6
Norco 10/325	Hydrocodone	10 mg	325 mg	12

is achieved. Long-acting narcotics, such as OxyContin®, are very effective in controlling pain, have a simple dosing schedule, and remove peaks and troughs of pain associated with intermittent narcotics. In patients not previously treated with narcotics, a dose of 10 mg every 12 h is a reasonable starting dose and can be titrated upward every 2–3 d until the most beneficial dose with the minimal side-effects is achieved. Patients previously on opiates can be started at a dose of 20 mg every 12 h and titrated accordingly. Patients must clearly understand that under no circumstances should a sustained-release narcotic tablet be broken, crushed, or chewed. This can result in the rapid release of a large dose of opioid, which can be life-threatening. The type and dose of narcotics prescribed must be individualized and take into account other sedative medications the patients currently take. Combining narcotics with anti-inflammatories, such as ibuprofen or Vioxx®, may decrease the narcotic dosage needed to achieve pain relief.

Referral to pain clinics knowledgeable in IC may be of benefit. Various narcotics or neuroleptics can be tried, along with nerve blocks or implantable pain pumps to treat the severe pain that can be associated with IC. In addition, many IC subjects complain of associated problems, such as fibromyalgia, irritable bowel syndrome, and vulvodynia. Referral to the appropriate specialist for treatment of these associated disorders is in order.

Intravesical Therapies

Intravesical therapies for IC have been a mainstay in treatment for many years *(51,52)*. Dimethylsulfoxide (DMSO) is the only FDA-approved intravesical therapy for this disease. DMSO (RIMSO®) is an unusual compound. It first was developed as an industrial solvent and may aid in delivering other compounds, such as steroids and heparin, into the detrusor muscle. Clinically, DMSO is thought to have anti-inflammatory properties and mast cell-stabilizing effects. Studies on DMSO have been poorly controlled because of the unique "garlic-like" odor that patients possess after being instilled with this medication. A "cocktail" of medication comprising 50 mL of DMSO, 100 mg of hydrocortisone, and 20,000 U of heparin is instilled in the bladder once a week for 6 to 8 wk and retained 15 to 20 min. Bladder symptoms may initially worsen; however, some IC patients will have symptomatic relief from this treatment. The symptom improvement is often short-lived and is best after the first course of DMSO. Subsequent treatments with this medication tend not to be as effective.

Intravesical heparin can be used in the treatment of IC *(53–58)*. Heparin is a glycosaminoglycan-type compound and binds tightly to the bladder mucosa. Similar to pentosan polysulfate, heparin may help rebuild the protective GAG layer of the bladder and improve bladder symptoms. Again, no controlled trials have been performed on this compound. Patients are taught intermittent self-catheterization and instill 25,000 U of heparin in their bladder in a 15-cc volume on a daily basis. The patients hold this medication until their next void. Only 1–3% of oral PPS is excreted in the urine, whereas heparin therapy delivers a large bolus of this GAG compound directly to the bladder mucosa. Daily intravesical heparin can be initiated in conjunction with beginning oral PPS. The heparin can be withdrawn after 8–12 wk and the patient maintained with oral therapy. This has the potential to shorten the time interval required to achieve a therapeutic effect from glycosaminoglycan therapy. If the patient cannot tolerate oral Elmiron®, intravesical heparin can be continued indefinitely. Heparin is not absorbed through the bladder mucosa; therefore, anticoagulation effects are not a concern.

Other intravesical therapies need to be performed under a general or regional anesthetic. These include sodium oxychlorosene *(59)* and silver nitrate. The utility of these treatments is in question, and their use has mostly fallen out of favor. These treatments are very caustic to the bladder and may lead to destruction of the bladder mucosa and formation of a new, more intact bladder lining. A voiding cystourethrogram should be performed to rule out vesicoureteral reflux before instilling these medications.

Intravesical bacillus Calmette Guerin (BCG) for the treatment of IC is in phase III clinical trials. A phase II double-blind, placebo-controlled trial demonstrated a 60% clinical response to BCG compared with a 27% placebo response rate *(60)*. Subjects who received a single 6-wk course of BCG and responded were followed for more than 2 yr, 90% continued to have marked clinical improvement in both pain and frequency symptoms despite no other therapy for their IC *(61)*. BCG is a weakened strain of the tuberculosis bacteria and has been used effectively for years in the treatment of superficial bladder cancer. The exact mechanism of action of BCG in bladder cancer is unknown but is thought to act by stimulating an immune response in the bladder. There is some evidence that IC may be secondary to an immune imbalance in the bladder *(62–69)*. Intravesical BCG may correct this imbalance, leading to long-term clinical improvement. Fifty milligrams of BCG diluted in 50 cc of normal saline is instilled in the bladder once a week for 6 wk. Patients are asked to retain the solution for as long as they can for up to 2 h. Bladder symptoms tend to worsen during the instillation period of BCG because of its irritative effects, and clinical improvement is not usually seen for at least 3 to 6 mo. PPS is known to tightly bind to BCG and may prevent attachment of the vaccine to the bladder lining, thus patients should not be receiving PPS while being treated with intravesical BCG.

Surgery for IC

Radical surgery for IC is rarely indicated and should be used as a last resort. Augmenting the bladder or diverting the urine while leaving the bladder in place is often doomed to failure. Removing the bladder with urinary diversion may be effective in very select, end-stage cases; however, this should not be considered the standard of care for IC. Patients choosing this mode of therapy need to be aware that this may not resolve the pain associated with IC *(70)*.

Sacral Neuromodulation

IC was thought to be a disease of the bladder, but in many patients it appears to be a syndrome involving the entire pelvic region with symptoms of urinary urgency, frequency, hesitancy, pelvic pain, bowel dysfunction, and vaginal discomfort. Chronic inflammation in a pelvic organ may lead to nerve upregulation to the spinal cord, affecting all pelvic structures. A new treatment that shows promise for refractory IC patients is sacral nerve modulation (Interstim® Medtronic, Inc). This technology is approved by the FDA for urinary urgency, frequency, urge incontinence, and idiopathic urinary retention. The benefit of sacral nerve stimulation is that a test can be performed before placing a permanent implant. The response to the test is assessed and if a patient experiences at least a 50% improvement in their symptoms and desires a permanent implant, the neurogenerator can be placed permanently in a subcutaneous pocket in the upper buttock. The device can be adjusted via an external programmer similar to a cardiac pacemaker, and the patient has his or her own external programmer to control the degree of stimulation. Early evidence suggests that temporary sacral nerve modulation may be very effective in treating refractory IC *(71,72)*. Recently, we reviewed our experience with sacral nerve modulation and found that greater than 85% of IC patients who had been refractory to on average six previous therapies responded to the Interstim. Of those implanted with a permanent generator, significant improvements were seen in urinary frequency, urgency, and pelvic pain and 95% would undergo the therapy again *(73)*. Further studies are needed to assess the utility of this technology for treating IC and to use these findings to study the pathophysiology of this disease.

CONCLUSIONS

The primary care physician has an integral role in identifying patients who may suffer from IC. Patients presenting with symptoms of urinary urgency, frequency, pelvic pain, bowel dysfunction, and vaginal pain should have IC in the differential diagnosis. Early recognition of IC usually results in more rapid control of symptoms. Recurrent urinary tract infection is the most common misdiagnosis of the IC patient. Urinary cultures should be performed prior to initiating antibiotic therapy and if cultures are negative, further evaluation should be considered. IC may present as a primary bladder disorder or may have associated conditions, such as fibromyalgia, chronic fatigue, vulvodynia, and irritable bowel. Multimodality therapy is most effective in controlling the symptoms of IC. Education about the disease is a mainstay in treatment. The patient must understand that this is a chronic condition and symptoms may wax and wane. Behavioral therapy, dietary modification, and stress reduction are integral in treating the symptoms of IC. There is a host of pharmaceutical therapies, including both oral and intravesical medications, that may improve the symptoms of IC. The pain associated with IC must be treated, which will allow the other standard therapies to be more effective. Sacral neuromodulation offers a new alternative to improve the symptoms if IC sufferers who are refractory to standard therapies. Finally, the IC patient must partner with the treating physician, be involved in directing therapy, and have reasonable expectations regarding symptom control.

REFERENCES

1. Hunner GL. A rare type of bladder ulcer in women: report of cases. Boston Med Surg J 1915; 172: 660–664.

2. Propert KJ, Schaeffer J, Brensinger CM, Kusek J, Nyberg LM, Landis JR. A prospective study of interstitial cystitis: results of longitudinal followup of the interstitial cystitis data base cohort. J Urol 2000; 163: 1434–1439.
3. Ratner V, Slade D, Greene G. Interstitial cystitis. A patient's perspective. Urol Clin North Am 1994; 21: 1–5.
4. Slade D, Ratner V, Chalker R. A collaborative approach to managing interstitial cystitis. Urology 1997; 49 (5A suppl): 10–13.
5. Slade DKA. Interstitial cystitis: a challenge to urology. Urol Nurs 1989; March: 5–7.
6. Alagiri M, Chottiner S, Ratner V, Slade D, Hanno PM. Interstitial cystitis: unexplained associations with other chronic disease and pain syndromes. Urology 1997; 49 (5A suppl): 52–57.
7. Nickel JC, Johnston B, Downey J, Barkin J, Pommerville P, Gregoire M, Ramsey E. Pentosan polysulfate therapy for chronic nonbacterial prostatitis (chronic pelvic pain syndrome category IIIA): a prospective multicenter clinical trial. Urology 2000; 56: 413–417.
8. Sant GR, Theoharides TC. Interstitial cystitis. Curr Opin Urol 1999;9: 297–302.
9. Novicki DE, Larson TR, Swanson SK. Interstitial cystitis in men. Urology 1998; 52: 621–624.
10. Berger RE, Miller JE, Rothman I, Krieger JN, Muller CH. Bladder petechiae after cystoscopy and hydrodistension in men diagnosed with prostate pain. J Urol 2001; 159: 83–85.
11. Gillespie L. Metabolic appraisal of the effects of dietary modification on hypersensitive bladder symptoms. Br J Urol 1993; 72: 293–297.
12. Bologna RA, Gomelsky A, Lukban JC. The efficacy of calcium glycerophosphate in the prevention of food-related flares in interstitial cystitis (abstract). Urology 2001; 57 (6A suppl): 122.
13. Rothrock NE, Lutgendorf SK, Kreder KJ, Ratliff T, Zimmerman B. Stress and symptoms in patients with interstitial cystitis: a life stress model. Urology 2001; 57: 422–427.
14. Keay SK, Zhang C, Shoenfelt J, et al.. Sensitivity and specificity of antiproliferative factor, heparin-binding epidermal growth factor-like growth factor, and epidermal growth factor at urine markers for intersitial cystitis. Urology 2001; 57 (6A suppl): 9–14.
15. Erickson DR. Urine markers of interstitial cystitis. Urology 2001; 57 (6A suppl): 15–21.
16. Shupp-Byrne D, Sedor JF, Estojak J, Fitzpatrick KJ, Chiura AN, Mulholland SG. The urinary glycoprotein GP51 as a clinical marker for interstitial cystitis. J Urol 1999; 161: 1786–1790.
17. Keay S, Zhang C-O, Hise MK, et al. A diagnostic in vitro urine assay for intersitial cystitis. Urology 1998; 52: 974–978.
18. Keay S, Zhang C-O, Kagen DI, Hise MK, Jacobs SC, Hebel JR, Gordon D, Whitmore K, Bodison S, Warren JW. Concentrations of specific epithelial growth factors in the urine of interstitial cystitis patients and controls. J Urol 1997; 158: 1983–1988.
19. Gillenwater JY, Wein AJ. Summary of the National Institute of Arthritis, Diabetes, Digestive and Kidney Diseases workshop on interstitial cystitis, National Institutes of Health, Bethesda, MD, August 28–29, 1987. J Urol 1988; 140: 203–206.
20. Hanno PM, Landis JR, Matthews-Cook Y, Kusek J, Nyberg L Jr. The diagnosis of interstitial cystitis: lessons learned from the National Institutes of Health interstitial cystitis database study. J Urol 1999; 161: 553–557.
21. Goin JE, Olaleye D, Peters KM, Steinert B, Habicht K, Wynant G. Psychometric analysis of the university of Wisconsin interstitial cystitis scale: implications for use in randomized clinical trials. J Urol 1998; 159: 1085–1090.
22. Keller ML, McCarthy DO, Neider RS. Measurement of symptoms of interstitial cystitis. A pilot study. Urol Clin North Am 1994; 21: 67–71.
23. O'Leary MP, Sant GR, Fowler FJ, Whitmore KE, Spolarich-Kroll J. The interstitial cystitis symptom index and problem index. Urology 1997; 49 (5A suppl): 58–63.
24. Bumpus HC Jr. Interstitial cystitis: its treatment by overdistension of the bladder. Med Clin N Am 1930; 13: 1495.
25. Dunn M, Ramsden PD, Roberts JBM, Smith JC, Smith PJB. Interstitial cystitis, treated by prolonged bladder distension. Br J Urol 1977; 49: 641–645.
26. Parsons CL. Interstitial cystitis. In: Ostegard D, Bent A, ed. Urogynecology and Urodynamics; Theory and Practice. Williams & Wilkins, New York, NY, 1996, pp. 409–425.
27. Messing EM, Stamey TA. Interstitial cystitis. Early diagnosis, pathology, and treatment. Urology 1978; 12: 381–392.

28. Waxman JA, Sulak PJ, Kuehl TJ. Cystoscopic findings consistent with interstitial cystitis in normal women undergoing tubal ligation. J Urol 1998; 160: 1663–1667.
29. Hanno P, Levin RM, Monson FC, et al. Diagnosis of interstitial cystitis. J Urol 1990; 143: 278–281.
30. Holm-Bentzen M, Søndergaard I, Hald T. Urinary secretion of a metabolite of histamine (1,4-methyl-imidazole-acetic-acid) in painful bladder disease. Br J Urol 1987; 59: 230–233.
31. Theoharides TC, Sant GR, El-Mansoury M, Letourneau R, Ucci AA, Jr, Meares EM, Jr. Activation of bladder mast cells in interstitial cystitis: a light and electron microscopic study. J Urol 1995; 153: 629–639.
32. Sant GR, Theoharides TC. The role of the mast cell in interstitial cystitis. Urol Clin North Am 1994; 21: 41–53.
33. Theoharides TC, Sant GR. Hydroxyzine therapy for interstitial cystitis. Urology 1997; 49 (5A suppl): 108–110.
34. Parsons CL. New concepts in interstitial cystitis. Int Urogynecol J Pelvic Floor Dysfunct 1997; 8: 1–2.
35. Parsons CL. Potassium sensitivity test. Tech Urol 1996; 2: 171–173.
36. Parsons CL, Zupkas P, Parsons JK. Intravesical potassium sensitivity in patients with interstitial cystitis and urethral syndrome. Urology 2001; 57: 428–432.
37. Chaiken DC, Blaivas JG, Blaivas ST. Behavioral therapy for the treatment of refractory interstitial cystitis. J Urol 1993; 149: 1445–1448.
38. Parsons CL, Benson G, Childs SJ, Hanno P, Sant GR, Webster G. A quantitatively controlled method to study prospectively interstitial cystitis and demonstrate the efficacy of pentosanpolysulfate. J Urol 1993; 150: 845–848.
39 Hanno PM. Analysis of long-term Elmiron therapy for interstitial cystitis. Urology 1997; 49 (5A suppl): 93–99.
40. Theoharides TC, Kempuraj D, Sant GR. Mast cell involvement in interstitial cystitis: a review of human and experimental evidence. Urology 2001; 57 (6A suppl): 47–55.
41. Simmons JC, Bunce PL. On the use of an antihistamine in the treatment of interstitial cystitis. Am Surg 1958; 24: 664.
42. Theoharides TC. Hydroxyzine for interstitial cystitis. J Allergy Clin Immunol 1993; 91: 686–687.
43. Knutton S, Baldwin T, Williams PH, McNeish AS. Actin accumulation at sites of bacterial adhesion to tissue culture cells: basis of a new diagnostic test for enteropathologenic and enterohemorrhagic *Escherichia coli*. Infect Immunol 1989; 57: 1290–1298.
44. Theoharides TC. Hydroxyzine in the treatment of interstitial cystitis. Urol Clin North Am 1994; 21: 113–119.
45. Hanno PM, Buehler J, Wein AJ. Use of amitriptyline in the treatment of interstitial cystitis. J Urol 1989; 141: 846–848.
46. Hanno PM. Amitriptyline in the treatment of interstitial cystitis. Urol Clin North Am 1994; 21: 89–91.
47. Renshaw DC. Desipramine for interstitial cystitis. JAMA 1988; 260: 341.
48. Rabin C, O'Leary A, Neighbors C, Whitmore K. Pain and depression experienced by women with interstitial cystitis. Women Health 2001; 31: 67–81.
49. Benedetti C, Butler SH. The Management of Pain. Lea & Febiger, Philadelphia, PA, 1990.
50. Brookoff D. The causes and treatment of pain in interstitial cystitis. In: Sant GR, editor. Interstitial Cystitis. Lippincott-Raven, New York, NY, 1997, pp. 177–192.
51. Sant GR. Intravesical 50% dimethyl sulfoxide (RIMSO-50) in treatment of interstitial cystitis. Suppl Urol 1987; 29: 17–21.
52. Parkin J, Shea C, Sant GR. Intravesical dimethyl sulfoxide (DMSO) for interstitial cystitis—a practical approach. Urology 1997; 49 (5A suppl): 105–107.
53. Hanno PM, Wein AJ. Medical treatment of interstitial cystitis (other than Rimso-50/Elmiron). Urology 1987; (29 suppl): 22–26.
54. Sant GR, LaRock DR. Standard intravesical therapies for interstitial cystitis. Urol Clin North Am 1994; 21: 73–83.
55. Parsons CL. The therapeutic role of sulfated polysaccharides in the urinary bladder. Urol Clin North Am 1994; 21: 93–100.

56. Bade JJ, Mensink HJA, Laseur M. Intravesical treatment of interstitial cystitis with a heparin analogue. Br J Urol 1995; 75: 260.
57. Nickel JC, Downey J, Morales A, Emerson L, Clark J. Relative efficacy of various exogenous glycosaminoglycans in providing a bladder surface permeability barrier. J Urol 1998; 160: 612–614.
58. Parsons CL, Housley T, Schmidt JD, Lebow D. Treatment of interstitial cystitis with intravesical heparin. Br J Urol 1994; 73: 504–507.
59. La Rock DR, Sant GR. Intravesical chlorpactin for refractory interstitial cystitis. Infect Urol 1995; September/October: 151–157.
60. Peters K, Diokno A, Steinert B, et al. The efficacy of intravesical Tice® bacillus Calmette-Guérin (BCG) in the treatment of interstitial cystitis (IC): a double-blind, prospective, placebo controlled trial. J Urol 1996; 157: 2090–2094.
61. Peters KM, Diokno AC, Steinert BW, Gonzalez JA. The efficacy of intravesical TICE® bacillus Calmette-Guérin (BCG) in the treatment of interstitial cystitis (IC): long-term follow-up. J Urol 1998; 159: 1483–1487.
62. Lotz M, Villiger P, Hugli T, Koziol J, Zuraw BL. Interleukin-6 and interstitial cystitis. J Urol 1994; 152: 869–873.
63. Liebert M, Wedemeyer G, Stein JA, et al. Evidence for urothelial cell activation in interstitial cystitis. J Urol 1993; 149: 470–475.
64. Christmas TJ, Bottazzo GF. Abnormal urothelial HLA-DR expression in interstitial cystitis. Clin Exp Immunol 1992; 87: 450–454.
65. Silk MR. Bladder antibodies in interstitial cystitis. J Urol 1970; 103: 307–309.
66. Keay S, Zhang C-O, Trifillis AL, Hebel JR, Jacobs SC, Warren JW. Urine autoantibodies in interstitial cystitis. J Urol 1997; 157: 1083–1087.
67. Ochs RL, Stein TW,Jr., Peebles CL, Gittes RF, Tan EM. Autoantibodies in interstitial cystitis. J Urol 1994; 151: 587–592.
68. Joustra B, Karrenbeld A, Mensink H. Specific auto-antibodies in interstitial cystitis patients sugge st an auto-immune etiology (abstract). J Urol 1996; 155: 431A.
69. Peters KM, Diokno AC, Steinert BW. A preliminary study on urinary cytokine levels in interstitial cystitis: does intravesical BCG treat IC by altering the immune profile in the bladder? Urology 1999; 54: 450–453.
70. Baskin LS, Tanagho EA. Pelvic pain without pelvic organs. J Urol 1992; 147: 683–686.
71. Maher CF, Carey MP, Dwyer PL, Schluter PL. Percutaneous sacral nerve root neuromodulation for intractable interstitial cystitis. J Urol 2001; 165: 884–886.
72. Zermann DH, Weirich T, Wunderlich H, Reichelt O, Schubert J. Sacral nerve stimulation for pain relief in interstitial cystitis. Urol Int 2000; 65: 120–121.
73. Peters KM. Neuromodulation for the treatment of refractory interstitial cystitis. MedReviews 2002; 4 (suppl. 1): S36–S43

10 Urinary Tract Infections in Adults

Joseph B. Abdelmalak, MD,
Sandip P. Vasavada, MD,
and Raymond R. Rackley, MD

CONTENTS

INTRODUCTION

Urinary tract infection (UTI) is a common health problem affecting millions of people each year. They are the most common nosocomial infections and are second in seriousness only to respiratory infections. UTIs account for more than 7 million physician visits every year in the United States alone *(1)*. They are the most common bacterial infection found in the elderly and the most frequent source of bacteremia *(2,3)*. The incidence ratio of UTIs in middle-aged women to men is 30:1. However, during later decades of life, the incidence of infection in women to men decrease. Women are especially prone to UTIs for reasons that are poorly understood. One factor may be that a woman's urethra is short, allowing bacteria quick access to the bladder. Also, a woman's urethral opening is near sources of bacteria from the anus and vagina. For many women, sexual intercourse seems to trigger an infection, although the reasons for this linkage are unclear *(4)*. In men, prostatitis syndromes account for about 25% of office visits for genitourinary tract infections *(5)*. Five percent of these men have bacterial prostatitis, 64% have nonbacterial prostatitis, and 31% suffer from pelviperineal pain syndrome *(6)*.

From: *Essential Urology: A Guide to Clinical Practice*
Edited by: J. M. Potts © Humana Press Inc., Totowa, NJ

Table 1
Functional and Structural Abnormalities of the Genitourinary Tract

Functional abnormalities	*Obstruction*	*Other*
• Vesicoureteral reflux	• Congenital abnormalities	• Diabetes mellitus
• Neurogenic bladder	• Renal cysts	• Renal failure
	• Pelviureteric obstruction	• Urinary diversions
Foreign bodies	• Ureteric and urethral strictures	• Urinary instrumentation
• Indwelling catheters	• Urolithiasis	
• Nephrostomy tubes	• Bladder diverticuli	
• Ureteric stents	• Tumors	

CLASSIFICATION/TERMINOLOGY

UTIs have been classified as acute or chronic, hospital-acquired (nosocomial) or community-acquired, uncomplicated or complicated, upper (renal) or lower (bladder, urethra, prostate), symptomatic or asymptomatic, and *de novo* or recurrent.

The term UTI refers to the invasion of the urinary tract by a nonresident infectious organism. Bacteriuria implies the presence of bacteria in the urine and may be symptomatic or asymptomatic. Pyuria signifies the presence of white blood cells in the urine, an inflammatory response to bacterial invasion. Complicated UTI indicates a UTI that occurs in a patient with a structural or functional abnormality of the genitourinary tract (Table 1). These abnormalities predispose a person to UTI through interference with the drainage of urine or through the formation of a nidus in which bacteria can grow.

ROUTES OF INFECTION

The infection spreads to the urinary tract either through the ascending route from the fecal reservoir through the urethra into the bladder particularly in patients with intermittent or indwelling catheters, hematogenous route secondary to staphylococcus aureus bacteremia, or direct extension route from adjacent organs via lymphatic as in case of retroperitoneal abscesses or severe bowel obstruction.

URINARY PATHOGENS

Escherichia coli is the most common infecting organism in patients with uncomplicated UTIs *(7)*. Other Gram-negative micro-organisms causing UTIs include *Proteus*, *Klebsiella*, *Citrobacter*, *Enterobacter*, and *Pseudomonas* spp. Gram-positive pathogens, such as *Enterococcus faecalis*, *Staphylococcus Saprophyticus*, and group B *Streptococci*, can also infect the urinary tract. Other micro-organisms called *Chlamydia* and *Mycoplasma* have been known to cause UTIs in both men and women, but these infections tend to remain limited to the urethra and reproductive system. These organisms may be sexually transmitted, so infections require treatment of both partners.

RISK FACTORS

The ureters and bladder normally prevent urine from backing up toward the kidneys, and the flow of urine from the bladder helps wash bacteria out of the body. In men, the prostate gland produces secretions that slow bacterial growth. In both sexes, immune defenses also prevent infection. Despite these safeguards, however, infections still occur. Some people are more prone to getting UTIs than others because of host factors such as alter urothelial mucosa adherence mucopolysacharide lining *(8)*. Any abnormality of the urinary tract that obstructs the flow of urine (e.g., kidney stone, enlarged prostate) sets the stage for an infection. In addition, catheters, tubes, or foreign bodies in the bladder are common sources of infection. This increases the risk of UTIs in unconscious, critically ill patients who often need a catheter that stays in place for a long time. People with diabetes also have a higher risk of UTIs because of changes in the immune system. Any such disorder that suppresses the immune system raises the risk of a UTI. Sexual intercourse *(4)* and women who use a diaphragm *(9)* have also been linked to an increased risk of cystitis. Hormonal changes and shifts in the position of the urinary tract during pregnancy make it easier for bacteria to travel up the ureters to the kidneys. For this reason, many doctors recommend periodic testing of urine in pregnant women.

DIAGNOSIS

UTIs may be asymptomatic. However, some patients report symptoms of incontinence and/or a general lack of well-being *(10)*. Pyelonephritis is a clinical syndrome characterized by flank pain, fever, chills, irritative voiding symptoms, and pyuria. Sometimes it presents with upper gastrointestinal symptoms, such as nausea, and vomiting. Cystitis and lower UTIs have the clinical manifestations of irritative voiding symptoms, including frequency, dysuria, urgency, and incontinence.

Urinalysis

Urine samples are collected in a sterile container through suprapubic aspiration, urethral catheterization especially in females, or by midstream voided urine after washing the genital area to avoid contamination. The sample is then tested for bacteruria, pyuria, and hematuria. Indirect dipstick tests are informative but are less sensitive than microscopic examination of the urine. About one-third of the women who have acute symptoms of cystitis have either sterile urine or some other cause for the symptom *(11)*. Many diseases of the urinary tract produce significant pyuria without bacteruria. These include staghorn calculi, tuberculosis, chlamydia, and mycoplasma. Microscopic hematuria is found in 40–60% of cystitis cases *(12)*. Associated gross hematuria should be evaluated further via imaging studies. Cystoscopy in those patients who are over 50 yr and/or have other risk factors for concomitant diseases, such as nephrolithes or transitional cell carcinoma (i.e., smoking).

Urine Culture and Sensitivity Test

Bacteria is cultured and tested against different antibiotics to determine the drug that best destroys the bacteria. It is important to bear in mind that a large percent of female with lower UTIs have been find to have sexually transmitted diseases. Additional cultures for *Gonococcus*, *Chlamydia*, urea plasma, and *Mycoplasma* should be considered.

Imaging Techniques

Radiologic studies are unnecessary for routine evaluation of patients with UTIs; however, they may be indicated to find out the cause of complicated cases. These are the

Table 2
Factors Influencing the Selection of Antimicrobial Agents in Treating UTI

Patient	*Drug*	*Organism*
• History of drug allergy	• Safety profile	• Gram's-stain
• Medical history (renal impairment, liver impairment)	• Spectrum of activity	• Special culture
• Concomitant medication	• Route of administration	
• Presence of urological abnormalities	• Costs	

cases where UTIs are associated with urinary calculi, ureteral strictures, ureteral reflux, urinary tract tumors, and urinary tract diversions. Helpful imaging techniques include the following:

- Plain x-ray film of the abdomen for detection of radiopaque calculi, or abnormal renal contour.
- Intravenous pyelogram that gives x-ray images of the bladder, kidneys, and ureters. An opaque dye visible on x-ray film is injected into the vein, and series of x-rays are taken. The films show an outline of the urinary tract, revealing even small changes in the structure of the tract. They are used to determine the site and extent of urinary tract obstruction.
- Voiding cystourethrogram for the evaluation of neurogenic bladder, urethral diverticulum, and to exclude or define presence of vesicoureteral reflux.
- Renal ultrasonography through the interpretation of the echo patterns of sound waves bounced back from internal organs. One can detect the presence of hydronephrosis, pyonephrosis, and perirenal abscesses. This technology poses no risk of radiation nor intravenous contrast.
- Computed tomography (CT), a more sensitive method to define renal as well as suprarenal pathology, especially when intravenous contrast is used. Spiral CT of the abdomen and pelvis with or without contrast are extremely sensitive in identifying calculi within the collecting system, and have become standard practice as part of acute flank pain protocol at Cleveland Clinic Foundation.
- Cystoscopy, through the use of fiberoptic, the urethra and the bladder can be inspected quickly and safely with local anesthetic on an office setting.

TREATMENT

General management of UTIs includes drinking plenty of water, which helps cleanse the urinary tract of bacteria. Taking cranberry juice and vitamin C (ascorbic acid) supplements inhibit the growth of some bacteria by acidifying the urine. Avoiding coffee, alcohol, and spicy foods is also useful. Heating pad and pain relief medication are helpful for pain management.UTIs are treated with antibacterial drugs. The choice of drug and length of treatment depend on several factors (Table 2). The sensitivity test is especially useful in selecting the most effective drug.

Acute Uncomplicated Cystitis

Patients with the symptoms of frequency, urgency, pyuria upon microscopic examination, and no known functional or anatomical abnormality of the genitourinary tract may be presumed to have acute uncomplicated cystitis. An empirical therapy with a 3-d regimen of trimethoprim/sulfamethoxazole (TMP-SMZ) or a fluoroquinolone without pretreatment culture and sensitivity testing is usually effective.

Recurrent Cystitis

Recurrent episodes of uncomplicated cystitis can be managed through several strategies. Behavioral therapy includes increasing fluid intake, urinating as soon as the need is felt as well as immediately after intercourse, and changing the method of contraception (for diaphragm-spermicide user). Long-term antimicrobial prophylaxis *(13)*, postcoital prophylaxes of a single-dose antibiotic *(14)*, or short-course (1 or 2 d) antibiotics for each symptomatic episode is recommended. For postmenopausal women, the use of vaginal estrogen cream may prove an effective preventive measure *(15)*.

Uncomplicated Pyelonephritis

Patients usually present with mild to severe flank pain, low- or high-grade fever, tenderness of the costovertebral angle on the infected side, or cystitis-like symptoms. Urine cultures and sensitivity tests are recommended followed by 10 to 14 d of appropriate oral antimicrobial therapy. If the patient presents with fever, nausea, and vomiting, one can be rehydrated and then given a single dose of a parenteral agent, after which an oral antimicrobial is prescribed. A urine culture should be obtained 1 to 2 wk after treatment to verify the cure.

Complicated UTIs

These patients present with signs of sepsis, hypotension, high temperature over 40°C, tender subcostal angle, or intractable nausea and vomiting. They are more likely to have functional, metabolic, or anatomic abnormalities of the urinary tract. Pretreatment cultures and sensitivity testing should be obtained, and a full course of appropriate antimicrobial therapy should be given. Severely ill patients may be hospitalized until they are able to ingest fluids and take medication on their own. Blood cultures should also be obtained. Complete investigations of the upper and lower urinary tract are recommended to assure no stones, hydronephrosis, or abscess. A follow-up urinalysis helps to confirm that the urinary tract is infection-free. Kidney infections generally require several weeks of antibiotic treatment.

Mycoplasma and Chlamydia Infections

Special cultures are needed to diagnose these infections. Longer treatment with tetracycline, TMP/SMZ, or doxycycline is necessary.

Catheter-Related Infections

Catheterization for more than 2 wk is usually associated with bacteruria. Prophylaxis antimicrobial therapy for UTI during short-term indwelling urethral catheterization is not recommended. Short-term antimicrobial therapy (5–7 d) is indicated only in symptomatic episodes, otherwise, the catheter should be removed if possible.

Prostatitis

Acute bacterial prostatitis presents with symptoms of frequency, urgency, dysuria, and obstructive voiding symptoms. It is usually associated with fever, chills, malaise, and myalgias. On examination, the prostate is warm, tender, swollen, and indurated. Culture and sensitivity of the voided urine is indicated, and blood cultures may be needed to isolate the pathogen. The causative organisms are primarily Gram-negative enteric bacteria, *Escherichia coli*, *Proteus*, *Klebsiella*, and *Pseudomonas*.

Prostate infections are harder to cure because antibiotics are unable to penetrate infected prostate tissue effectively. For this reason, men with prostatitis often need long-term treatment (at least 30 d) with a carefully selected antibiotic. Severely ill patients need hospitalization and parenteral antimicrobial agents, such as an aminoglycoside–penicillin combination. Mild and moderate cases respond well to fluoroquinolones or TMP/SMZ, which have a cure rate of 60–90% *(16)*. Chronic bacterial prostatitis has episodes of recurrent bacteriuria with the same organism between asymptomatic periods.

Asymptomatic Bacteruria

Treatment of asymptomatic bacteruria is indicated in pregnant women and in those requiring urological surgery *(17)*. Preoperative treatment reduces postoperative complications, including bacteremia *(18)*.

Infections in Pregnancy

The presence of asymptomatic bacteruria in a pregnant woman should be treated with a 7-d treatment of ampicillin or nitrofurantoin promptly to avoid the risk of premature delivery of the baby, low birth weight, pyelonephritis, and high blood pressure *(19)*.

UTI With Renal Failure

When creatinine clearance is significantly impaired, antibiotic dosage adjustments should be made because the renal blood flow is decreased and the perfusion of antimicrobial agents into the renal tissue and urine is impaired. Ampicillin, TMP/SMZ, and fluoroquinolone are all effective in the treatment of UTI in uremic patients *(19,20)*. Nitrofurantion and tetracyclines are contraindicated for treatment of UTI in uremic patients.

Prophylaxis

Antimicrobial prophylaxis is recommended to ensure sterility of urine for those who appear prone to develop infections. These include immunocompromised patients, heart-diseased patients, people with a prosthetic heart valve, and patients who are scheduled for a procedure (cystoscopy). Oral or vaginal estrogen administration to postmenopausal women also reduces the symptoms of cystitis *(17,21)*.

SUMMARY

UTI is one of the most common health problems affecting all ages. It is the most common nosocomial, bacterial infection in the elderly. Women are especially prone to UTIs for reasons that are poorly understood, while prostatitis syndromes account for 25% of male office visits for genitourinary tract infections. Acute cystitis or pyelonephritis in adult patients should be considered uncomplicated if there are no known functional or anatomic abnormalities of the genitourinary tract. Most of these infections are caused by *E. coli*. A 3-d regimen with TMP/SMZ is an effective treatment, but alternative regimens, such as nitrofurantoin (7-d regimen), a fluoroquinolone, or an oral third-generation cephalosporin may have a better result. For acute uncomplicated pyelonephritis, a 10- to 14-d regimen is recommended. Men with prostatitis often need long-term treatment (at least 30 d) with a carefully selected antibiotic. Longer treatment with tetracycline, TMP/SMZ, or doxycycline is necessary for patients with *Mycoplasma* or *Chlamydia* infections. Complicated UTIs will not be treated unless the underlying abnormality is corrected.

REFRENCES

1. Patton JP, Nash DB, Abrutyn E. Urinary tract infection: economic consideration. Med Clin North Am 1991; 75: 495–513.
2. Mulholland SG. Urinary tract infection. Clin Geriatr Med 1990; 6: 43–53.
3. Esposito AL, Gleckman RA, Cram S, Crowley M, McCabe F, Drapkin MS. Community-acquired bacteremia in elderly: analysis of 100 consecutive episodes. J Am Geriatr Soc 1980; 28: 315–319.
4. Storm BL, Collins M, West SL, Kreisberg J, Weller, S. Sexual activity, contraceptive use and other risk factors for symptomatic and asymptomatic bacteriuria: a case control study. Ann Intern Med 1987; 107: 816–823.
5. Lipsky BA. Urinary tract infection in men. Ann Intern Med 1989; 110: 138–150.
6. Brunner H, Weinder W, Scheifer HG. Studies of the role of ureaplasma urealyticum and mycoplasm hominis in prostatitis. J Infect Dis 1983; 147: 807–813.
7. Johnson JR. Virulence factors in *Escherichia coli* urinary tract infection. Clin Microbiol Rev 1991; 4: 80–128.
8. Schaeffer AJ, Rajan N, Cao Q, et al. Host pathogenesis in urinary tract infections. Int J Antimicrob Agents 2001; 17(4): 245–251.
9. Fihn SD, Latham RH, Roberts P, et al. Association between diaphragm use and urinary tract infection. JAMA 1985; 254: 240–245.
10. Boseki JA, Caboose WD, Abrutyn E, Running K, Stamm WE. Lack of association between bacteriuria and symptoms in the elderly. Am J Med 1986; 81: 979–982.
11. Johnson JR, Stamm WE. Diagnosis and treatment of acute urinary tract infection. Infect Dis Clin North Am 1987; 1: 773–791.
12. Stamm WE, Counts GW, Wagner KF, et al. Antimicrobial prophylaxis of recurrent urinary tract infections: a double-blind, placebo-contracted trial. Ann Intern Med 1980; 92: 770–775.
13. Harding GK, Ronald AR, Nicolle LE, et al. Long-term antimicrobial prophylaxis for recurrent urinary tract infection in women. Rev Infect Dis 1982; 4: 438–443.
14. Stapleton A, Latham RH, Johnson C, Stamm WE. Postcoital antimicrobial prophylaxis for recurrent urinary tract infection: a randomized, double-blind, placebo-controlled trial. JAMA 1990; 264: 703–706.
15. Raz R, Stamm WE. A controlled trial of intravaginal estriol in post-menopausal women with recurrent urinary tract infections. N Engl J Med 1993; 329: 753–756.
16. Meares EM Jr. Infection stones of the prostate gland, laboratory diagnosis and clinical management. Urology 1974; 4: 560–566.
17. Zhanel GG, Harding GK, Guay DR. Asymptomatic bacteruria: which patient should be treated? Arch Intern Med 1990; 150: 1389–1396.
18. Andriole VT, Patterson TF. Epidemiology, natural history, and management of urinary tract infections in pregnancy. Med Clin North Am 1991; 75: 359–373.
19. Bennett WM, Craven R. Urinary tract infections in patients with sever renal disease. Treatment with ampicillin and trimethoprim-sulfamethoxazole. JAMA 1976; 236: 946–948.
20. Kunin CM, Craig WA, Uehling DT. Trimethoprim therapy for urinary tract infection. Long-term prophylaxis in uremic patient. JAMA 1978; 239: 2588–2590.
21. Parsons CL, Schmidt JD. Control of current lower urinary tract infection in the postmenopausal women. J Urol 1982; 128: 1224–1226.

11 Evaluation and Treatment of Benign Prostatic Hyperplasia

Elroy D. Kursh, MD

CONTENTS

INTRODUCTION

Benign prostatic hyperplasia (BPH) is the most common tumor known to humankind. Moreover, bladder outflow obstruction (BOO) secondary to BPH is a very prevalent problem in aging men. The number of men in the United States aged 55 to 64 years is expected to increase by 50% in the next decade, from 11.4 million to almost 17 million. Additionally, the number of men with symptoms secondary to BPH was estimated at approx 25 million in 2000 and is expected to grow to 34 million by 2110. It is evident from numerous reports that only a fraction of men with symptoms secondary to BPH are currently being managed with any form of therapy.

NEW TERMINOLOGY

For decades, the group of symptoms associated with BPH have been known as "prostatism," which was subdivided into "obstructive" and "irritative" voiding symptoms. Unfortunately, these terms are largely meaningless. They are neither gender-specific, because women may experience similar symptoms, nor disease-specific, because a wealth of data demonstrate that lower urinary tract symptoms in older men are often unrelated to either BPH or BOO demonstrated by pressure-flow studies.

The old terminology needs to change, not only because the terms are nonspecific but also because patients may not be treated appropriately if diagnoses are based on a

From: *Essential Urology: A Guide to Clinical Practice*
Edited by: J. M. Potts © Humana Press Inc., Totowa, NJ

history of symptoms and physical findings alone. To advise patients correctly and offer them the best possible outcome, physicians should adopt the new terminology proposed at the International Consensus Conference on BPH in Monaco in 1995 and evaluate patients according to their lower urinary tract symptoms (LUTS), their prostate status, and their voiding characteristics. What follows are the more specific terms developed at the conference:

1. LUTS replaces the term prostatism because LUTS occur in both sexes and have many causes, such as an overactive bladder (detrusor instability) and bladder hypersensitivity, in addition to bladder outlet obstruction.
2. Voiding symptoms, previously called "obstructive voiding symptoms," include a decreased force of urinary stream or slow urinary stream, intermittency, dribbling, hesitancy, and the need to strain to void. The new term is preferred because these symptoms may be associated with detrusor (bladder) underactivity, decompensation, or acontractility and are not necessarily related to obstruction.
3. The term storage symptoms replaces "irritative voiding symptoms" because irritative connotes inflammation, which is not responsible for these symptoms in most men. Storage symptoms include frequency, nocturia, urgency, incontinence, and bladder discomfort. There is increasing evidence that nocturia, which traditionally has been considered to be one of the most reliable symptoms of BOO, is very prevalent in aging men and women. The prevalence of both nocturnal polyuria related to the absence of the circadian rhythm of argenine vasopressin secretion and nocturnal detrusor overactivity make nocturia a less reliable symptom in the overall symptomatic assessment of BOO.
4. BPH is retained to describe a characteristic prostatic histologic pattern present in more than 70% of men over age 70, but only about one-half of these men have gland enlargement, and only one-quarter experience LUTS.
5. Benign prostatic enlargement (BPE) indicates enlargement in the size of the prostate detected by either digital rectal examination (DRE) or transrectal ultrasound.
6. BOO is the urodynamically accepted term for proven obstruction.
7. Benign prostatic obstruction (BPO) refers to BOO in association with BPE.

PATHOPHYSIOLOGY OF LUTS

As already emphasized, the concept that symptoms in the aging male population are typically caused by the BOO arising from an enlarged prostate is a gross oversimplification. It is now widely recognized that not all men who present with LUTS have BPH and that the pathophysiology of those symptoms may not even be related to the prostate. The paradigm is shifting because symptoms frequently present in the absence of an enlarged prostate and because woman present with LUTS as often as men.

A major cause of LUTS related to BOO is the associated bladder dysfunction. BOO causes an increase in bladder mass, a decrease in urinary flow, a decrease in bladder compliance, and incomplete voiding. The increased muscle mass in the bladder is initially a compensatory adaptive reaction that permits most adults to void completely. The increased bladder mass is predominately the result of hypertrophy (increased size of the smooth muscle cells) rather than hyperplasia (increased number of smooth muscle cells). Compensated bladder function is characterized by a relatively constant bladder mass. The shift to decompensated bladder function is a state in which the ability of the bladder to empty efficiently and completely is impaired. This results in a reduced contractile response of the bladder smooth muscle cells and is characterized by progressive deterioration in the contractile and functional status of the bladder, a rapid increase in bladder mass, and a progressive decrease in the volume fraction of smooth muscle elements. The end-stage of a decompensated bladder is characterized by either an organ with a thick fibrous wall, low capacity, poor compliance, and little or no contractile function or a dilated bladder with a thin fibrous wall, large capacity, and little or no contractile function.

The current theory on the shift from compensation to decompensation is that the dysfunctions are directly related to specific cellular and subcellular alterations in the neuronal, mitochondrial, and sarcoplasmic reticulum compartments. Electromicroscopic data supports the hypothesis that ischemia is a major factor in the etiology of bladder dysfunction in obstruction. BOO induces hypoxia within the bladder wall and the bladder smooth muscle and autonomic nerves appear to be the most vulnerable tissues in the bladder.

Certain patients, despite relatively severe symptomatology, remain in a compensated state for an indefinite period. Alternatively, some patients progress at varying rates from a compensated to a decompensated state. Further studies are required to determine the stage during decompensation at which relief of obstruction enables the bladder to regain its normal structural and functional characteristics. Basic laboratory studies in animals support the need for early treatment of partial BOO.

EVALUATION OF BPH

A thorough history should be obtained in men presenting with LUTS. A history includes assessment of voiding and storage symptoms as outlined previously. It is advisable to request that the patient complete the American Urologic Association Symptom Index (AUASI) form (Table 1). The AUASI consists of seven symptoms (straining, incomplete voiding, frequency, intermittency, stream force, urgency, and nocturia), each of which is graded on a severity scale of 0 to 5. Thus, the total score range is from 0 to 35 (most severe). Although the AUASI has excellent test reliability and predictive validity, it is used only 7.5% of the time, even by practicing urologists.

It is also helpful to complete a Quality of Life Symptom Assessment Form, which is based on five questions with different weightings (Table 2). Probably the most important question in this form (question 4) asks the patient, “If you were to spend the rest of your life with your prostate symptoms just as they are now, how would you feel about that?” (Table 2). Therefore, some standard forms used in an urological practice only ask question 4 in addition to the AUASI. Another form that can also be completed is the Problems Due to Symptoms Index, which consists of seven questions, each scored 0 to 4. The value of completing the Quality of Life Scale and the Problems Due to Symptoms index is that recent epidemiological studies indicate that worry and embarrassment reflect quality of life issues that appear to be most important in influencing patients who seek treatment for LUTS. Prevalent urinary symptoms alone do not influence a man’s health care-seeking behavior. Men with bother scores greater than predicted from their symptom scores tended to seek treatment, and those patients with heightened bother were older, poorer, more anxious and had lower physiological well-being scores.

A DRE is performed, and prostate size is estimated on a 0 to 4 scale. Each plus of enlargement is considered to represent 25 cm^3 or 25 g of prostate growth. For example, a 2+ enlarged gland is considered to be 50 cm^3 or 50 g in size. It is helpful to palpate for the presence of a median sulcus, which is apparent when the gland is generally 25 cm^3

Table 1
American Urological Association (AUA) Symptom Index

Questions to be answered	*Not at all*	*Less than 1 time in 5*	*Less than half the time*	*About half the time*	*More than half the time*	*Almost always*
1. Over the past month, how often have you had a sensation of not emptying your bladder completely after you finish urinating?	0	1	2	3	4	5
2. Over the past month, how often have you had to urinate again less than 2 h after you finished urinating?	0	1	2	3	4	5
3. Over the past month, how often have you found you stopped and started again several times when you urinate?	0	1	2	3	4	5
4. Over the past month, how often have you found it difficult to postpone urination?	0	1	2	3	4	5
5. Over the past month, how often have you had a weak urinary stream?	0	1	2	3	4	5
6. Over the past month, how often have you had to push or strain to begin urination?	0	1	2	3	4	5
7. Over the past month, how many times did you most typically get up to urinate from the time you went to bed at night until the time you got up in the morning?	0	1	2	3	4	5
	(None)	(1 time)	(2 times)	(3 times)	(4 times)	(5 times)

Sum of the seven circled numbers (AUA Symptom Score): ________
Scoring: Mild: 0 to 7 Moderate: 8 to 19 Severe: 20 to 35

Table 2
Quality of Life Symptom Assessment

1. Over the past month, how much physical discomfort did any urinary problems cause you?
   - 0 = none
   - 1 = only a little
   - 2 = some
   - 3 = a lot
2. Over the past month, how much did you worry about your health because of any urinary problems?
   - 0 = none
   - 1 = only a little
   - 2 = some
   - 3 = a lot
3. Overall, how bothersome has any trouble with urination been during the past month?
   - 0 = not at all bothersome
   - 1 = bothers me a little
   - 2 = bothers me some
   - 3 = bothers me a lot
4. If you were to spend the rest of your life with your prostate symptoms just as they are now, how would you feel about that?
   - 0 = delighted
   - 1 = pleased
   - 2 = mostly satisfied
   - 3 = mixed (about equally satisfied & dissatisfied)
   - 4 = mostly dissatisfied
   - 5 = unhappy
   - 6 = terrible
5. Over the past month, how much of the time has any urinary problem kept you from doing the kinds of things you usually do?
   - 0 = none of the time
   - 1 = a little of the time
   - 2 = some of the time
   - 3 = most of the time
   - 4 = all of the time

Total: ________

or less. The median sulcus is usually obliterated when the gland reaches 50 cm^3 or an estimated size of 2+ or more. Recent data indicates that the DRE underestimates true prostate size measured by transrectal ultrasonography or magnetic resonance imaging by 20 to more than 30%. The magnitude of underestimation increases with increasing prostate volume.

The prostate is also assessed for the presence of prostate nodules. The presence of any indurated or hard areas within the prostate is highly suggestive of possible prostate cancer. A soft nodular area that has the same consistency as the rest of the gland may represent a lobular area of BPH. Although induration within the prostate may be caused by pathologic conditions other than prostate cancer, such as prostatic calcifications, it is imperative to rule out a diagnosis of prostate cancer if questionable areas of induration are detected. Therefore, patients with suspicious areas of induration should be referred for urological consultation to rule out a possible diagnosis of prostate cancer. It is advisable to obtain a prostate-specific antigen (PSA) value annually in all men starting at age 50 until approximately age 70 years. Data indicate that the PSA is more accurate and has greater sensitivity in detecting early prostate cancer than the DRE. Obviously, any patient with a suspicious nodule on DRE should have a PSA ordered. Recent data indicates that PSA is a useful surrogate marker for prostate volume and that patients with larger prostates have higher PSA values. Additionally, PSA increases as men age and it may be a better predictor of men at risk for acute urinary retention than other parameters.

Before beginning therapy, it is helpful to obtain a few objective studies to better quantify the degree of problem that the patient is experiencing. These basic studies are uroflowmetry and measurement of a postvoid residual (PVR).

There are a variety of simple means of measuring uroflowmetry, and the study is almost universally available in practicing urologists' offices. The test should be performed with a minimum voided volume of 125 mL. The most important measurement obtained during uroflowmetry is the maximum flow rate (Q_{max}), which normally is greater than 15 mL/s. The average flow rate is also recorded. Studies have demonstrated that there is variability in the outcome of this test and variability is increased among men with LUTS secondary to BPH. Theoretically, a pressure flow study is a more sophisticated urodynamic means of accurately detecting obstruction. Various nomograms have been devised as a standard means of plotting data. Unfortunately, controversy exists among urologists about where on the nomogram to place the borders of delineating obstruction, the equivocal zone, and no obstruction. Additionally, studies have shown that there is not much difference between the sensitivity of uroflowmetry and pressure flow studies in predicting success. Although I recommend obtaining the more sophisticated pressure flow studies in complex cases, I do not feel that it is necessary to obtain this study in all patients with LUTS.

Measurement of the PVR is usually obtained in the urologist's office with the use of abdominal ultrasound to measure the residual volume in the bladder after the patient completes voiding. In the past, this was usually done by catheterizing the patient after the patient completely emptied his bladder. Studies have demonstrated that measurement of the PVR has substantial within-patient variability. Therefore, some urologists recommend repeating the test. It has been shown that there is no correlation between the volume of PVR and the presence of urinary tract infections as was thought to be the case in the past. Theoretically, patients should be able to empty their bladders relatively completely. Because of variability, there is no particular volume of PVR that is considered to be abnormal. The major value of recording the PVR is that an abnormal test is a sign of bladder function abnormality rather than merely evidence of BOO. Patients with consistently large PVRs greater than several hundred milliliters (e.g., 300 mL) may have a decompensated bladder secondary to BOO, in which case surgical relief of the obstruction is advisable.

In summary, physicians frequently recommend medical therapy without the benefit of a simple flow study or measurement of a PVR. I have observed an increasing number of patients inappropriately managed with medical therapy who had huge PVRs in the vicinity of 1000 mL secondary to decompensated bladders. In most instances, appropriate therapy for these patients is transurethral resection of the prostate (TURP) to completely remove the obstruction in an attempt to preserve bladder function and prevent further bladder decompensation.

TREATMENT

There are a variety of treatments available for managing BOO secondary to BPH, including observation, phytotherapy, medical treatment, minimally invasive treatment and TURP, or open surgical removal of the prostate. The decision of whom and when to treat relies more on the art than the science of medicine. One must consider which patient is likely to develop problems and/or progress and what the patient's values are. Because every treatment has potential side effects against which the benefits of treatment should be considered, there is no universal rule or algorithm approach to the management of BPH. The selection of treatment and the recommendation for surgery is a result of a negotiation between the physician and patient. Some patients tolerate their symptoms well and are willing to put up with annoying symptoms rather than face surgery,whereas others welcome surgery as a definitive resolution of their symptoms.

Observation

Many patients with LUTS secondary to BOO can be managed with observation. Most patients with AUASI scores in the mild range (<7) are best managed conservatively with observation. In approx 50% of these patients, the symptoms remain stable and do not progress. Patients are reassured that treatment is not advisable at this time. It is recommended that the patient status be monitored annually for possible progression. Observation may also be appropriate for patients with AUASI scores in the moderate range (8 to 19) if they are tolerating the symptoms well and if the symptoms are not worrisome or bothersome. Of course, patients with higher AUASI scores are generally more bothered by their LUTS.

It is important to note that patients with decompensated bladders often have fewer symptoms. Annoying LUTS secondary to BOO is usually related to an hypertrophied bladder and associated symptoms of bladder instability which, as already mentioned, is a compensatory response to BOO. These patients may experience annoying frequency, urgency, and even urgency incontinence, and they are anxious to have relief of their symptoms. Alternatively, patients with varying degrees of bladder decompensation have fewer symptoms because the bladder capacity may be very large. Such a patient may have little or no urinary frequency and nocturia and is often reluctant to undergo treatment despite the fact that the bladder may be severely decompensated. Such patients generally have large residuals (>500 mL). Therefore, as already emphasized, it is advisable to obtain a PVR to rule out patients with bladder decompensation before recommending observation or medical therapy.

Phytotherapy (Herbal or Alternative Therapy)

For many patients, herbal medicine provides an attractive alternative to conventional treatment because the medication is easy to purchase; available in the local pharmacy, health food store, or over the Internet; and a prescription by a physician is not required. Other reasons for their popularity are that phytotherapies are perceived to be as natural and therefore healthier, and they are purported to have virtually no side effects. The Food and Drug Administration (FDA) and US health care professionals have been reluctant to advocate their use, primarily because their reported efficacy and safety have not been substantiated by randomized, double-blind, placebo-controlled studies. Most studies of this form of therapy are open-label, retrospective studies with no placebo control or poorly conducted placebo control and data are often conflicting and inconclusive. Prospective, randomized, placebo-controlled studies are essential when evaluating treatments for the management of BPH because a placebo effect of 40–60% has been observed in controlled studies.

The most common phytotherapies for BPH are saw palmetto (*Serenoa repens*), African plumb (*Pygeum africanum*), and South African Star Grass (*Hypoxis rooperi*). Saw palmetto is the most frequently used phytotherapy for LUTS. Permixon, a liposterolic extract of *S. repens* (extracted from the dwarf palm indigenous to the southeastern United States and West Indies) is the preparation most studied. The exact mechanism of action of *S. repens* remains uncertain. However, a recent study demonstrated epithelial contraction, especially in the transition zone, indicating a possible mechanism of action, but a change in prostate volume or PSA has not been observed. Available information on saw palmetto extract consists largely of in vitro experiments and European trials, of which many have limited value as noted by various observers.

Similar limitations have been observed in the few studies assessing the other forms of alternative therapy. There are no data from well-designed, long-term, randomized, placebo-controlled studies to suggest that any alternative therapy has an effect on long-term outcome or disease progression.

Because the effectiveness of phytotherapy has not been adequately investigated, a general recommendation for its use cannot be made. There are some patients with mild symptoms (AUASI < 7) who appear to respond to these preparations. For these patients, phytotherapy may be an alternative to conservative treatment or observation. Saw palmetto, African plumb, and phytosterols appear to be slightly better than placebo, although further long-term studies are needed before definitive conclusions can be drawn.

In general, I do not recommend phytotherapy for patients with moderate to severe LUTS (AUASI ≤7), a truly enlarged prostate (>25 mL), or clinically evident BOO because the data indicate that there are more effective alternatives, including α-adrenergic receptor blockers, 5α-reductase inhibitors, and surgery.

Medical Therapy

α-Adrenergic Receptor Blockers

The rationale for the use of α-adrenergic receptor blockers in the management of BPH is based on research indicating that prostate smooth muscle is partially responsible for BOO via an α-adrenergic receptor-mediated mechanism. Therefore, the α-adrenergic receptor antagonist relaxes prostate smooth muscle leading to a reduction in LUTS associated with BOO. The α_1-adrenergic receptor subtype, in particular, has been found to mediate smooth muscle contraction in the prostate, bladder base, and proximal urethra.

The selective, long-acting, α_1-adrenergic receptor blockers marketed in the United States include terazosin (Hytrin), doxazosin (Cardura), and tamsulosin (Flomax). All of these agents have comparable, well-established efficacy in regard to the management of LUTS. Selective α_1-adrenergic receptor blockers provide rapid symptom relief, with partial symptom relief observed in as little as 1 wk. Full therapeutic benefit is observed after 2–3 mo of therapy. Use of these agents is recommended for all patients who seek immediate symptom relief, including men with small prostates. In general, men with BPH treated with any of these products experience a 30 to 40% symptom reduction and a 16 to 25% improvement in Q_{max} with mean Q_{max} improvement in the vicinity of 3 mL/s. Additionally, all of these agents have a sufficient half-life to permit convenient once-daily dosing, but terazosin and doxazosin must be titrated to avoid first-dose effects (e.g., dizziness, syncope). Terazosin is initiated at 1 mg daily doses at bedtime and titrated to 5 or 10 mg per day over a period of 1 to 2 wk to achieve desired improvement. Doxazosin can be initiated with 1-mg per day doses and titrated over a period of 1 to 2 wk to a maximum dose of 8 mg per day. Titration reduces the risk for first-dose cardiovascular effects. Statistically and clinically significant changes in blood pressure reduction were observed in hypertensive men, however, no change in blood pressure is observed for normotensive men in most studies. The most commonly reported side effects are dizziness and asthenia.

Although these agents have comparable efficacy, there are differences among the cardiovascular safety intolerability profiles of these α_1-adrenergic receptor blockers. In general, those agents that are more effective for treating hypertension (i.e., doxazosin, terazosin) are a little more likely to effect blood pressure in normotensive men with BPH than tamsulosin. In controlled studies, drop-out rates for tamsulosin are comparable to placebo, whereas the drop-out rates were slightly higher for patients managed with doxazosin and terazosin, in the vicinity of 4 to 10% greater than placebo-treated men. Another advantage of tamsulosin is that it does not require titration. If a patient finds one particular side effect intolerable, another agent may be considered. In general, switching between different α_1-adrenergic receptor blockers to enhance efficacy is not recommended and not likely to produce a different response.

In summary, each of these $\alpha_1$adrenergic blocking agents have similar efficacy with slightly different side effect profiles. When choosing between the various agents, the physician should consider the expense of the various agents, the presence of accompanying medical conditions, such as hypertension, and the side-effect profile.

5α-Reductase Inhibitors, Finasteride (Proscar)

Dihydrotestosterone (DHT) is the predominant androgen in the prostate and an important regulator of prostate growth. The enzyme 5α-reductase converts testosterone to the more potent androgen DHT. A reduction in serum testosterone but not DHT is associated with intolerable sexual side effects, particularly erectile dysfunction and decreased libido. Therefore, treatment with the 5α-reductase inhibitor, finasteride, results in a reduction in DHT within the prostate and subsequent reduction in prostate volume without causing sexual side effects.

The Proscar Long-Term Efficacy and Safety Study (PLESS) is the largest clinical trial to investigate finasteride for the management of BPH. In this multicenter, double-blind, placebo-controlled study, more than 3000 men with moderate to severe urinary symptoms and an enlarged prostate at baseline were randomized to 5 mg finasteride per day ($n = 1513$) or placebo ($n = 1503$) after a 1-mo placebo run in. All participants were monitored for 4 yr. The mean AUASI score decreased by 3.3 and 1.3 points in the finasteride and placebo arms, respectively ($p < 0.001$). Statistically significant symptom improvements were observed beginning at about 8 mo and continuing throughout the study end point. Similarly, Q_{max} improved by 1.9 mL/s and 0.2 mL/s at the study end point for the finasteride and placebo arms, respectively ($p < 0.001$).

Significant improvement in urinary flow over placebo was evident beginning within 4 mo and was maintained through the end of the study. Supporting the hypothesis that 5α-reductase has an effect on disease progression, finasteride decreased baseline prostate volume by 18% compared with a 14% increase for placebo ($p < 0.001$).

Men with baseline prostate volumes greater than 40 mL are more likely to respond to finasteride treatment than men with smaller prostates. Others have demonstrated that men with larger prostates experience greater improvement in total symptom severity and Q_{max} with finasteride. Because PSA is a surrogate predictor of prostate volume, men with higher baseline PSAs (PSA ≥ 1.4 ng/mL) were found to experience greater improvement with finasteride treatment. Additionally, analysis of the PLESS study data revealed that finasteride significantly reduced the risks of developing acute urinary retention or the need for BPH-related surgery.

Finasteride has a predictable effect on PSA values. Men treated with this drug have PSA levels of approximately half of those of matched, untreated men and a patient's PSA value is expected to decrease to approximately half of the original value after starting treatment. With this knowledge in mind, a physician can follow a patient's PSA value who is treated with finasteride over time, observing for changes in PSA levels in order to exclude a diagnosis of prostate cancer. In a large cooperative VA study, the efficacy of placebo, terazosin (10 mg daily), finasteride (5 mg daily), and a combination of both drugs was compared in men with BPH. In this study, treatment with terazosin was effective whereas finasteride was not, and the combination of terazosin and finasteride was no more effective than terazosin alone. Although this study suggests that the treatment with finasteride offers no benefit and that the α_1-adrenergic blocking agent, terazosin, is more effective than finasteride, the mean prostate volume in the patient's evaluated in this study was less than 40 cm^3. Therefore, the lack of response in the finasteride arm of the study may have been related to the fact that smaller prostates were treated in this study.

In summary, treatment with finasteride results in approximately a 20% reduction in prostate volume and subsequent reduction in urinary symptoms and improved urinary flow rates. The use of finasteride should be confined to patients who have larger prostates greater than 40 cm^3. Alternatively, men with smaller prostates are best treated medically with one of the α_1-adrenergic blocking agents.

Minimally Invasive Treatment

Currently, there are a number of competing minimally invasive technologies for management of BOO secondary to BPH. Virtually all of these technologies provide energy or heat to the prostate to produce varying degrees of coagulation necrosis in the prostate, thereby reducing the size of the prostate and attempting to relieve obstruction. The most frequently used competing technologies include transurethral microwave thermotherapy (TUMT), transurethral needle ablation (TUNA), and interstitial laser coagulation (ILC).

TUMT is performed in the office setting with the use of a special catheter that contains a microwave antenna. Cold water is circulated through the catheter to attempt to cool the urethra and avoid urethral injury and reduce pain. Rectal temperatures are monitored via thermosensors placed on a rectal probe. Likewise, thermosensors in the catheter record urethral temperature. When the temperature reaches a certain threshold in the urethra or rectum, the energy is automatically turned off by the computer that controls the entire treatment. An advantage of TUMT is that it is performed in the office setting without general or regional anesthesia. Sedation is usually administered because patients generally have some discomfort, sense the heating process, or complain of a strong urge to void.

Radiofrequency is the energy source used in TUNA. The operation is performed endoscopically using the transurethral approach. Although TUNA may be performed in the office setting using local anesthesia, at times it is preferable to use a more formal anesthetic and perform the procedure in the operating room. The radiofrequency energy is applied through two needle electrodes, which are inserted into the prostate transurethrally and a protective sleeve is passed over the electrodes for a short distance to protect and avoid thermal injury to the urethra.

ILC of the prostate is also performed transurethrally. Generally, ILC is performed in an ambulatory surgical setting under general or spinal anesthesia, although local anesthesia with a prostate block has been used. A laser fiber is inserted into the prostate and laser energy radiates heat in all directions through a 1-cm long diffuser tip at a low power (20 W). The heat produces an olive-shaped area of coagulation necrosis of about 2 × 2.5 cm or a volume of approx 4 cm^3. To reduce damage to the urethra, the fiber is inserted into the interstitium of the prostate. The location and number of punctures of the laser fiber vary according to the size of the prostate.

There are advantages and disadvantages to each of these technologies. A satisfactory outcome is achieved in only a subset of patients using each of these modalities and no procedure is clearly superior to the other. Patients often require a catheter for 2 to 7 d after any of these therapies because the application of thermal energy to the prostate results in prostatic edema and an inability to void. After treatment, patients do not experience relief of their symptoms or improved voiding until 6 to 8 wk have elapsed and resorption of some of the prostate parenchyma occurs.

I believe that the minimally invasive treatment of BPH will continue to evolve and that an effective minimally invasive procedure that is performed in the physician's office will be developed. It is likely that the development of an effective minimally invasive approach will have profound impact on the management of BOO secondary to BPH.

TURP and Open Surgical Removal of the Prostate

TURP remains the most commonly used surgical treatment with superior improvement in objective evaluation parameters such as improved flow rate, making it the gold standard form of treatment. Also, TURP remains the treatment to which all new therapies are compared. TURP requires a general or spinal anesthetic and hospitalization for 1 or 2 d and may be associated with complications, such as incontinence (1%), bleeding, and water intoxication. Technical advances over the years, including improved instrumentation and optics, better light sources (fiberoptics), and use of video have enhanced the urologist's ability to safely perform TURP.

Open surgical removal (suprapubic or retropubic prostatectomy) may be required for very large prostates with prostate volumes in the vicinity of 100 cm^3. The urologist may elect to perform transrectal ultrasound to more accurately assess prostate volume before making a definitive recommendation on the type of surgery to be performed.

SUMMARY

The management of BPH has undergone tremendous change in the last decade. In the past, the problem has almost exclusively been the domain of urologists with surgery being the primary form of therapy. Today, BPH is more likely to be initially treated by a primary care physician and internist (49% of cases), whereas urologists provide primary treatment in only a little more than one-third of men with symptomatic BPH.

Pharmacotherapy has developed into the dominant first line of therapy. It is popular among patients and physicians because clinically significant subjective improvement can be obtained with fewer side effects. Although TURP remains the gold standard form of surgical therapy for BPH, less-invasive minimally invasive treatment options are being developed. The minimally invasive treatments are mostly heat-based therapies that cause coagulation necrosis in the prostate and attempt to reduce prostate volume. Reflecting the shift toward pharmacotherapy and minimally invasive treatment, fewer prostatectomies are being performed. Furthermore, basic research has led to a better understanding of the pathoetiology and pathophysiology of BPH and the effect that BOO has on bladder function. It is anticipated that continued research should enhance the physician's armamentarian for managing this prevalent problem.

SELECTED READINGS

Jepsen JV, Bruskewitz RC. Comprehensive patient evaluation for benign prostatic hyperplasia. Urology 1998; 51 (suppl 4A): 13–18.

Gosling JA, Kung LS, Dixon JS, Horan P, Whitbeck C, Levin RM. Correlation between the structure and function of the rabbit urinary bladder following partial outlet obstruction. J Urol 2000; 163: 1349–1356.

Lepor H, Williford WO, Barry MJ, et al. The efficacy of terazosin, finasteride, or both in benign prostatic hyperplasia. N Engl J Med 1996; 333: 533–539.

McConnell JD, Bruskewitz R, Walsh P, et al for the Finasteride Long-Term Efficacy and Safety Study Group. The effect of finasteride on the risk of acute urinary retention and the need for surgical treatment among men with benign prostatic hyperplasia. N Engl J Med 1998; 338: 557–563.

12 Prostatitis/Chronic Pelvic Pain Syndrome

Jeannette M. Potts, MD

CONTENTS

INTRODUCTION

Approximately 2 million men in the United States are diagnosed and treated for prostatitis each year. It is estimated that 35–50% of men will experience pain or discomfort attributed to prostatitis at some time during their lifetime. Recent epidemiological studies suggest that 5–9% of unselected men in the community experience prostatitis symptoms at any given time. The prevalence of self-reported prostatitis among health professionals was 16% and correlated with greater odds with history of sexually transmitted disease and stress reported at home or at work.

The most common form of prostatitis, accounting for greater than 90% of cases, is chronic abacterial prostatitis, also described as chronic pelvic pain syndrome (CPPS) (National Institutes of Health [NIH] Category III Prostatitis). The focus of this chapter will be placed on this form of prostatitis; however, diagnosis and treatment for the other NIH categories of prostatitis will be included (Table 1).

From: *Essential Urology: A Guide to Clinical Practice*
Edited by: J. M. Potts © Humana Press Inc., Totowa, NJ

NIH CATEGORY I PROSTATITIS (ACUTE BACTERIAL PROSTATITIS)

Diagnosis

Acute prostatitis is the easiest of the prostatitis syndromes to recognize. Patients present with moderate to severe lower urinary tract symptoms (LUTS) characteristic of bladder infection, associated with fever, chills, malaise, perineal, rectal, lower back pain, and sometimes generalized arthralgias/myalgias. On physical exam, patients may have urinary retention, and the prostate gland is typically exquisitely tender. Urinalysis and cultures are usually positive; the most common organism cultured in this setting is *Escherichia coli* (80%). Other pathogens include *Pseudomonas aeruginosa, Serratia, Klebsiella, Proteus,* and enterococci.

Treatment

Fluoroquinolones remain the mainstay of therapy. Initial therapy should be administered intravenously. Antibiotic alternatives for acute bacterial prostatitis are ampicillin/gentamycin combination, doxycycline, and trimethoprim-sulfa. Treatment duration should total 4–6 wk and can be completed using oral regimens after acute symptoms subside to prevent chronic bacterial prostatitis and/or prostatic abscess. In men with urinary retention, urethral catheterization may increase the likelihood of prostatic abscess formation; therefore, one should consider suprapubic catheter placement in these patients.

NIH CATEGORY II PROSTATITIS (CHRONIC BACTERIAL PROSTATITIS)

Diagnosis

This form of prostatitis is more commonly found in older men as a relapsing disease with occasional exacerbations. Patients typically have a history of recurring urinary tract infections, but asymptomatic bacteriuria may also be the presenting sign. In this form of prostatitis, the prostate serves as a reservoir for bacteria. Bacterial localization cultures using the Meares-Stamey or 4-glass technique are necessary to confirm the diagnosis and identify the culpable organism (Table 2). A modification of this technique is the pre-post massage test, which may be more feasible in a busy clinic setting. Recurrent infection caused by the same organism is considered one the hallmarks of this disease.

Treatment

Despite therapy, cure rates for chronic bacterial prostates are less than optimal. Prescribing antibiotics that can achieve adequate concentrations in prostatic fluid is essential; fluoroquinolones have been shown to be most efficacious. Other antibiotic alternatives include carbenicillin, doxycycline, and cephalexin. Treatment duration may vary from a minimum of 4 wk up to 4 mon. Weidner and colleagues *(1)* demonstrated the eradication of pathogens from expressed prostatic secretions (EPS) in 92% of patients 3 mo after a 4 wk course of ciprofloxacin. After 12–24 mo, 70–80% of patients remained "cured." The presence of prostatic calculi did not influence treatment outcome in this study. In patients with frequent or serious recurrences, suppressive antibiotic regimens

Table 1
NIH Prostatitis Classification

Category		
Category	I	Acute bacterial
Category	II	Chronic bacterial
Category	III	Chronic abacterial/ chronic pelvic pain syndrome a. Inflammatory: elevated white blood cell count in EPS, VB3, or semen b. Noninflammatory (formerly, prostatodynia)
Category	IV	Asymptomatic: histological or andrological identification

Table 2
Localization Cultures

VB1	Initial urine 10 mL	Representative of urethral flora
VB2	Midstream urine	Representative of Bladder milieu
EPS	Prostatic secretions Retrieved by prostate Massage	Microscopic evaluation for white blood cells and microorganisms
VB3	Post massage urine 10 mL	Representative of prostatic flora

should be prescribed using low doses of TMP-sulfa, nitrofurantoin, or tetracycline on a daily basis. Transurethral resection of the prostate may afford cure in about one third of patients with well-documented chronic bacterial prostatitis.

NIH CATEGORY III PROSTATITIS (CHRONIC PELVIC PAIN SYNDROME)

Diagnosis

A comprehensive history must be obtained with special attention to risk factors for predisposing factors for this condition (urethral stricture, prior sexually transmitted disease, genitourinary surgery, trauma, stressful life events, co-morbid conditions associated with Functional Somatic Syndromes) or that would cause LUTS(Calculi, neurological disorders, systemic diseases, neoplasm). Review of systems should include psychosocial assessment, that is, sexual history, occupation, social support, physical activity, and exercise habits.

The physical examination must include a thorough evaluation of the pelvic floor, which is best conducted while the patient is in the supine lithotomy position, which allows the examiner to access the perineum, anal sphincter, and the pelvic floor musculature by digital rectal exam. The internal examination is performed methodically by carefully palpating the coccyx, the Levator ani muscles, the ischial tuberosities, the internal obturator muscles, and finally the prostate. Attempts to reproduce the pain or identify trigger points that are tight and spastic should be the goal of this exam. This evaluation also provides valuable education for the patient in terms of differentiating pelvic pain from the discomfort often associated with digital exam of the prostate.

Prostate massage and the retrieval of expressed prostatic secretions and/or post-massage urine specimen for culture should be performed to exclude possible bacterial etiologies. Specific cultures may be required to rule out infections caused by sexually transmitted organisms, such as *Chlamydia trachomatis* and *Ureaplasma urealyticum*.

In some men, further testing may be required to rule out other urological, colorectal, or neurological conditions related to the patient's presentation. These may include endoscopic examinations, radiological studies, and often urodynamic testing.

Treatment

Little evidence exists to support the use of antibiotics and/or α-blockers in this setting; however, most practitioners prescribe these medications empirically always or almost always. Attempts should be made to provide symptomatic relief while establishing diagnosis and awaiting confirmatory test results. Anti-inflammatories may be prescribed to patients in whom there exist no contraindications. We have had much success managing CPPS by means of physical therapy incorporating specific stretching and strengthening exercises, biofeedback, and progressive relaxation. In some instances, additional therapy by means of myofascial release or soft tissue mobilization is provided by means of external and internal massage.

I have found that many patients welcome this fresh approach, which avoids ingestion of medication and invasive interventions. This strategy also provides much-needed empowerment to a group of patients who have experienced frustration and helplessness in association with their diagnosis. Evidence from other subspecialties also supports counseling patients about management of their condition rather than cure. Setting reasonable expectations with our patients further serves to assuage potential frustration as we implement new treatments.

NIH CATEGORY IV PROSTATITIS (ASYMPTOMATIC PROSTATIC INFLAMMATION)

Diagnosis

Identification of category IV prostatitis is typically incidental as patients are asymptomatic. Evaluation of asymptomatic men with elevated prostate-specific antigen (PSA), 42% had evidence of prostatitis upon examination of expressed prostatic secretions. After these men were treated with a 4-wk course of antibiotics, PSA levels normalized in nearly half of the men, obviating need for subsequent prostate biopsy. Histologically, prostatic inflammation has been observed in 50–90% of specimens from prostate biopsies and prostatectomies. Leukocytospermia may be identified in some men undergoing fertility evaluations.

Treatment

Men with this form of prostatitis are usually not treated with antibiotics unless they develop symptoms, have positive semen or EPS cultures, or are subjects in an empiric trial in the setting of unexplained infertility or in men in whom prostatitis is the suspected cause for elevated PSA level.

RATIONALE FOR THE EVALUATION AND TREATMENT OF CHRONIC PELVIC PAIN SYNDROME

Background

It is well recognized that only 5–7% of patients diagnosed with prostatitis have positive bacterial cultures, yet urologists and primary care physicians continue to prescribe antibiotics to patients presenting with LUTS attributed to prostatitis. Ironically, physicians who were more likely to prescribe antibiotics were also less likely to perform prostate massage and obtain appropriate cultures. Not surprising, treatment outcomes have been unsatisfactory, leading to the emergence of other therapies (α-blockers alone or with antibiotics, finasteride, saw palmetto, quercetin, nonsteroidal anti-inflammatory drugs, allopurinol, anticholinergics, antidepressants, and microwave therapy), illustrating the confusion over the etiology and ultimately obscuring the optimal treatment for chronic abacterial prostatitis.

Unfortunately, there continues to exist paucity in evidence based medical research in this area. The quality of published research is limited because of short-term follow-up, inconsistent inclusion criteria, and lack of prospective study designs. The recent establishment of a diagnostic consensus and a symptom score index are promising steps toward understanding the etiology of abacterial prostatitis and testing efficacy and durability of therapies with greater accuracy.

The constellation of symptoms associated with this disorder are not unique to a urological diagnosis, sharing characteristics with similar chronic pain syndromes seen in other medical subspecialties. Furthermore, symptoms attributed to chronic abacterial prostatitis and prostatodynia may be caused by a disorder unrelated to the prostate gland!

Initially, it is important to point out contradictions that exist in terms of the definition of prostatitis. Identifying and quantifying white blood cells in the EPS, VB3, or semen, for example, has been shown to vary significantly in the same patient, regardless of absence or presence of symptoms; correlating only with the clinical course of acute bacterial prostatitis, but not category II or III prostatitis. Although evidence of inflammation may be observed in the EPS of up to 52% of patients with chronic abacterial prostatitis/CPPS, EPS from asymptomatic men with elevated PSA levels demonstrated similar rates of inflammation (45%). The presence of inflammatory cells in EPS correlate poorly with the presence of inflammatory cells in semen as well.

Correlation of symptomology and histological changes cannot support the diagnosis of clinical prostatitis. Recently, True and colleagues *(2)* found histological evidence of inflammation in only 5% of symptomatic men; meanwhile, greater than 50% of biopsy specimens from asymptomatic men with elevated PSA have demonstrated significant inflammatory changes. Earlier pathology references indicate that greater than 90% of prostatectomy specimens contain evidence of chronic and acute inflammatory changes.

A form of chemical (noninfectious) prostatitis had been proposed as a sequelae to urinary reflux into the prostatic ductules. Kirby *(3)* and later Persson and colleagues *(4)* observed evidence of urinary reflux in men with abacterial prostatitis symptoms but not among asymptomatic controls. This led to the use of allopurinol in the treatment of category III prostatitis because it could lower levels of urate in the urine and prostatic fluid, as these were considered to be the culprits. Considering the cause of the reflux, however, may be the key to deciphering the complicated presentation of most of the patients seeking consultation for this disorder.

A plausible cause for urinary reflux is the nonrelaxation of the external sphincter, known as pseudo dyssynergia. Kaplan and colleagues *(5)* concluded that voiding dysfunction, including pseudo-dyssynergia, is often misdiagnosed as chronic prostatitis. In a later study, involving only those patients with urodynamic evidence of dyssynergia, a treatment regimen combining behavioral modification and biofeedback was successful in significantly ameliorating symptoms in 83% of patients. The association between prostatitis and voiding dysfunction has been observed by other investigators who describe acquired urinary changes and sphincter "incoordination," reported in 64–81.6% of patients with prostatitis.

Looking outside the box, or outside the prostate as the case may be, allows us to understand that voiding dysfunction is one of the manifestations of CPPS rather than a misdiagnosis. Only a few investigators have considered etiological factors outside the prostate gland. In 1977, Segura and colleagues *(6)* described pelvic floor myalgia in men who were previously diagnosed with chronic prostatitis. In 1988, Miller *(7)* considered emotional stressors as precipitants of prostatitis symptoms and prescribed stress management alone to 110 of his patients, which resulted in 86% favorable response rate. Berghuis and colleagues *(8)* observed higher levels than controls of hypochondriasis, depression, hysteria, and somatization among the prostatitis cohort. And finally, Zermann and colleagues *(9)* reported their observations correlating anal sphincter muscle incoordination and associated pelvic pain syndromes. They also described chronic abacterial prostatitis as a myofascial pain syndrome.

Gynecologists are often confronted with patients suffering from chronic pelvic pain. The myriad of names given to the condition has been described as "figments of our frustration" *(10)*. It is estimated that 30–76% of diagnostic laparoscopies for pelvic pain reveal normal tissue and that 12% of hysterectomies are performed solely because of pelvic pain.

In one series of 183 patients with negative laparoscopic findings, 60% were diagnosed with a somatoform disorder. Similar studies have concluded that stress and anxiety are significant contributing factors in the presentation of chronic pelvic pain. Concurrent diagnoses observed by gynecologists, included dysmenorrhea, urethral syndrome, irritable bowel syndrome, (IBS), and abdominal bloating. Abnormal muscle tension and nerve root hypersensitivity, both manifested as trigger points, have been implicated as the cause of chronic pelvic pain in women. These have been addressed with a combination of exercise, biofeedback and anesthetic trigger point injections, with promising results.

Colleagues in colorectal surgery have more than a dozen names to describe pelvic pain and chronic intractable rectal pain. Investigators rarely identify an organic cause to explain the patients' symptomology. Likewise, patients also possess similar comorbidities, such as IBS, depression, and unspecified genitourinary complaints. Internal massage of pelvic floor muscles along with exercise has been employed by investigators in three series, with success rates ranging from 67 to 93%.

Patients suffering from fibromyalgia (FM) also share many of the characteristics of patients diagnosed with NIH category III prostatitis, and up to 40% of FM patients have a history of chronic pelvic pain. Comorbid conditions often associated with FM include migraines, chronic fatigue syndrome, IBS, depression, restless leg syndrome, and myofascial pain syndromes. Treatment strategies involve exercise, counseling, antidepressant medications, and nonsteroidal anti-inflammatory drugs. Unfortunately, compliance rates for prescribed treatment regimens, especially exercise, are quite low.

In 2001, Aaron *(11)* compared 127 twins diagnosed with chronic fatigue and their healthy cotwin for prevalence of functional somatic syndromes (FSS) including chronic prostatitis. The comorbid conditions were identified with significantly greater frequency among the fatigued twins. These observations support an environmental, rather than a genetic factor, which may predispose some individuals to such syndromes.

Table 3
Functional Somatic Syndromes (FSS)

Atypical, noncardia chest pain	Multiple chemical sensitivity
Chronic headache	Nonulcer dyspepsia
Chronic fatigue syndrome	Premenstrual syndrome
Fibromyalgia	Temporomandibular joint syndrome
Globus syndrome	Urinary urgency-frequency syndrome
IBS	

The features of chronic prostatitis share characteristics of FSS, defined as symptoms that "cannot be explained in terms of a conventionally defined medical disease" *(12)*. Wessely and colleagues postulate the existence of specific somatic syndromes as largely an artifact of medical subspecialization. They observed a high prevalence of emotional distress among patients with FSS as well as a higher number of comorbid conditions, usually other FSS (Table 3). We evaluated 86 consecutive patients previously diagnosed with chronic abacterial prostatitis and identified FSS in 65.1% of the men. These findings are especially impressive because the lifetime prevalence for somatization disorders in the general population in only 0.5%. Psychosocial disturbances were observed in 47.9% of patients, consistent with 25–62% prevalence rates reported by gynecologists, colorectal surgeons, and other specialists treating chronic pelvic pain.

Although it is paramount to bear in mind the psychosocial aspects of CPPS, it is important to avoid compartmentalizing the patient once again into a solely psychological diagnosis. Unfortunately, the terminology used to describe this possible unifying syndrome as functional and somatic implies that the disorder has no physiological basis, which is not the case. Neuroendocrine alterations have been identified in patients suffering from chronic pain syndromes. Substance P measured in cerebrospinal fluid was higher in patients with FM when compared with levels in controls. Elevation of Substance P has been associated with sleep deprivation and increased pain perception. Disruption of the serotonergic pathway has been implicated in nonulcer dyspepsia, IBS, chronic fatigue syndrome, and premenstrual syndrome.

Exciting research in the field of pain medicine has revealed complex neurobiological mechanisms that transduce exteroreceptive and interoreceptive stimuli into memory, which may predispose patients to subsequent "amplified" pathological responses. The amplified pathological responses may be induced by psychological stress or trauma and be manifested as "limbically augmented pain syndromes."

CONCLUSIONS

Appropriate management of men with prostatitis requires accurate identification of the category of prostatitis with the aid of the NIH classification system. Chronic forms of this disease are rarely associated with bacteria. In this setting, antibiotic therapy should be prescribed only after cultures prove that bacteria are localized to the prostate gland. Underlying pelvic floor muscle dysfunction and/or FSS should be considered as causes or significant contributors of symptoms. A multidisciplinary approach, incorporating methods of pain medicine and physical therapy, may prove to be most beneficial for patients suffering from NIH category III prostatitis/CPPS.

SELECTED READINGS

Alexander RB, Ponniah S, Hasday J, Hebel R. Elevated level of proinflammatory cytokines in the semen of patients with chronic prostatitis/chronic pelvic pain syndrome. Urology 1998; 52: 744–749.

Anderson RU. Management of chronic prostatitis-chronic pelvic pain syndrome. Urol Clin North Am 2002; 29: 235–239.

Combs AJ, Glassberg AD, Gerdes D, Horowitz M. Biofeedback therapy for children with dysfunctional voiding. Urology 1998; 52: 312–315.

Costello K, Myofascial syndromes. In: Steege J, Metzger D, Levy B, eds. Chronic Pelvic Pain: An Integrated Approach. W.B. Saunders, Co., Philadelphia, PA, 1998.

Doble A. An evidence based approach to the treatment of prostatitis: is it possible? Curr Urol Rep 2000; 1: 142–47.

Grant SR, Salvati EP, Rubin RJ. Levator syndrome: an analysis of 316 cases. Dis Colon Rectum 1975; 18: 161–163.

Kellner R. Psychosomatic syndromes, somatization and somatoform disorder. Psychother Psychosom 1994; 61: 4–24.

King Baker P, Steege JF, Metzger DA, Levy BS. Musculoskeletal problems. In: Steege J, Metzger D, Levy B, eds. Chronic Pelvic Pain: An Integrated Approach. W.B. Saunders, Co., Philadelphia, PA, 1998.

Krieger JN, McGonagle LA. Diagnostic considerations and interpretation of microbiological findings for evaluation of chronic prostatitis. J Clin Microbiol 1989; 27: 2240–2244.

McNaughton Collins M, Fowler FJ Jr, Elliott DB, Albertsen PC, Barry MJ. Diagnosing and treating chronic prostatitis: do urologists use the four-glass test? Urology 2000; 55: 403–407

Collins MM, Meigs JB, Barry MJ, Walker Corkery E, Giovannucci E, Kawachi I. Prevalence and correlates of prostatitis in the health professionals follow-up study cohort. J Urol 2000; 167: 1363–1366.

Mason E, McLean P, Cox J. Psychosocial aspects of the urethral syndrome in women. J Ir Med Assoc 1977; 70: 11.

Meares EM, Stamey TA. Bacteriologic localization patterns in bacterial prostatitis and urethritis. Invest. Urol. 1968; 5: 492–518.

Millea PJ, Holloway R. Treating fibromyalgia. Am Family Physician 2000; 62: 1575–1582.

Nickel JC. The pre and post massage test (PPMT): a simple screen for prostatitis Tech Urol 1997; 3: 38–43.

Nickel JC, Downey J, Johnston B, Clark J, Group TC, for the Canadian Prostatitis Research Group . Predictors of patient response to antibiotic therapy for the chronic prostatitis/chronic pelvic pain syndrome: a prospective multicenter study. J Urol 2001; 165: 1539–1544.

Nickel JC, Nyberg LM, Hennenfent M. Research guidelines for chronic prostatitis: Consensus report from the first national institutes of health international prostatitis collaborative network. Urology 1999; 54: 229–233.

Pasqualotto FF, Sharma RK, Potts JM, Nelson DR, Thomas AJ Jr, Agarwal A. seminal oxidative stress in chronic prostatitis patients. Urology 2000; 55: 881–885.

Potts JM. Prospective identification of National Institutes of Health category IV prostatitis in men with elevated prostate specific antigen. J Urol 2000; 164: 1550–1553.

Potts JM, O'Dougherty E. Pelvic floor physical therapy for patients with prostatitis. Curr Urol Rep 2000; 1: 155–158.

Potts JM, Sharma RK, Pasqualotto FF, Nelson DR, Agarwal A. Association of *Ureaplasma urealyticum* infection with abnormal seminal reactive oxygen species and absence of leukocytospermia. J Urol 2000; 163: 1775–1778.

Reiter R, Gambone J. Nongynecologic somatic pathology in women with chronic pelvic pain and negative laparoscopy. J Reprod Med 1991; 36: 253–259.

Rome HP, Rome JD. Limbically augmented pain syndrome (LAPS): kindling, corticolimbic sensitization, and the convergence of affective and sensory symptoms in chronic pain disorders. Pain Med 2000; 1: 7–23.

Schaeffer AJ. Prostatitis: US perspective Int'l J Anti Micro Ag 1998; 10: 153–159.

Schover LR. Psychological factors in men with genital pain. Cleve Clin J Med 1990; 57: 697–700.
Sinaki M, Merritt JL, Stillwall GK. Tension myalgia of the pelvic floor. Mayo Clinic Proc 1997; 55: 717–722.
Stamey, TA. Prostatitis, prostatosis and prostatodynia. Urology 1981; 25: 439–443.
Thiele GH. Coccygodynia: cause and treatment. Dis Colon Rectum 1963; 6: 422.
Travell JG, Simons DG. Myofascial Pain and Dysfunction: The Trigger Point Manual. Williams & Wilkins, Baltimore, MD, 1983.
Weiss JM. Pelvic Floor myofascial trigger points: manual therapy for interstitial cystitis and the urgency-frequency syndrome. J Urol 2001; 166: 2226–2231.

REFERENCES

1. Weidner W, Ludwig M, Brahler E, Schiefer HG. Outcome of antibiotic therapy with ciprofloxacin in chronic bacterial prostatitis. Drugs 1999; 58 (suppl 2): 103–106.
2. True LD, Berger RE, Rothman I, Ross SO, Krieger JN. Prostate histopathology and chronic prostatitis/chronic pelvic pain syndrome: a prospective biopsy study. J Urol 1999; 162: 2014–2018.
3. Kirby RS, Lowe D, Bultitude MI, Shuttleworth KE. Intra-prostatic urinary reflux: an aetiological factor in abacterial prostatitis. Br J Urol. 1982; 54(6): 729–731.
4. Persson BE, Ronquist G, Ekblom M. Ameliorative effect of allopurinol on nonbacterial prostatitis: a parallel double-blind controlled study. J Urol 1996; 155: 961–964.
5. Kaplan SA, Santarosa RP, D'Alisera PM, et al. . Pseudodyssynergia (contraction of the external sphincter during voiding) misdiagnosed as chronic non-bacterial prostatitis and the role of biofeedback as a therapeutic option. J Urol 1997; 157: 2234–2237.
6. Segura JW, Opitz JL, Greene LF. Prostatosis, prostatitis or pelvic floor tension myalgia? J Urol 1979; 122(2): 168–169.
7. Miller HC. Stress prostatitis. Urology 1988; 32: 507–10.
8. Berghuis JP, Heiman JR, Rothman I, Berger RE. Psychological and physical factors involved in chronic idiopathic prostatitis. J Psychosom Res 1996; 41: 313–325.
9. Zermann DH, Ishigooka M, Doggwiler R, Schmidt RA. Chronic prostatitis: a myofascial pain syndrome? Infect Urol 1999; 12: 84–88.
10. Slocumb JC. Neurological factors in chronic pelvic pain: trigger points and the abdominal pelvic pain syndrome. Am J Obstet Gynecol 1984; 149: 536–543.
11. Aaron LA, Herrell R, Ashton S, Belcourt M, Schmaling K, Goldberg J, Buchwald D. Comorbid clinical conditions in chronic fatigue: a co-twin control study. Gen Intern Med 2001; 16: 24–31.
12. Wessely S, Nimnuin C, Sharpe M. Functional somatic syndromes: one or many? Lancet 1999; 354: 936–939.

13 Erectile Dysfunction

Drogo K. Montague, MD
and Milton M. Lakin, MD

CONTENTS

INTRODUCTION

Before the early 1970s, impotence was almost always considered to be the result of psychological causes, and its treatment usually consisted of empiric testosterone administration or referral to a psychiatrist *(1)*. Three sentinel events mark the modern history of impotence treatment. These include the invention of the inflatable penile prosthesis in 1973 *(2)*, the introduction of penile injection therapy in the early 1980s *(3,4)*, and the launch of the first significantly effective systemic agent, sildenafil citrate, in 1998 *(5)*. The first two of these sentinel events established urologists as the primary caregivers for men with impotence; however, since 1998, the availability of effective systemic therapy has shifted the focus for the initial treatment of this disorder away from the urologist and toward the primary care physician (PCP). Indeed, according to Pfizer, Inc, the manufacturers of sildenafil citrate, PCPs write more than 60% of the prescriptions for this medication (data on file; Pfizer, Inc., New York, NY).

At the first National Institutes of Health Consensus Development Panel on Impotence in 1993, it was suggested that the term erectile dysfunction (ED) should replace the term impotence, which was imprecise and carried negative connotations. This consensus panel defined ED as the inability to attain and/or maintain penile erection sufficient for satisfactory sexual performance *(6)*.

Some form of sexual dysfunction affects 10 to 52% of men and 25 to 63% of women *(7,8)*. These disorders have a significant impact on quality of life, and many of them can be effectively treated in the primary care setting. The Massachusetts Male Aging Study

From: *Essential Urology: A Guide to Clinical Practice*
Edited by: J. M. Potts © Humana Press Inc., Totowa, NJ

showed that 52% of men between the ages of 40 and 70 have ED if mild, moderate, and severe degrees of this disorder are considered together. Between the ages of 40 and 70, the prevalence of mild ED remains relatively constant; however, the prevalence of moderate and severe ED increases with each decade with the combined total rising from about 40% at age 40 to almost 70% at age 70 *(7)*. Although the incidence of this disorder increases with age, ED should not be considered an inevitable or natural consequence of aging. One recent study reported that one-third of men over the age of 70 reported no difficulties with erection *(9)*.

There are, however, changes in sexual function that normally occur with aging. For erections to occur, there is an increased need for direct stimulation of the external genitalia. It may take longer to reach orgasm, and there is often a decrease in the force and volume of the ejaculate. Also, there is an increase in the refractory period or the time after orgasm before a man can obtain another erection *(10)*. In all likelihood, the increase in the incidence of ED with age is caused by age-related disorders, such as vascular disease.

Reasons for PCP Involvement in the Management of ED

Why should the PCP be interested in the management of this disorder? In addition to being a problem that is likely to be present in many of the PCP's male patients, ED has a significant impact on the quality of life of these patients and their partners being associated with decreased self-esteem, depression, poor self-image, poor relationships, and increased anxiety *(8)*. Furthermore, ED may be a presenting manifestation of underlying disease; for example, one study showed that 15% of apparently healthy men presenting with ED had abnormal glucose tolerance *(11)*. Risk factors and other underlying diseases associated with ED are shown in Table 1. Routine questioning about men's sexual health may not only uncover problems the PCP can effectively treat; it may also provide valuable clues as to men's health. Furthermore, the involvement of the PCP in the management of this disorder provides another opportunity to encourage the patient to improve lifestyle factors, such as obesity, lack of exercise, poor diet, smoking, and alcohol abuse *(12)*.

Identifying Patients With Sexual Problems

During routine examinations, PCPs should ask whether their patients are sexually active and whether they are having any problems. If the patient indicates a problem is present, the PCP should enquire as to whether the patient is interested in pursuing possible treatment. Because of time constraints, it may be necessary to make another appointment for the evaluation of this newly identified problem. In some cases the appropriate initial management may be referral to a urologist, gynecologist, sex therapist, or psychiatrist. In many cases, however, the PCP is the most appropriate person to do the initial evaluation and begin treatment. In this review we consider male sexual dysfunctions in general, ED in particular, and the role of the PCP in the management of ED.

Male Sexual Dysfunction

Most male sexual dysfunction falls into three areas: decreased libido, orgasm and ejaculatory disorders, and ED. Libido or sexual drive has many determinants. Serum testosterone and possibly prolactin should be measured in men suffering from low libido to see if hypogonadism is present. Other possible causes of low libido include depression

Table 1
Risk Factors and Diseases Associated With Erectile Dysfunction

Alcohol and drug abuse	Medications
Chronic illness (e.g., chronic renal failure)	Neurological disease (e.g., multiple sclerosis)
Coronary artery/vascular disease	Obesity/low levels of physical activity
Depression	Peyronie's disease
Diabetes mellitus	Smoking
Hyperlipidemia	Surgery (prostate, bladder, rectal, vascular)
Hypertension	Thyroid disease (hyper / hypothyroidism)
Hypogonadism / hyperprolactinemia	Trauma (spinal cord, pelvic, perineal)

and relationship problems. In some cases, low libido develops as a consequence of ED; the man eventually loses interest in sexual activity because of repeated failures. Low libido is also often associated with chronic illness and with the use of medications such as antiandrogens and central nervous system depressants. If possible, treatment for low libido should be directed to the underlying cause.

Premature ejaculation is the most common form of male sexual dysfunction, affecting approx 30% of men with a similar prevalence across age groups *(8)*. In some cases, premature ejaculation develops as a response to ED; in these cases, the ED should be treated first. When premature ejaculation exists by itself, treatment may be either pharmacological or behavioral. Traditional treatment for this disorder has been behavioral as suggested by Masters and Johnson *(10)*. Pharmacological treatment for this disorder became possible when it was noted that drug treatment for depression in men sometimes resulted in retarded ejaculation or inability to reach orgasm *(13)*. Off-label use of some antidepressant medications in low doses either on a daily or prn basis has been shown to be effective in the treatment of premature ejaculation *(14–18)*. Topical use of anesthetic creams or ointments has also been suggested as treatment for this disorder *(19)*.

ERECTILE DYSFUNCTION

ED may either be primary, existing since first sexual experience, or secondary (acquired). In terms of etiology, ED traditionally has also been classified as being psychogenic, organic, or mixed organic and psychogenic. As previously stated, it was once believed that almost all ED was caused by psychological factors. Now, it is generally recognized that more than 80% of cases of ED are associated with one or more significant underlying organic disorders *(20)*. In almost all cases of "organic ED," there are also associated psychological factors and thus most ED is of mixed organic and psychogenic etiology. ED as a result of psychogenic factors alone may occur in otherwise healthy men; this is particularly true in younger men.

Sildenafil citrate is effective in ED of diverse etiologies, including psychogenic and various subcategories of organic ED *(21)*. Thus, it is no longer as important to classify ED into psychogenic, organic, and mixed categories as it once was. For almost all men with ED initial treatment will be with an oral agent, and because the PCP in many cases will prescribe this agent, it is appropriate to examine what the PCP should do to evaluate the man with ED and how oral agents should be prescribed.

Table 2
Medications Associated With Erectile Dysfunction[a]

Alcohol	Digoxin
Antiandrogens	H_2-receptor blockers
Antidepressants	Illicit drugs
Antihypertensives	Ketoconazole
Antipsychotics	Lipid-lowering agents
Cytotoxic drugs	

[a]Modified from Maurice *(50)* and Miller *(9)*.

Work-Up of ED

Medical History

ED is often associated with significant underlying organic disorders and may in some cases be the presenting manifestation of one of these disorders. The history should be directed toward uncovering possible evidence of the disorders listed in Table 1. Men often relate the onset of ED to taking a new medication. Many of the medications associated with ED are listed in Table 2. When the onset of ED coincides with a new medication, stopping the medication if possible or substituting another should be considered. Many times, however, the ED will persist despite these measures.

Sexual History

If the PCP elicits a complaint suggesting ED, further questioning should take place. Was the onset of the problem sudden or gradual? How long has the problem been present? Does the man have difficultly achieving an erection, maintaining it, or both? Is the erection curved and if so how long has it been curved? Does the man experience normal erections during the night, on arising in the morning, or with masturbation? In general the sudden onset of ED in the absence of a precipitating event suggests a psychogenic etiology; so does the history of normal erections in some circumstances but not in others. Other questions the PCP should determine include the following: Can the man reach orgasm and does he ejaculate? Does ejaculation occur too soon? Are orgasm/ejaculation painful? How is the man's interest in sex or libido? Other than ED does the man have any relationship difficulties with his partner or partners? Have there been any significant stressors such as job, family, or financial problems?

Physical Examination

The PCP should note the following on the physical exam. Does the man appear either acutely or chronically ill? Does his affect suggest possible depression? Are secondary sex characteristics normal; is gynecomastia present? Peripheral pulses should be examined particularly the femoral pulses and those in the lower extremities. Examination of the external genitalia should note whether any obvious plaques or nodules suggestive of Peyronie's disease are present. The size and consistency of the testes should be noted. During the rectal examination of the prostate the anal sphincter tone should be noted; if it is decreased, the bulbocavernosus reflex may be absent. Decreased anal sphincter tone and decreased sensation in the genital area (saddle sensation), an absent bulbocavernosus reflex, and an abnormal gait are neurological findings sometimes associated with ED and with neurogenic bladder and rectal disorders.

Laboratory Studies

Serum studies should be conducted to assess the man's general state of health and to uncover occult disorders listed in Table 1. These might include a complete blood count, complete metabolic panel, fasting blood sugar or hemoglobin A1C, and a serum testosterone.

Treatment of ED

If ED occurs in the setting of a relationship problem, it is usually best to address the relationship problem before prescribing ED treatment. This may require referral for marital therapy. If ED occurs in a man where depression is also present, it is best to initiate treatment for depression first or to treat both disorders simultaneously because they may be interdependent. As mentioned, changing medication may be appropriate, and finally lifestyle modifications should be recommended when appropriate.

First-Line ED Therapy: The Phosphodiesterase Inhibitors

Penile flaccidity is a state of relatively high sympathetic tone. Smooth muscle in the corpus cavernosum is in a state of contraction, and blood flow into the corpora cavernosa is relatively low with equal venous outflow. Sexual stimulation results in a nonadrenergic, noncholinergic neurally mediated release of nitric oxide. Nitric oxide combines with the enzyme guanylate cyclase in the smooth muscle cell to produce cyclic GMP (cGMP); this in turn results in smooth muscle relaxation making erection possible. cGMP is broken down in a process involving the enzyme phosphodiesterase type 5 (PDE 5). This is performed to prevent the penis from remaining permanently erect *(22)*.

Sildenafil citrate (Viagra) is a potent PDE 5 inhibitor. By inhibiting this enzyme, sildenafil citrate results in larger concentrations of cGMP, improved smooth muscle relaxation, and erections provided that sexual stimulation is present in the first place.

In a multicenter study, sildenafil citrate led to 69% of all attempts of sexual intercourse being successful compared with 22% in men receiving placebo. The mean number of successful attempts at sexual intercourse per month was 5.9 for sildenafil citrate vs 1.5 for placebo. Headache, flushing, nasal congestion, and dyspepsia were side effects seen in 6 to 18% *(5)*. In higher doses (100 mg and above) transient visual (brightness and color) changes were observed in some patients *(23)*.

Sildenafil citrate results in a mild reduction in systolic blood pressure, as do organic nitrates. When given together, there may be a significant synergistic blood pressure lowering, and thus use of sildenafil citrate is contraindicated in any man taking organic nitrates in any form (Sildenafil package insert; Pfizer, Inc., New York, NY, 1999). Current package labeling suggests using caution when prescribing sildenafil citrate to patients who have had myocardial infarction, stroke, or life-threatening arrhythmia within the last 6 mo. Caution is also advised when prescribing sildenafil citrate to men with blood pressure less than 90/50 mmHg or greater than 170/110 mmHg, men with cardiac failure or unstable angina, and men with retinitis pigmentosa *(24)*. The safety of sildenafil citrate in men with stable coronary artery disease has been repeatedly demonstrated *(25,26)*.

Sildenafil citrate has three dosage forms (tablets): 25 mg, 50 mg, and 100 mg. For most men, the initial appropriate dose is 50 mg; if this is not effective, the dose may be increased to 100 mg. Men should be instructed to take the medication in anticipation of sexual activity. If the stomach is empty, the onset of action may be as early as 30 min.

If it is taken after a fatty meal, absorption is delayed and may take an hour or more. The half-life of the drug is 4 h, and thus there is a window of opportunity after drug ingestion from 30 min to 8 to 12 h (two to three half lives). Men should be cautioned not to take this medication more than once in 24 h. The 25-mg dose should be considered as the initial dose in the elderly or in men taking drugs metabolized by the same liver enzyme as sildenafil citrate (cytochrome P450 isoform 3A4). These drugs included cimetidine, ketoconazole, erythromycin, and protease inhibitors such as ritonavir.

Men should understand that taking sildenafil citrate by itself does nothing to promote or enhance libido, orgasm, or ejaculation. Indeed, an erection ordinarily will not occur unless the man receives sexual stimulation. Anxiety may prevent this medication from working in men who would otherwise respond to it. Many men are assumed to be nonresponders to this medication when in reality they have not had an adequate clinical trial. It has been shown that it may take as many as eight attempts before this medication demonstrates its effectiveness *(27)*. Usually doses higher than 100 mg result in a higher incidence of side effects without a corresponding increase in efficacy.

Sildenafil citrate has shown efficacy across a wide spectrum of erectile dysfunction etiologies. Because sexual stimulation is necessary for this drug to be effective, its effectiveness is less after non-nerve-sparing prostatectomy *(28)* and in diabetes mellitus *(29)*. In general, however, there is no absolute predictor of response to sildenafil citrate; consequently, a treatment trial should be considered in most men with ED unless there is a contraindication.

Future Systemic Agents to Treat ED

A new PDE 5 inhibitor, Vardenafil (Bayer Corporation), has just received Food and Drug Administration (FDA) approval, and another PDE 5 inhibitor, tadalafil (Lilly-ICOS), is awaiting FDA approval. A centrally acting agent, sublingual apomorphine, is available in Europe, but its application for FDA approval was withdrawn and its future availability in the United States at this time is uncertain. Other systemic agents with different mechanisms of action are under development; once they are available, combination therapy with more than one agent may possibly be effective in some men with ED who are nonresponsive to a single agent.

Second-Line Treatment Options for ED

If first-line systemic therapy fails or is contraindicated, second-line treatment options should be considered. These include the use of a vacuum constriction device, penile injection therapy, and intraurethral medication. Although some PCPs may choose to administer second-line treatments in their practices, most will refer men who fail systemic therapy to a urologist who specializes in ED treatment.

Vacuum. These devices have existed for about 75 yr and have been an accepted option in the treatment of ED since the early 1980s. A vacuum erection device consists of a vacuum chamber, a pump to create a vacuum, and one or more constriction bands or rings (Fig. 1). The patient uses a water-soluble lubricant to lubricate his penis and the open end of the chamber. He then places the chamber over his flaccid penis and activates the manual or battery-operated pump. The vacuum draws blood into the penis, producing an erection-like state. The constriction band or ring is then displaced onto the base of the penis to maintain the erection, and the chamber is removed. The man has coitus with ring in place; the ring should not be left on for more than 30 min.

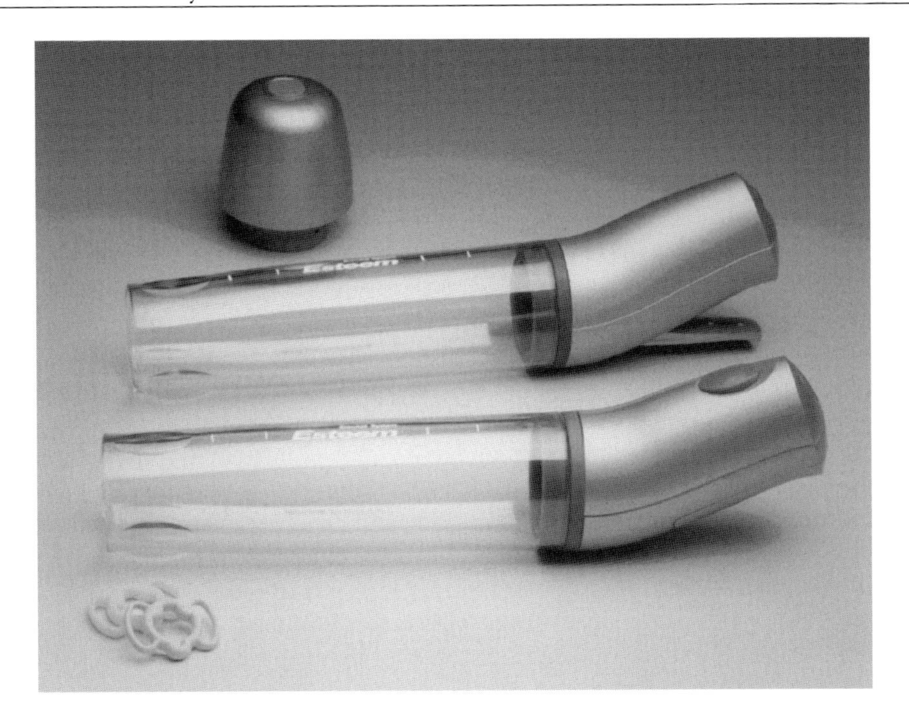

Fig. 1. Osbon ErecAid® Esteem™ vacuum system. Courtesy of Timm Medical Technologies, Inc., Eden Prairie, MN.

The erection produced by these devices has a larger circumference than normal but is pivoted at the base. The skin temperature is approx 1°C lower than normal *(30)*. Bruising and petechiae may occur, and the ejaculate may or may not be trapped by the constriction ring. Pain may also occur on creation of the vacuum or use of the constriction band *(31)*. Despite these negative issues, an erection-like state sufficient for coitus is created in more than 90% of uses. Patient and partner acceptance of the use of these devices to treat ED is not high; Jarow showed that when 377 men were presented a variety of treatment options for ED, only 12% chose a vacuum erection device *(32)*. There are few contraindications to the use of these devices; men taking anticoagulants may use these devices with care *(33)*. Serious complications are rare; they include Peyronie's disease *(34,35)*, skin necrosis *(34,36)*, and Fournier's gangrene (seen in a man using a constriction ring; ref. *37*).

Penile Injection Therapy. Penile injection therapy to treat ED was introduced in the early 1980s *(3,4)*. The patient uses a small needle (27 to 30 gauge) to inject a vasoactive drug or drug mixture into one of his corpora cavernosa. Because the septum between the two corporeal bodies is incomplete, a substance injected into one corpus cavernosum reaches both erectile bodies. There are two FDA-approved drugs for penile injection therapy: alprostadil (Caverject, Pharmacia & Upjohn) and alprostadil as an alfadex complex (Edex, Schwarz Pharma). Both are forms of prostaglandin E1. Papaverine hydrochloride and phentolamine mesylate have also been used off label for penile injection therapy. These drugs may be used in combination; and when prostaglandin E1, papaverine, and phentolamine are injected together, the therapy is commonly known as "trimix."

In 1996, the Alprostadil Study Group reported that 87% of injections in 683 men produced erections suitable for coitus *(38)*. In a study using trimix in 116 patients, a success rate of 92% was reported *(39)*. Complications of penile injection therapy include prolonged erections, pain, and penile fibrosis. The goal with penile injection therapy is to find a drug or drug mixture and a dose that produces an erection lasting about 1 h. Prolonged erections left untreated may result in ischemic damage to cavernosal smooth muscle and a significant worsening of the ED. If an erection does not subside within 3 h, pharmacological reversal with injection of a sympathomimetic drug, such as phenylephrine, is required. Penile pain, not from the injection *per se* but after the injection, is most likely to occur with prostaglandin E1 monotherapy. Penile fibrosis may require cessation of penile injection therapy *(40,41)*. Despite the high success rates with penile injection therapy, patient dropout rates are often 50% or greater *(42)*.

Intraurethral Medication. Some men have a fear of needles or reluctance to inject medication into their penises. Intraurethral medication for ED was developed to deliver vasoactive medication to the erectile bodies through vascular communications between the corpus spongiosum and the adjoining corpora cavernosa *(43)*. A small pellet of medication is inserted via a disposable applicator into the distal urethra. At the present time, there is one FDA-approved intraurethral medication to treat ED: intraurethral alprostadil (MUSE, Vivus). In general, this form of therapy has a lesser success rate than penile injection therapy *(44–46)*; however, it offers for some men an alternative to penile injection therapy. Penile pain is present in 24% of patients *(46)*. This form of ED treatment is contraindicated when pregnancy is desired or during pregnancy unless a condom is used.

Third-Line Therapy: Penile Prosthesis Implantation

When systemic therapy fails and when second-line therapies either fail or are rejected, third-line therapy in the form of penile prosthesis implantation should be considered. Penile prostheses are broadly classified as being either semirigid or inflatable. The goal of penile prosthesis implantation should be to provide penile flaccidity and erection that come as close as possible that which occurs through natural mechanisms. Today's three-piece inflatable penile prostheses with length and girth expanding cylinders, a small scrotal pump, and a large volume abdominal fluid reservoir (Fig. 2) come closest to meeting this ideal *(47)*.

Penile prosthesis implantation is usually performed under spinal or general anesthesia. Immediate complications include infection and erosion; either complication usually requires removal of the device. Initial success rates for penile prosthesis implantation are on the order of 95%. The principal long-term complication of penile prosthesis implantation is mechanical failure of the device. Today's three-piece inflatable penile prostheses have 5-yr actuarial survival rates free of mechanical failure of 93 to 94% *(48,49)*.

SUMMARY

ED is a common problem in the male patients of PCPs, affecting 52% of those between the ages of 40 and 70. ED may be a presenting manifestation of significant underlying organic disease. Furthermore, its presence gives the PCP another reason for recommending improved lifestyles for their male patients. For most men with ED, the most appropriate first-line therapy is with the systemic phosphodiesterase inhibitor, sildenafil citrate.

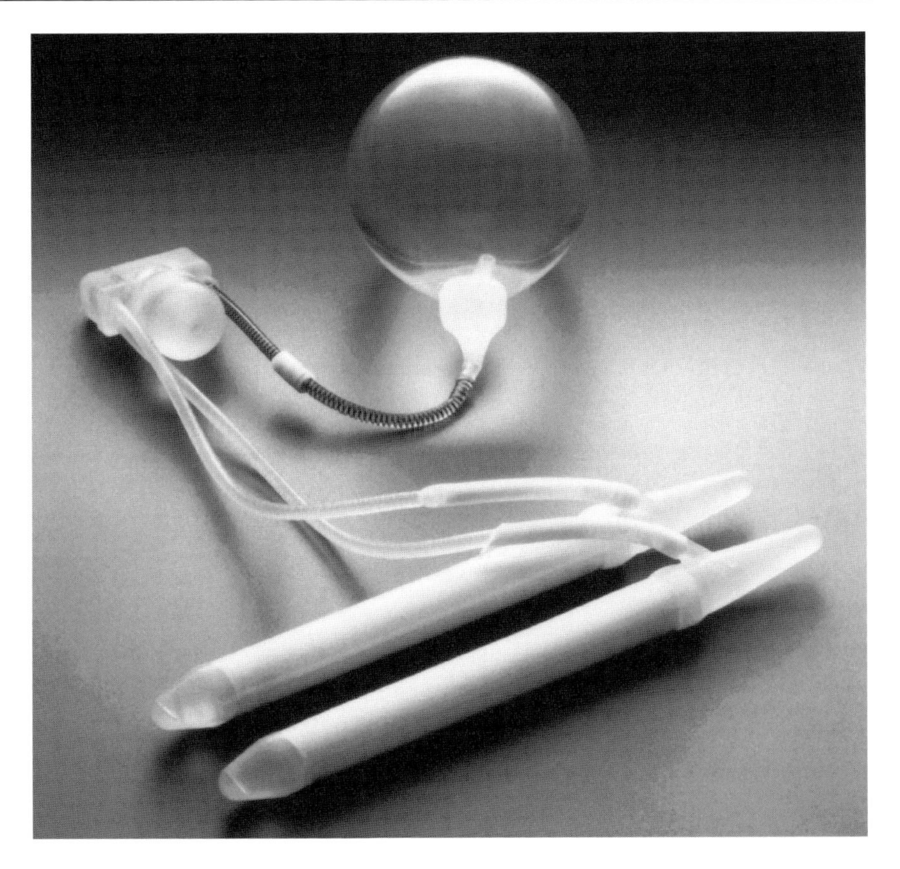

Fig. 2. AMS 700 Ultrex Plus™ Penile Prosthesis. Courtesy of American Medical Systems, Inc. Minnetonka, MN.

When men fail to respond to this first-line treatment, referral to a urologist should be considered for possible second-line therapies (vacuum constriction devices, penile injection therapy, or intraurethral medication). If second-line therapies are either ineffective or unacceptable, men with ED may benefit from penile prosthesis implantation.

REFERENCES

1. Smith DR, ed. General Urology. 5th Ed. Lange Medical Publications, Los Altos, CA, 1966
2. Scott FB, Bradley WE, Timm GW. Management of erectile impotence: use of implantable inflatable prosthesis. Urology 1973; 2: 80–82.
3. Virag R. Intracavernous injection of papaverine for erectile failure. Letter to the editor. Lancet 1982; 2: 938.
4. Brindley GS. Cavernosal alpha-blockade: a new technique for investigating and treating erectile impotence. Br J Psychiatry 1983; 143: 332.
5. Goldstein I, Lue TF, Padma-Nathan H, et al: Oral sildenafil in the treatment of erectile dysfunction. Sildenafil Study Group (*see* comments) [published erratum appears in N Engl J Med 1998; 339: 59]. N Engl J Med 1998; 338:1397–1404.
6. NIH Consensus panel on impotence: impotence. JAMA 1993; 270: 83–90.
7. Feldman HA, Goldstein I, Hatzichristou DG, et al. Impotence and its medical and psychosocial correlates: results of the Massachusetts Male Aging Study. J Urol 1994; 151: 54–61.

8. Laumann EO, Paik A, Rosen RC. Sexual dysfunction in the United States: prevalence and predictors. JAMA 1999; 281: 537–544.
9. Miller TA. Diagnostic evaluation of erectile dysfunction. Am Family Phys 2000; 61: 95–104.
10. Masters WH, Johnson VE. Human Sexual Inadequacy. Little, Brown and Company, Boston, MA, 1970.
11. Dewire DM. Evaluation and treatment of erectile dysfunction. Am Family Phys 1996; 53: 2101–2108.
12. Sadovsky R. Integrating erectile dysfunction treatment into primary care practice. Am J Med 2000; 109(suppl 9A): 22S-28S.
13. Waldinger MD, Berendsen HH, Blok BF, et al. Premature ejaculation and serotonergic antidepressants-induced delayed ejaculation: the involvement of the serotonergic system. Behav Brain Res 1998; 92: 111–118.
14. Kara H, Aydin S, Yucel M, et al. The efficacy of fluoxetine in the treatment of premature ejaculation: a double-blind placebo controlled study (*see* comments). J Urol 1996; 156: 1631–1632.
15. Kim SC, Seo KK. Efficacy and safety of fluoxetine, sertraline and clomipramine in patients with premature ejaculation: a double-blind, placebo controlled study. J Urol 1998; 159: 425–427.
16. Seagraves RT, Seagraves K, Maguire E. Clomipramine versus placebo in the treatment of premature ejaculation: a pilot study. J Sex Marital Ther 1993; 19: 198–200.
17. McMahon CG, Touma K. Treatment of premature ejaculation with paroxetine hydrochloride as needed: 2 single-blind placebo controlled crossover studies. J Urol 1999; 161: 1826–1830.
18. Waldinger MD, Hengeveld MW, Zwinderman AH, et al. Effect of SSRI antidepressants on ejaculation: a double-blind, randomized, placebo-controlled study with fluoxetine, fluvoxamine, paroxetine, and sertraline. J Clin Psychopharmacol 1998; 18: 274–281.
19. Choi HK, Jung GW, Moon KH, et al. Clinical study of SS-cream in patients with lifelong premature ejaculation. Urology 2000; 55: 257–261.
20. Benet AE, Melman A. The epidemiology of erectile dysfunction. Urol Clin North Am 1995; 22: 699–709.
21. Jarow JP, Burnett AL, Geringer AM. Clinical efficacy of sildenafil citrate based on etiology and response to prior treatment (*see* comments). J Urol 1999; 162: 722–725.
22. Wallis RM, Corbin JD, Francis SH, et al. Tissue distribution of phosphodiesterase families and the effects of sildenafil on tissue cyclin nucleotides, platelet function, and the contractile responses of trabeculae carnae and aortic rings in vitro. Am J Cardiol 1999; 83: 3C–12C.
23. Morales A, Gingell C, Collins M, et al. Clinical safety of oral sildenafil citrate (VIAGRA) in the treatment of erectile dysfunction. Int J Impot Res 1998;10: 69–73; discussion 73–64.
24. Mittleman MA, Glasser DB, Orazem, J, et al. Incidence of myocardial infarctin and death in 53 clinical trials of Viagra (sildenafil citrate). J Am Coll Cardiol 2000; 35 (A suppl): 302.
25. Conti CR, Pepine CJ, Sweeney M. Efficacy and safety of sildenafil citrate in the treatment of erectile dysfunction in patients with ischemic heart disease. Am J Cardiol 1999; 83: 29C–34C.
26. Herrmann HC, Chang G, Klugherz BD, et al. Hemodynamic effects of sildenafil in men with severe coronary artery disease. N Engl J Med 2000; 342: 1622–1626.
27. Levine LA. Diagnosis and treatment of erectile dysfunction. Am J Med 2000; 109 (9A suppl): 3S–12S.
28. Zippe CD, Jhaveri FM, Klein EA, et al. Role of Viagra after radical prostatectomy. Urology 2000; 55: 241–245.
29. Price DE, Gingell JC, Gepi-Attee S, et al. Sildenafil: study of a novel oral treatment for erectile dysfunction in diabetic men. Diabetic Med 1998; 15: 821–825.
30. Nadig PW, Ware JC, Blumoff R. Noninvasive device to produce and maintain an erection-like state. Urology 1986; 27: 126–131.
31. Levine LA, Dimitriou RJ. Vacuum constriction and external erection devices in erectile dysfunction. Urol Clin North Am 2001; 28: 335–341.
32. Jarow JP, Nana-Sinkam P, Sabbagh M, et al. Outcome analysis of goal directed therapy for impotence. J Urol 1996; 155: 1609–1612.
33. Limoge JP, Olins E, Henderson D, et al. Minimally invasive therapies in the treatment of erectile dysfunction in anticoagulated cases: a study of satisfaction and safety. J Urol 1996; 155: 1276–1279.

34. Ganem JP, Lucey DT, Janosko EO, et al. Unusual complications of the vacuum erection device. Urology 1998; 51: 627–631.
35. Kim JH, Carson CCD: Development of Peyronie's disease with the use of a vacuum constriction device. J Urol 1993; 149: 1314–1315.
36. Meinhardt W, Kropman RF, Lycklama AA B, et al. Skin necrosis caused by use of negative pressure device for erectile impotence. J Urol 1990; 144: 983.
37. Theiss M, Hofmockel G, Frohmuller HG. Fournier's gangrene in a patient with erectile dysfunction following use of a mechanical erection aid device (*see* comments). J Urol 1995; 153: 1921–1922.
38. Linet OI, Orginc FG, Group AS. Efficacy and safety of intracavernosal alprostadil in men with erectile dysfunction. N Engl J Med 1996; 334: 873–877.
39. Bennett AH, Carpenter AJ, Barada JH. An improved vasoactive drug combination for a pharmacological erection program. J Urol 1991; 146: 1564–1565.
40. Lakin MM, Montague DK, Mendendorp SV, et al. Intracavernous injection therapy: analysis of results and complications. J Urol 1990; 143: 1138–1141.
41. Chen RN, Lakin MM, Montague DK, et al. Penile scarring with intracavernous injection therapy using prostaglandin E1: A risk factor analysis. J Urol 1996; 155: 138–140.
42. Casabe A, Bechara A, Cheliz, G. et al. Drop-out reasons and complications in self-injection therapy with a triple vasoactive drug mixture in sexual erectile dysfunction. Int J Impot Res 1998; 10: 5–9.
43. Vardi Y, Saenz de Tejada I. Functional and radiologic evidence of vascular communication between the spongiosal and cavernosal compartments of the penis. Urology 1997; 49: 749–752.
44. Fulgham PF, Cochran JS, Denman JL, et al. Disappointing initial results with transurethral alprostadil for erectile dysfunction in a urology practice setting (*see* comments). J Urol 1998; 160: 2041–2046.
45. Shabsigh R, Padma-Nathan H, Gittleman M, et al. Intracavernous alprostadil alfadex is more efficacious, better tolerated, and preferred over intraurethral alprostadil plus optional actis: a comparative, randomized, crossover, multicenter study. Urology 2000; 55: 109–113.
46. Werthman P, Rajfer J. MUSE therapy: preliminary clinical observations. Urology 1997; 50: 809–811.
47. Montague DK, Lakin MM. Early experience with the controlled girth and length expanding cylinder of the AMS Ultrex penile prosthesis. J Urol 1992; 148: 1444–1446.
48. Milbank AJ, Montague DK, Angermeier KW, et al. Mechanical failure with the AMS Ultrex IPP: Pre- and Post-1993 structural modification. Presented at the Meeting of the Sexual Medicine Society of North America, Charleston, SC, December 7–9, 2001.
49. Wilson SK, Cleves MA, Delk JR 2nd. Comparison of mechanical reliability of original and enhanced Mentor Alpha I penile prosthesis. J Urol 1999; 162: 715–718.
50. Maurice WL. Sexual Medicine in Primary Care. Mosby, St. Louis, MO, 1999.

14 Complementary Medications in Urology

Elliot Fagelman, MD, *Bridgit Mennite,*
and Franklin C. Lowe, MD, MPH

CONTENTS

COMPLEMENTARY THERAPY AND PROSTATE CANCER

Prostate cancer is the most common malignancy in men and the second leading cause of cancer related deaths among American males. In general, curative treatments, including radical prostatectomy, brachytherapy, and external beam radiation, are used in those with localized disease and a life expectancy of 10 or more years. Androgen deprivation has been and still is the first-line therapy in those with metastatic disease. However, in those with metastatic disease, the duration of response is limited, and the cancer eventually becomes hormone refractory. In those with hormone-refractory

From: *Essential Urology: A Guide to Clinical Practice*
Edited by: J. M. Potts © Humana Press Inc., Totowa, NJ

prostate cancer, chemotherapy and secondary hormonal manipulation are systemic treatments used. Currently, complimentary medications have been used and are undergoing evaluation in the prevention and treatment of prostate cancer.

SELENIUM

The beneficial role of selenium in reducing the incidence or risk of death from prostate cancer has been suggested by several studies. In the United States, lower age-specific death rates for some cancers have been seen in those states with higher selenium levels. In a double-blind placebo-controlled study, yeast containing 200 μg of selenium or placebo was given to individuals with a history of nonmelanoma skin cancer and no affect on skin cancer recurrence was found. However, individuals receiving selenium had a decreased incidence of prostate cancer, lung cancer, and colorectal cancer. One potential draw back of the study was that it was not designed to detect a change in prostate cancer incidence. The Health Professionals study evaluated the association between the risk of prostate cancer and the prediagnostic level of selenium in toenails (marker for long-term selenium consumption). There was reduced risk of advanced prostate cancer in those with higher selenium levels.

At this time, trials are underway to gain a better understanding of the role of selenium in prostate cancer. The Selenium Vitamin E Comparison Trial (SELECT) is a multicenter randomized double-blind study assessing the role of vitamin E (400 mg) and selenium (200 μg) in preventing prostate cancer. Until the results of further studies are obtained, specific recommendations regarding utility of selenium are difficult to make.

VITAMIN E

Vitamin E refers to a family of compounds (tocopherols and tocotrienals). α-Tocopherol is the most abundant natural form of vitamin E and has the highest bioactivity. Vitamin E normally consumed as a nutritional supplement or with foods. Good sources of vitamin E include plant-derived oils, avocados, nuts, eggs, peanut butter, soybeans, and whole-grain breakfast cereals. Vitamin E appears to be a safe compound. Dosages from 100 to 800 IU/d have been used. One potential drug interaction is with warfarin. Large vitamin E doses increase the vitamin K requirement of the body. α-Tocopherols can decrease platelet aggregation. Owing to the potential of bleeding complications, vitamin E should be stopped before prostate biopsy or radical prostatectomy. In one clinical trial, the α-tocopherol β-carotene (ATBC) trial, there was a slightly higher but not statistically significant incidence of hemorrhagic stroke seen in those randomized to Vitamin E.

Numerous mechanisms have been proposed as being beneficial in preventing cancer. These include antioxidant effects, antiprostaglandin, cell cycle inhibition, proapoptotic, cellular signaling, anticarcinogen, antiproliferative, and hormonal effects.

Observational trials have suggested a beneficial role in vitamin E supplementation and the development of prostate cancer. In a case-control study, a protective trend was observed in those who used vitamin E with a 24% reduction in prostate cancer risk. In a prospective cohort study, vitamin E levels were measured and at 17-yr follow-up, low vitamin E levels were significantly associated with prostate cancer death among smokers. The beneficial effect of vitamin E in smokers was seen in another large cohort study. Smokers who used supplemental vitamin E experienced a 56% reduction in fatal or metastatic prostate cancer.

The ATBC trial was a randomized double-blind clinical trial in which male smokers received vitamin E, β-carotene, both, or none. The study was designed to determine whether lung cancer could be prevented, not prostate cancer. After 5 yr, a 33% decrease in prostate cancer was seen, and at 7 yr, a 41% reduction in prostate cancer deaths was reported.

These results must be interpreted with caution because the ATBC trial was not designed to evaluate prostate cancer. In addition, the beneficial results in smokers may be to the result of an interaction of smoking and vitamin E, not vitamin E alone.

Further studies being conducted should provide further information. A phase III multicenter trial in Canada is evaluating the effect of vitamin E (800 IU/d) in those with high-grade prostatic intraepithelial neoplasia. High-grade prostatic intraepithelial neoplasia is associated with a high rate of prostate cancer on repeat biopsy. The end point of the study is the development of invasive prostate cancer. A second study is the SELECT trial, in which vitamin E and selenium are being evaluated in preventing prostate cancer.

TOMATO PRODUCTS AND LYCOPENE

Epidemiological studies have suggested that the consumption of tomato products may decrease the risk of prostate cancer. Lycopene is the major carotenoid in tomato products and has been suggested to be of benefit with regard to prostate cancer. Lycopenes have been shown to cause in vitro inhibition of prostate cancer cell growth. No specific recommendations can be made at this time with regard to how much lycopene or the quantity of tomato products should be consumed to help prevent prostate cancer. Further studies are needed to define their role in protecting against prostate cancer. Miller et al.'s *(1)* recently published review on the subject is recommended for more comprehensive review.

PC-SPES

PC-SPES (Botaniclab, Brea, CA) is a combination of eight herbal compounds that is no longer commercially available because of product impurities. PC-SPES has been used to treat prostate cancer in China and has been used in the United States as well. The mechanism of action is not exactly known, however, there is likely estrogenic activity. PC-SPES has been studied in vitro and in animal models and has shown the ability to inhibit the growth of both androgen sensitive and androgen independent cell lines. PC-SPES has been used by patients with prostate cancer on the advice of friends or prostate cancer support groups without physician involvement.

PC-SPES has been evaluated in patients with androgen-dependent prostate cancer. In patients with androgen-dependent prostate cancer, prostate-specific antigen (PSA) response (>50% decline in PSA after treatment) rates range from 45 to 100 %. Small et al. *(2)* evaluated 33 patients with androgen-dependent prostate cancer who used nine PC-SPES capsules per day. Of the patients, 32 were evaluable and all had a 80% or greater decline in PSA, with the median duration of decline over 57 wk; 97% had castrate levels of testosterone while being treated. Also of importance, two patients with a positive bone scan showed improvement as well as one patient with a bladder mass on computed tomography scan.

PC-SPES has shown activity in hormone-refractory prostate cancer (HRPCA). PSA response rates have ranged from 52 to 81%. Responses were seen in patients who had undergone secondary hormonal treatment and chemotherapy. The median time to progression in the study by Small et al. was 16 wk. The study by Oh et al. *(3)* showed that the median duration of PSA response was 2.5 mo.

Although an herbal therapy, there are significant toxicities associated with the use of PC-SPES. The most common side effects include breast tenderness, impotence, loss of libido, and thrombosis. Thrombotic events have been seen in 4 to 6% of patients. These include deep vein thrombosis, pulmonary embolism, and precipitation of angina.

PC-SPES is an expensive therapy, costing more than $300 for a 1-mo supply. In general, insurance companies do not cover this therapy.

In summary, PC-SPES is an herbal therapy with activity against androgen sensitive and HRPCA. It is important for physicians to ask patients with prostate cancer it they are taking this herbal medication because it can influence the interpretation of results of treatment. In addition, patients taking PC-SPES should be warned about the risk of life-threatening thrombotic events.

VITAMIN D

The active form of vitamin D is calcitriol. Epidemiological evidence suggests that calcitriol may decrease the risk of prostate cancer and/or prostate cancer death. Age, African-American race, and residence in northern regions are risk factors for prostate cancer and are associated with low vitamin D levels. Prostate cancer mortality is higher in northern counties of the United States. In one case-control study by Corder et al. *(4)* using stored sera, men who developed prostate cancer were found to have lower vitamin D levels than controls. In men older than 57, lower vitamin D levels were associated with poorly differentiated and palpable prostate cancer. An association was not seen in those with low-grade nonpalpable tumors. It is important to note that not all studies have shown an associated of vitamin D levels and prostate cancer.

In vitro calcitriol has been shown to control the proliferation of hormone-responsive cancer cell lines. There have been reports that calcitriol may work in synergy with chemotherapeutic agents (cisplatin and carboplatin) to inhibit the growth of androgen-dependent and -independent prostate cancer cell lines. In vivo, growth of human tumors grafted into mice have been inhibited by calcitriol. The exact mechanism of action is not known; however, it may involve cell-cycle arrest.

There have been a limited number of clinical studies evaluating the effects of calcitriol on prostate cancer. Dosages in the range of 1.5 μg/d to 2.5 μg have been used. In a small phase II study in patients with HRPCA, there were no objective responses, and no patient showed a PSA decline of 50% or more. In patients with increasing PSA levels after radical prostatectomy or radiation with no evidence of metastatic disease, calcitriol increased the doubling time of the PSA rise. Side effects seen with calcitriol treatment include hypercalcemia and hypercalciuria. Administering steroids may be beneficial in limiting the toxicity of calcitriol.

In summary, calcitriol may be beneficial in preventing and treating prostate cancer. Further studies need to be completed before reaching any definitive conclusion regarding the utility of calcitriol in preventing and treatment of prostate cancer.

SOY PHYTOESTROGENS

Interest in soy comes from epidemiological evidence that there is a lower incidence of prostate cancer in populations with a diet high in soy products. Japanese and Chinese men have a lower incidence of prostate cancer than Americans. When Asian men move to the United States, their incidence of prostate cancer rises. Soy products are a more abundant in the Asian diet when compared with the average American diet. Phytoestrogens are plant compounds with weak estrogenic activity. Lignans, flavonoids, and isoflavanoids are three major classes of phyoestrogens. Soy products contain isoflavanoids. Genestein and daidzein are isoflavanoids and have been evaluated for their utility in preventing and treating prostate cancer. Of these two compounds, genistein has been more extensively studied.

Several mechanisms of action have been proposed. An estrogenic effect on prostate cancer cells has been proposed; however, there may be other mechanisms at work. In vitro studies have evaluated the effect of genestein on signal transduction pathways. Genestein may inhibit prostate cancer by inhibiting epidermal growth factor stimulated growth. Augmentation of transforming growth factor I, through synthesis or secretion, may also inhibit cellular growth. In vitro studies have also demonstrated inhibition of angiogenesis. Prostate cancer and benign prostatic hyperplasia (BPH) tissue obtained from transurethral resection of the prostate and radical prostatectomy has been studied in histoculture. Genestein demonstrated an inhibitory effect on both BPH and prostate cancer tissue.

In summary, epidemiological and in vitro studies suggest a beneficial effect of dietary soy. However, there is a lack of clinical data to support the routine use of soy products in the prevention or treatment of prostate cancer.

GREEN TEA

Green tea is comes from the dried unfermented plant leaves of Camellia sinensis. Green tea contains many compounds, including flavonols or catechins. Epigallocatechin-3-gallate is a major component of green tea. Interest in green tea in the development of prostate cancer comes from epidemiological studies. Similar to soy, green tea is a regular part of the diet seen in Japanese and Chinese populations, where there is a low incidence of prostate cancer. Japanese and Chinese men who move to the Untied States show an increase in prostate cancer.

Mechanism of action of action, evaluated in vitro, include effects of the androgen receptor, androgen responsive genes, the regulatory enzyme ornithine decarboxylase, and apoptosis.

The potential role of treatment of prostate cancer has been evaluated in vivo in mice. One study demonstrated a reduction in the size of human prostate cancer xenografts implanted in mice using intraperitoneal injections of epigallocatechin-3-gallate.

In summary, in vitro and in vivo animal studies suggest a possible beneficial role of green tea with regard to prostate cancer. However, clinical studies are needed before recommendations, in the prevention and treatment of prostate cancer, can be made.

HERBAL MEDICATIONS IN THE TREATMENT OF BPH

Phytotherapeutic agents are very popular in the treatment of BPH. They are popular in Europe in the treatment of lower urinary tract symptoms (LUTS) associated with BPH. In the United States, these agents are readily obtained through health food stores, vitamin shops, and the Internet. More than 30% of patients seeing urologists for BPH/LUTS may be taking these medications. It is important to note that the amounts of extracts are variable because of differences in extraction procedures and the natural variability of plants. Because of this variability, a product comparison is not possible. The following is a summary of the more popular plant extracts used in the treatment of BPH/LUTS. This subject has been extensively reviewed in recent years.

Serenoa repens
(Saw Palmetto Berry Extract)

Saw palmetto berry (SPB) extract is the most popular phytotherapeutic agent used to treat BPH/LUTS. Mechanisms proposed include antiandrogenic effects, inhibition of 5-α-reductase, inhibition of growth factors, an anti-inflammatory effect, an antiestrogenic effect, and an antiedema effect. In vitro studies used to evaluate these effects often used supraphysiological doses; thus, the significance of the findings is not known.

Marks et al. *(5)* evaluated the clinical and tissue effects of SBP in men with symptomatic BPH. Forty-four patients were randomized to treatment with 106 mg of SPB lipoidal extract and other herbs three times a day for 6 mo or placebo. There were no significant differences in any of the clinical parameters evaluated. Histological evaluation of prostate tissue revealed an increase in the percentage of atrophic glands in those treated with SPB.

SPB (Permixon) was compared with finasteride in a 6-mo, randomized, double-blind, study of 1098 patients. Symptom scores were improved to an equal extent in both groups (37% with Permixon vs 39% with finasteride). Peak flow improved in both groups to a similar extent. In those taking Permixon, there was less sexual dysfunction. Conclusions regarding the efficacy of Permixon cannot be made from this study as there was no placebo group. The improvement may have been secondary to the placebo effect.

Braeckman et al. *(6)* performed a double-blind, placebo-controlled study on the efficacy of an extract of *Serenoa repens* (prostserene 160 mg twice a day) vs placebo (twice a day) over 3 mo. Two-hundred five patients were compared (99 placebo group and 106 in the treatment group). There were statistically significant improvements in the patients' symptoms and quality of life. Compared with baseline, there was a decrease in prostate volume in the treated group. Side effects were seen in 8.3% of patients in the placebo group and 9.1% in the treatment group. Side effects reported in the treatment group included gastrointestinal changes, sexual dysfunction, allergic reaction, headache, increase in blood pressure, important fatigue, insomnia, and fixation on the urinary problems.

A beta analysis of placebo-controlled studies for Permixon brand SPB demonstrated an improvement in symptoms and an increase in peak flow rate. Nocturia was the only symptom evaluated in all studies. There was an increase in peak flow by 1.5 mL/s and a decrease in nocturia by 0.5 times per night. The clinical significance of these improvements is limited.

In summary, the current evidence suggests a possible benefit of SPB in the treatment of LUTS caused by BPH. However, the effect, if any appears to be small.

Pygeum africanum
(African Plum)

Pygeum africanum is used commonly in France under the trade name Tadenan. The extract comes from the bark of the African plum tree. In the United States, it is frequently sold over the counter in health food stores in combination with other agents, including SPB. The exact mechanism of action is not known. In vitro studies have demonstrated several effects, including inhibition of fibroblast growth factors, antiestrogenic effects, and the inhibition of chemotactic leukotrienes and other 5-lipooxygnease metabolites. In addition, there may be a beneficial effect on the bladder.

There has been a limited amount of clinical data regarding the use of Tadenan. A 2-mo open-label trial using 100 mg of Tadenan daily demonstrated a 40% decrease in symptom scores and improvement in mean peak urinary flow rates. No side effects were reported. This was an uncontrolled study so no conclusions can be drawn. The frequency of dosing has been evaluated a once daily dose of 100 mg was compared with 50 mg twice day. There was similar efficacy and safety between the two regimens. In summary, the lack of clinical data limits any specific recommendations regarding the use of Tadenan.

Hypoxis rooperi
(South African Star Grass)

The extract from the South African star grass contains mainly β-sitosterol with lesser amounts of other sterols. The major active component is thought to be β-sitosterol. The extract of β-sitosterol has been marketed as Harzol and Azuprostat. Both of these agents have been studied in clinical trials.

Harzol has been studied in a double-blind placebo-controlled trial. There were improvements in symptom score, flow rates, and residual urine volume in the group treated with Harzol when compared with the placebo group. During an 18-mo follow-up study, the 38 patients who continued Harzol maintained their improvement.

Azuprostat has been evaluated in a randomized, double blind, placebo-controlled clinical trial as well. Improvements were seen in symptom scores, flow rates, and residual urine. In summary, studies of β-sitosterol products have promising results. If duplicated, these products may have a role in the medical management of BPH/LUTS.

Other Phytotherapeutic Agents

Urtica docita (stinging needle), *Secale cerale* (rye pollen), and combinations of phytotherapeutic agents are used as well. There are limited data on these agents and combinations of agents.

CLINICAL MANAGEMENT OF PHYTOTHERAPEUTIC AGENTS AND BPH

There is no standard of care for the management of patients taking phytotherapeutic agents for LUTS/BPH. If a patient presents while taking these medications, they are usually symptomatic, otherwise they would not be seeking care. At presentation, the patient should be informed that the efficacy, safety, and side effects are not known. If a patient refuses traditional medical therapy, such as α-blockers and 5-α-reductase inhibitors, phytotherapeutic agents are a reasonable alternative as long as the patient understands the limitations and unknown risks of taking these agents.

Treatment of BPH/LUTS is usually directed at decreasing a patient's symptoms. In patients whose symptoms do not improve with these agents or in whom the symptoms are severe, traditional medical therapy should be undertaken. In patients with complications secondary to BPH, such as urinary retention, bladder calculi, urinary tract infections, deterioration of renal function, or hematuria, the use of phytotherapeutic agents should be discouraged. In these situations, more aggressive medical and surgical treatment are warranted.

PHYTOTHERAPY IN THE TREATMENT OF CHRONIC PROSTATITIS

Chronic nonbacterial prostatitis (NBP) and prostatodynia are poorly understood diseases. The proposed etiologies of NBP include "spastic" dysfunction of the bladder neck and prostatic urethra, resulting in urinary reflux into the intraprostatic and ejaculatory ducts; tension myalgia of the pelvic floor; nonspecific inflammation; infection with fastidious organisms; and psychogenic causes.

Possible mechanisms of action of plant extracts in the treatment of chronic prostatitis include the following: anti-inflammatory effect on prostaglandin synthesis, 5-α-reductase activity (decreased prostatic secretions), α-adrenergic blockade (decreased bladder neck tone), bladder contractility (decreased bladder irritability), psychological mechanisms (placebo effect), and unknown mechanisms.

Rye pollen extract and the bioflavonoid quercetin have been evaluated in the treatment of NBP. In an uncontrolled study, 78% of men without complicating factors (e.g., strictures, bladder neck fibrosis, prostatic calculi) demonstrated improvement.

Quercetin was evaluated in a prospective, double-blind, placebo-controlled study; 67% of patients treated with quercetin improved whereas only 20% of those taking placebo showed improvement.

In summary, the limited literature available suggests there may be a role for these agents in the treatment of NBP. Further work needs to be performed in this area before recommending these medications routinely in the management of NBP/Prostatodynia.

VARIABILITY OF ACTIVE INGREDIENTS IN NUTRITIONAL SUPPLEMENTS FOR PROSTATE DISEASE

In 2002, Fleshner et al. *(7)* reported on the reliability of the active ingredients in various brands of nutritional supplements for prostate disease. Vitamin E, vitamin D, selenium, lycopene, and Saw Palmetto were evaluated. The measured dose in the products was compared with the dose on the product label. Samples of vitamin E fell in a range of –41% to +57%. Selenium fell in a range of –19% to + 23%. Samples of vitamin D fell within 15% of the stated dose. SPB fell in a range of –97% to + 140%. Lycopene brands were between –38% to + 143%. In summary, there is a wide variation in the actual dose of nutritional supplements making prescribing these supplements difficult.

CRANBERRY JUICE AND URINARY TRACT INFECTIONS

Over the years it has been "known" by the general public that urinary tract infections (UTIs) can be prevented by consuming cranberry juice. For years, it was felt that the mechanism of action was the result of urinary acidification. However, it is likely that inhibition of bacterial adherence to urothelial cells is the mechanism of action of any potential or actual benefit of cranberry juice in preventing UTIs. In one study, subjects consumed up to 4 L of cranberry juice per day. The urine became slightly more acidic ranging from +0.1 to –0.5. None of the urine samples possessed antibacterial activity against *Escherichia coli* at the pH at which they were voided.

Bacterial adherence to urothelial cells is important in the pathogenesis of UTIs. In vitro studies have demonstrated the ability of cranberry juice to prevent bacterial adherence to urothelial cells. Proanthocyanidins are compounds in cranberries that likely possess the ability to prevent bacteria from adhering to urothelial cells.

Clinical studies have suggested a benefit in reducing the incidence of bacteruria and UTIs. Studies to date have suggested a benefit of decreasing the incidence of bacteriuria in nursing home patients and a decrease in UTIs in sexually active women. However, there was no change in the frequency of UTIs or bacteriuria in children with neurogenic bladder using intermittent catheterization.

In summary, there may be a beneficial role of cranberry juice supplements in preventing UTIs by reducing bacterial adherence to the urinary tract. A three-arm trial comparing antibacterial prophylaxis to cranberry juice to placebo will be necessary to further define the benefit of cranberry juice in preventing UTIs.

USE OF COMPLEMENTARY MEDICATIONS IN BLADDER CANCER

A combination of high doses of vitamin A, vitamin B_6, vitamin C, and vitamin E has been shown in a double-blind randomized clinical trial to reduce the recurrence of transitional cell carcinoma of the bladder. Sixty-five patients were randomized to receive the recommended daily allowance of multiple vitamins or the recommended daily allowance plus 40,000 IU of vitamin A, 100 mg of vitamin B_6, 2000 mg of vitamin C, and 400 IU of vitamin E. The 5-yr estimates of disease recurrence were 91% in the recommended daily allowance arm and 41% in the megavitamin arm. Nausea was the most common side effect in the high-dose arm. Increased fluid intake and selenium may beneficial in preventing bladder cancer as well as the vitamins just mentioned.

SUGGESTED READINGS

Castle EP, Thrasher JB. The role of soy phytoestrogens in prostate cancer. Urol Clin N Am 2002; 29: 71–81.

Clinton SK. Lycopene: chemistry biology and implications for human health and disease. Nutr Rev 1998; 56: 35–51.

Fagelman E, Lowe FC. Herbal medications in the treatment of benign prostatic hyperplasia. Urol Clin N Am 2002; 29: 23–29.

Fleshner NE. Vitamin E and prostate cancer. Urol Clin N Am 2002; 29: 67–70.

Giovannuci E. Epidemiologic characteristics of prostate cancer. Cancer 1995; 75: 1766–1777.

Gupta S, Mukhtar H. Green tea and prostate cancer. Urol Clin N Am 2002; 29: 49–57.

Kamat AM, Lamm DL. Chemoprevention of bladder cancer. Urol Clin N Am 2002; 29: 157–168.

Konety BR, Getzenberg RH. Vitamin D and prostate cancer. Urol Clin N Am 2002; 29: 95–106.

Lowe FC, Fagelman E. Cranberry juice and urinary tract infections: what is the evidence? Urology 2001; 57: 407–413.

Lowe FC, Fagelman E. Phytotherapy for chronic prostatitis. Curr Urol Rep 2000; 1: 164–166.

Marks LS, Partin AW, Epstein JI, et al. Effects of saw palmetto herbal blend in men with symptomatic benign prostatic hyperplasia. J Urol2000; 163: 1451–6.

Moyard MA. Potential lifestyle and dietary supplement options for the prevention and postdiagnosis of bladder cancer. Urol Clin N Am 2002; 29: 31–48.

Nelson MA, Reid M, Duffeld-Lillico AJ, Marshall JR. Prostate cancer and selenium. Urol Clin N Am 2002; 29: 67–70.

Oh W, Small E. PC-SPES and prostate cancer. Urol Clin N Am 2002; 29: 59–66.

REFERENCES

1. Miller EC, Giovannucci E, Erdman JW, Bahnson R, Schwartz SJ, Clinton SK. Tomato products, lycopene, and prostate cancer risk. Urol Clin N Am 2002; 29: 83–93.

2. Small E, Frohlich M, Bok R, et al. A prospective trial of the herbal supplement PC-SPES in patients with progressive prostate cancer. J Clin Oncol 2000; 18: 3595–603.
3. Oh W, George D, Hackmann K, Manola J, Kantoff PW. Activity of the herbal combination, PC-SPES, in the treatment of patients with androgen independent prostate cancer. Urology 2001; 57: 122–126.
4. Corder EH, Guess HA, Hulka BS, et al. Vitamin D and prostate cancer; a prediagnostic study with stored sera. Cancer Epidemiol Biomarkers Prev 1993; 2: 467–72.
5. Marks LS, DiPaola RS, Nelson P, et al. PC-SPES: herbal formulation for prostate Cancer. Urology 2002; 60: 369–377.
6. Braeckman J, Denis L, de Leval J, et al. A double-blind, placebo-controlled study of the plant extract *Serenoa repens* in the treatment of benign hyperplasia of the prostate. Euro J Clin Res 1997; 9: 247–259.
7. Fleshner NE, Feifer A, Klotz LH. Analytical precision and reliability of commonly used nutritional supplements in prostate disease (Abstract 117). J Urol 2002; 167 (suppl):29.

Index